An Introduction to
Behavioral Endocrinology

An Introduction to
Behavioral Endocrinology

ALAN I. LESHNER

Bucknell University

New York
Oxford University Press   1978

Library of Congress Cataloging in Publication Data

Leshner, Alan I   1944-
    An introduction to behavioral endocrinology.

    Bibliography: p.
    Includes index.
    1. Psychology, Physiological.   2. Endocrinology—
Psychosomatic aspects.   I.   Title.
QP360.L465   152   77-13230
ISBN 0-19-502266-1
ISBN 0-19-502267-X pbk

to Agi and Sarah

PREFACE

This book is an overview of the field of behavioral endocrinology, the study of the relationship between hormones and behavior. There has been only one other single-authored, comprehensive survey of the field, the classic published by Frank Beach in 1948 and titled *Hormones and Behavior*, although there have been a few collections of readings and essays that discuss some of the important findings in the area.

Although this book is designed to stand on its own as the basis for a course in behavioral endocrinology, it also is intended to be useful as a supplement in some other, broader courses, such as physiological psychology, animal behavior, zoology, and any of a variety of medical school courses. It also might be useful as a first reader for the professional interested in learning about the relationship between hormones and behavior in general, or about the relationship between hormones and a particular class of behaviors.

The book is organized, functionally, into sections. The first chapter provides a basic introduction to the field and considers some general theoretical issues and the major techniques of study. The second chapter is concerned with the role of hormones in what have been called regulatory behaviors—those behaviors which seem to serve primarily in the maintenance of the internal economy of the organism. The third and fourth chapters consider the relationship between hormones and some social behaviors, includ-

viii *Preface*

ing agonistic behaviors and pheromonal and ultrasonic communication. Chapters 5 and 6 examine the role of hormones in reproductive behaviors, specifically sexual and parental responses. Chapters 7 and 8 are concerned with emotion, emotionality, and mood states. Finally, Chapter 9 integrates some of the earlier discussions and reconsiders some of the theoretical issues introduced in Chapter 1 and discussed in later chapters. At the back of the book, there is an appendix which is designed to provide the less advanced reader with some of the general principles of endocrinology and neuroendocrinology.

I am grateful to the many colleagues and students who read and criticized sections of earlier versions of the manuscript. Among these are M. F. Breen, W. E. Bridson, C. S. Carter, J. W. Davenport, S. M. Essock, O. R. Floody, R. W. Goy, Tj. B. van Wimersma Greidanus, J. A. Politch, K. E. Roche, S. M. Schwartz, and G. N. Wade. I also wish to thank D. K. Candland, W. I. Smith, and R. M. Tarpy for their advice and encouragement throughout this project. I am particularly grateful to F. A. Beach and D. A. Goldfoot, who kindly read and commented on an earlier draft of the entire book. I have benefited greatly from their council.

This project was finished while I was a Visiting Scientist at the Wisconsin Regional Primate Research Center and was supported by National Research Service Award #HD05394 from NICHD. I am very grateful to R. W. Goy and the staff of the Primate Center for their support and for the many discussions that have greatly increased the quality of this work. Finally, I wish to thank Marcus Boggs and Brenda Jones of Oxford University Press for their editorial assistance.

Alan I. Leshner
August, 1977

CONTENTS

An Introduction to
Behavioral Endocrinology

Chapter 1

INTRODUCTION AND BASIC ISSUES

Although behavioral endocrinology has only recently been emerging as a distinct discipline, we have known for centuries that endocrine function and behavior are related. Aristotle may not have known in detail about hormones and their functions, but he did know that endocrine glands are important both to physiology and behavior. He described in detail the effects of castration in birds and compared these effects to those known to occur in man (Turner & Bagnara, 1971). Probably the first formal study in behavioral endocrinology was conducted in 1849 by the Swedish scientist Berthold, who studied the effects of castration on reproductive activity of birds. As a part of that study, Berthold replaced one testis in the body cavity and observed that this treatment restored the castrated bird's behavior to normal. On the basis of the study, Berthold proposed that a substance particular to the testes was involved in the control of reproduction (Beach, 1975).

The early controversies over the sequence of physiological and behavioral events in emotion spurred another type of investigation into the relationship between hormones and behavior. In 1924, Marañon injected human subjects with epinephrine (adrenalin) in the hope of inducing genuine emotional states by purely physiological means. However, no subjects reported experiencing genuine emotions, although some did report feeling "as if they were afraid."

The real impetus to the study of hormone–behavior interactions came during the second quarter of this century with the classic work of Frank Beach and W. C. Young on the role of reproductive hormones in sexual behavior and that of Curt Richter on the role of hormones in running activity and in dietary self-selection. In 1948, Beach published his classic monograph *Hormones and Behavior*, which stood as the only comprehensive text in the field until the late 1960s. In 1967, Whalen published a compendium of important papers in a book titled *Hormones and Behavior*, and in the last few years, some additional edited volumes have appeared, such as Levine's *Hormones and Behavior* (1972) and Eleftheriou and Sprott's *Hormonal Correlates of Behavior* (1975).

SOME THEORETICAL ISSUES

We shall begin our discussion of hormone–behavior interactions in Chapter 1 on a very general level. Each of the subsequent chapters considers the role of hormones in a specific class of behaviors. However, some behavioral endocrinologists have been interested in whether generalizations can be made that are appropriate to all classes of hormone–behavior interactions. Toward that end, the following section is devoted (1) to a consideration of how hormones and behavior can be related, and (2) to a consideration of some models proposed as general descriptions of the role of endocrine function in behavior. An additional objective is to provide a theoretical framework around which our later discussions will be organized.

Questions of Mediation

How are hormones and behavior related? We know that hormones can affect behavioral responses and that, conversely, endocrine function can be modified if the subject has certain experiences and engages in specific behaviors. In addition, we know that the endocrine system, along with the nervous system, is one of the major signaling systems of the body, and that hormones act as chemical messengers, affecting the rates and directions of ongoing physiological reactions throughout the organism. However, in spite of their pervasive actions, hormones usually cannot make muscles move (the case of oxytocin's effects on the uterus may be one exception), and muscle movements do not directly affect endocrine secretions. Therefore, it is more likely that hormones and behavior are related indirectly, through mediating mechanisms.

HOW CAN HORMONES AFFECT BEHAVIOR? Hormones exert at least two kinds of effects on behavior. In adulthood, the hormonal state of the individual can affect both the form and intensity of its behavioral responses. This relationship will be referred to as that between the *baseline hormonal state* and behavior; the effects of the baseline hormonal state are similar to what have often been called the "activational" effects of hormones (Young, 1961). However, the hormonal environment during early stages of development also has dramatic effects on the way an individual will respond to certain stimuli in adulthood. In this way, hormones can exert rather distant *organizing* effects on behavior, and this temporally distant relationship will be referred to as that between the *early hormonal state* and behavior (Goy & Goldfoot, 1973). Because mediation of the two types of relationships might be different, it seems best to treat them separately here.

The baseline hormonal state. Before considering the mechanisms by which hormones affect behavior, we should make clear exactly what is meant by the concept "baseline hormonal state." The term is used here to denote the hormonal state of an individual as it enters a situation. The individual's hormonal state is constantly changing, and, if hormones affect behavior, we would expect to see behavioral changes accompanying those hormonal fluctuations.

For example, as a female's hormonal state changes across a reproductive cycle, such changes are considered to be alterations in her baseline hormonal state. Then, if the gonadal hormones affect behavior, we would expect to see behavioral changes that coincide with these fluctuations in gonadal hormone levels. Similarly, there are circadian rhythms in the levels of some hormones, and we might expect to see behavioral changes that accompany those hormone changes.

It should be made clear, however, that the concept of the baseline hormonal state is not meant to be restricted only to the precise point in time that the individual enters the test situation; in some cases the baseline hormonal state must include the recent hormonal history. For example, we know that some hormones, such as the adrenal glucocorticoids and the androgens are released in pulses, and, therefore, that the animal's hormonal state can change from moment to moment. Yet, we do not really expect to see changes in behavior corresponding to those frequent changes in hormone levels. The amount of time that a particular hormonal state must be in effect before behavior is affected can vary from behavior to behavior and from hormone to hormone; those questions can be determined empirically. However, a term like "baseline hormonal state" is needed to characterize the individual's *functional* hormonal state as it enters a situation.

Because their physiological effects are so pervasive, hormones can affect behavior in many ways: by altering the general metabolic state of the organism, the state of the effectors, the state of sensory receptor areas, or the state of the central neural mechanisms that are responsible for interpreting sensory information and/or organizing behavior patterns (Beach, 1948, 1974).

Because hormones have dramatic effects on metabolic processes, it seems reasonable that some hormones might affect behavior by affecting the general state of the organism. For example, because the thyroid hormones have such important effects on carbohydrate metabolism, they might affect some behaviors, such as voluntary exercise, by modifying the amount of carbohydrates available to supply the energy needed to support these behaviors (Leshner & Walker, 1973). Or, since ACTH has been shown to affect the amplitude of muscle contraction (Strand, Stoboy & Cayer, 1974), this pituitary hormone could modify the amplitude of behavioral responses that involve muscle contraction.

Hormones also might affect behavior through their effects on the state or sensitivity of peripheral sensory receptor areas. Adjustment or modification of the state of the sense organs alters the probability of a stimulus eliciting a perceptual response (Horn, 1965), and some hormones have been shown to modify the state of peripheral receptor areas. For example, increasing estrogen levels in rats increases the size of the receptive field around the vagina (Komisaruk, Adler & Hutchinson, 1972; Kow & Pfaff, 1974), which could increase the responsiveness of the female to stimulation provided by a male. In addition, olfaction is an important sense modality in many types of social interaction, and changes in both adrenal and gonadal hormone levels have been reported to affect olfactory sensitivity (LeMagnen, 1952; Vernikos-Danellis, 1972). Thus, hormones could affect social responses by altering the individual's sensory responses to olfactory stimuli. However, we do not know whether such effects are exerted at the level of the peripheral receptor or at the central neural mechanisms involved in the perception of olfactory stimuli.

Many behavioral effects of hormones appear to be mediated at the central nervous system circuits directly involved in the perception of stimuli and the integration of behavioral responses. Two kinds of evidence support this view: First, many of the brain areas implicated in the control of specific behavior patterns are particularly sensitive to those hormones which also affect behaviors when injected systemically. Second, many studies have shown that direct injection of hormones into restricted brain sites can reverse the behavioral changes that are produced by removing those hormones from the general circulation. Thus, although manipulating circulating hormone levels modifies behavioral responding, in many cases the neural rather than the peripheral effects of these hormones are critical to the normal display of the behavior. For example, male sexual responding is greatly reduced following the withdrawal of the androgens by castration. Systemic injections of androgens can restore the sexual responding of castrates to normal levels, but so can implants of androgens restricted to the preoptic area of the hypothalamus. Significantly, this brain area has been implicated in the control of male sexual responding. Thus, although castration results in a reduction in androgen levels throughout the body, one need only restore androgen levels in the brain in order to restore the behavior to normal levels (Davidson, 1972; Lisk, 1973).

Hormones can modify brain function and, thereby, behavior in many ways: by altering the general metabolic state of brain cells, by altering the electrical characteristics of specific neuronal elements and, thereby, the excitability of specific systems, or by modifying the states of the relevant neurotransmitter systems so that some circuits are sensitized and others are desensitized. All of these are likely possibilities and will be discussed in later chapters (also see the excellent reviews in Lissák, 1973).

It should be made clear that hormones can affect behavior in more than one way—i.e., a single hormone can exert multiple effects on a particular behavior. For example, even though one effect of estrogens on female sexual behavior could result from an increase in the size of the receptive field around the vagina, the estrogens could also directly affect the state of the relevant brain circuits. A single hormone can affect any behavior in any of several ways.

The early hormonal state. Manipulations of the early hormonal environment can have dramatic effects on the development and display of a wide range of adult behavior patterns. Many of these effects depend on the hormonal state during specific developmental stages or *critical periods* (e.g., Goy, Bridson & Young, 1964), and these temporally delayed reactions to the early hormonal environment tend to be relatively permanent and irreversible (Beach, 1974). The effects of the early hormonal state can mediate adult behavior by modifying the adult's general metabolic state, the functioning of particular endocrine subsystems in adulthood, or the state of critical central nervous system circuits.

Manipulation of many hormones, such as those of the thyroid and the adrenal, during early developmental stages appears to have lasting effects on metabolic processes carrying over into adulthood. For example, the human cretin, who has suffered from thyroid insufficiency during the perinatal period, seems to have reduced levels of oxygen consumption (decreased metabolic rate) in adulthood, and often appears lethargic and slow to learn (Levine & Mullins, 1966). Some of the behavioral effects of early thyroid deficiency— e.g., lethargy in adulthood—might be the result of this lasting change in metabolic rate.

Changes in the early hormonal environment also can produce lasting changes in the functioning of the adult endocrine system. Therefore, some early hormonal manipulations might affect adult behavior patterns because they produce changes in the adult hormonal characteristics on which those behaviors depend. For example, early adrenal manipulations appear to alter adult levels of avoidance responding (Nyákás & Endröczi, 1972). In addition, such manipulations alter the responsiveness of the pituitary-adrenal axis to stress in adulthood (Joffe, Milkovic & Levine, 1972). Because adult levels of pituitary-adrenal functioning are important to avoidance responding, the effects of adrenal manipulations made early in development on adult avoidance behavior might be mediated by the altered pituitary-adrenal responsiveness that these manipulations produce.

The effects of the early hormonal state on adult behavior also could be mediated by changes in the brain. Changes in the early hormonal environment appear to alter permanently both the anatomical characteristics of the brain and the sensitivity of specific neural sites to the circulating hormones on which behaviors depend. Perhaps the most dramatic, or at least the most studied, manipulations are those that affect adult reproductive physiology and behavior. There are marked gender differences in morphology, physiology, and behavior, many of which can be partially reversed by early manipulations of the levels of the sex hormones. The relative permanence of the effects of the early hormonal environment on adult sexual behavior, despite attempts to counteract them with adult hormone therapy, has led to the suggestion that the early hormonal state is involved in the *organization* of sex differences in the brain circuits that mediate reproductive physiology and behavior (see Phoenix et al., 1959). Proponents of this suggestion argue that neural effects of the sex hormones during the critical developmental period are the most important factors in their effects on adult behavior, and the data support this view. For example, implants of testosterone restricted to the hypothalamus of newborn female rats can accomplish much of the same kind of masculinization as do systemic androgen injections (Nadler, 1973). In addition, male rats that have been castrated during the neonatal period exhibit less neural sensitivity to androgens in adulthood than intact rats, and they are behaviorally feminized (McEwen, Pfaff & Zigmond, 1970). Female rats androgenized during infancy appear to exhibit less hypothalamic sensitivity to circulating ovarian hormones than nonandrogenized females, and their behavior is masculinized (Dunlap, Preis, & Gerall, 1972).

Many other effects of the early hormonal state also may be mediated by neural mechanisms. For example, thyroid deficiency leads to a decrease in the number of synapses in the brain (Balász, Potel & Hajós, 1975), and this change in brain structure could mediate the effects of neonatal thyroid deficiency on learning abilities (Davenport & Dorcey, 1972). Which particular effects of the early hormonal state are mediated by what changes in brain functioning, and related changes in behavior, will be considered in greater detail in later chapters.

HOW CAN BEHAVING OR HAVING EXPERIENCES MODIFY ENDOCRINE FUNCTIONS? Many kinds of experience and many forms of behaving result in changes in endocrine function. For example, male rats exhibit a rise in the levels of testosterone, luteinizing hormone (LH), and prolactin following copulation. In fact, mere exposure to a female can cause these hormonal changes in sexually experienced males (Kamel et al., 1975). However, in the same way that hormones usually cannot make muscles move, muscular movement cannot directly cause changes in endocrine function. Therefore, the effects of behaving or experience on endocrine function probably are indirect—mediated by some other mechanism.

Muscular exertion causes changes in the levels of the circulating metabolites, such as lipids and carbohydrates, and changes in the levels of these substances could trigger hormonal secretion. For example, the pancreatic secretion of insulin is responsive to the circulating levels of sugar in the blood. Therefore, as muscles move, glucose is released into the bloodstream, and insulin will be released in response to the relative hyperglycemia that results.

However, there probably is more to behavior (and certainly to experience) than muscle movements, and most endocrine subsystems are controlled by the central nervous system, rather than directly by levels of metabolites in the blood. Therefore, it seems most probable that the effects of experiences on endocrine function are mediated through the central nervous system, which is sensitive to the state of the peripheral receptors and also integrates the functioning of the endocrine system (see Whalen, 1967).

For example, experiences in competitive situations produce dramatic changes in the state of the central nervous system circuits which control endocrine function. Defeat has a significant effect on protein synthesis in the brain (Eleftheriou, 1971) and alters the state of the brain neurotransmitter systems. Daily fighting experiences lead to increases in central catecholamine and serotonin levels (Modigh, 1973; Welch & Welch, 1969), and these increases are more pronounced in some brain areas than in others (Eleftheriou & Church, 1968; Welch & Welch, 1971). This altered neurotransmitter activity in particular brain areas, like the limbic system and the hypothalamus, should be reflected in altered levels of the hormones of both the pituitary-adrenocortical and pituitary-gonadal axes, since these endocrine subsystems are ultimately under the control of precisely these neural areas (Antelman & Brown, 1972; Ryzhenkov, 1973; Sawyer & Gorski, 1971). Thus, it is possible that agonistic experiences modify endocrine function through the effects of these experiences on brain function. Specific examples from other classes of experience and behavior will be discussed in later chapters.

Long-Chain Hormone–Behavior Interactions

Although the effects of hormones on behavior and those of experiences or behaving on endocrine function have been studied as if they were separate relationships, most students of hormone–behavior interactions agree that they are not separate. Living organisms are dynamic, and so are their interactions with their environments. Although an individual may enter a situation in one baseline hormonal state and, therefore, respond in a particular way initially, its experiences in that situation can change its hormonal state. As its hormonal state changes, so should its behavior. This dynamic view of hormone–behavior interactions combines the two relationships of hormonal effects on behavior and the effects of experiences on endocrine function; this type of combined relationship will be referred to as a *long-chain hormone–behavior interaction* to distinguish it from what might be called "short-chain" hormone–behavior interactions: the effects of hormones on behavior or those of experiences on endocrine function studied separately.

It might be useful to point out here that the existence of a long-chain hormone–behavior interaction does not imply that the same hormone must be involved at all points in the chain. One could have an interaction of this class where, first, one hormone affects the individual's initial responses. Then, engaging in that behavior leads to a change in the level of a second hormone, which, then, feeds back and alters the level or form of responding.

Lehrman's classic description of the parental behavior of ring doves provides a clear example of long-chain hormone–behavior interactions. According to his description "participation in courtship appears to induce the secretion of hormones which facilitate the building of a nest; participation in nest building under these conditions contributes stimulation of the secretion of the hormone(s) which induce the birds to sit on eggs. Stimulation arising from the act of sitting on the eggs induces the further secretion of a hormone which (a) induces the birds to continue incubating, and (b) helps bring the birds into a condition of readiness to feed young when they hatch" (Lehrman, 1965, p. 370).

Models of Hormone–Behavior Interactions

Most investigators now share this long-chain view of hormone–behavior interactions, and Beach summarized it in what he termed a "simplified model" of the sequence of relationships: "(1) External Stimulus I elicits the release of Hormone A into the bloodstream. (2) Hormone A renders the individual sensitive to Stimulus II. (3) The behavior evoked by Stimulus II gives rise to interoceptive Stimulus III. (4) Stimulus III results in release of Hormone B, which in turn increases the individual's responsiveness to environmental Stimulus IV, and so on" (Beach, 1965, pp. 561-562).

In his 1967 collection of readings, Whalen proposed a somewhat more complex model of hormones and behavior that is reproduced in Figure 1-1. It connotes the same general relationships as the "simplified model" proposed by Beach, but it also includes some of the mediational relationships discussed above. Whalen's model

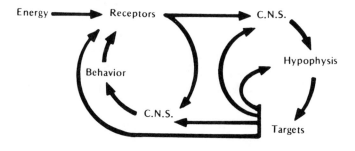

FIG. 1-1

Whalen's model of hormone–behavior interactions (from Whalen, *Hormones and Behavior*. New York: D. Van Nostrand Company, 1967, p. 4, by permission).

consists of two separate but interrelated loops. The loop on the left shows a sequence of events dealing with stimuli (energy), the nervous system, and behavior. The loop on the right is concerned with the secretion of hormones. The two loops are connected both by hormones and by the behaviors that lead to later changes in hormone levels. According to this model, physical energies or stimuli impinge on receptors and these stimuli are integrated by the central nervous system and cause behavior. The stimuli, both from the outside world and from behaving, cause hormone secretion through the mediation of the central nervous system. This hormonal secretion then causes changes in behavior both by modifying the state of the sensory receptors and by altering the activity of the central nervous system circuits that are responsible for the perception of stimuli and the integration of responses.

These kinds of models have been very useful because they have provided a framework from which many later investigations have proceeded. However, for providing a general description of the role of hormones in behavior that includes all aspects of hormone–

behavior interactions, these models are incomplete. For example, they do not include the possible role of the baseline hormonal state in determining behavioral reactions. Rather, they begin with the hormonal responses to stimulation. Second, they only include some of the possible physiological mediating mechanisms discussed here. Specifically, the possibility that hormones affect behavior by altering the individual's general metabolic state is not considered. Third, they do not include the organizing effects of hormones present early in development on adult behavior patterns. Fourth, another, recently suggested, behaviorally-related function of hormones—that on an animal's quality as a stimulus affecting the behavior of other animals (see Leshner, 1975, and discussion below)—is not included.

Thus, if we are interested in visualizing the multifaceted relationship between hormones and behavior that includes all aspects to be discussed in this book, we must develop yet another model. Such a model is presented in Figure 1-2. It is based on an earlier model proposed by Leshner (1975) to summarize the relationship between hormones and agonistic behavior, but his model also was missing some important elements, which are included here.

According to the model suggested in Figure 1-2, the hormonal state during early critical periods organizes the states of the mechanisms that will be important in the determination of adult responses. These mechanisms include the sensory receptors, the general metabolic state, the important brain circuits, and the adult baseline hormonal state. Then, in adulthood, the baseline hormonal state further prepares or presets those potential mediating mechanisms. In this way, both kinds of hormonal effects discussed in this book are included: those of hormones present early in development and those of the baseline hormonal state.

The individual then enters the situation and is exposed to relevant exciting stimuli. Those stimuli impinge on the sensory receptors, and that information is integrated in the central nervous system. That neural activity, then, determines whether, in what

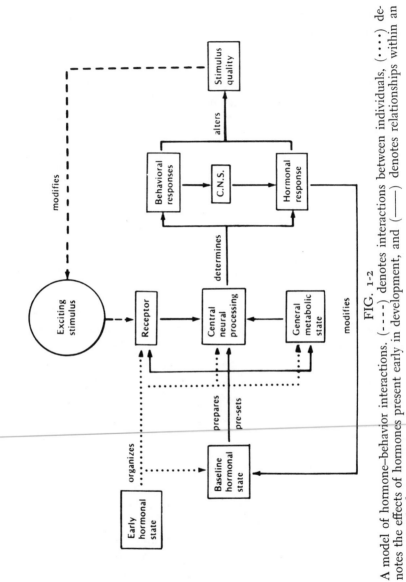

FIG. 1-2

A model of hormone–behavior interactions. (- - -) denotes interactions between individuals, (·····) denotes the effects of hormones present early in development, and (——) denotes relationships within an adult individual.

way, and how intensely the individual will react to the exciting stimuli, including both behavioral and hormonal reactions. In this model, an individual's behavioral and hormonal responses to stimulation are seen as a direct consequence of neural activity. However, the nature of that neural activity depends not only on the nature of the exciting stimulus, but also on the individual's hormonal state early in development and on its baseline hormonal state prior to entering the situation (acting via the effects of these hormonal factors on the general metabolic state, the sensory receptors, and the brain itself).

Both the experiences of the individual and the behaviors in which it engages produce changes in its hormonal state, probably through the effects of these experiences and actions on neural activity. (As discussed in an earlier section of this chapter, behavioral responses can only lead to hormonal change through the mediation of the central nervous system; hence the "second brain" in the model.) Then, because these changes in the individual's hormonal characteristics really represent changes in its baseline hormonal state at the next point in time, its behavioral reactions to the same exciting stimuli should change. In this way, the hormonal responses to stimulation feed back and modify the individual's reactions in the same or future similar situations—what we have called a long-chain hormone–behavior interaction.

This model also incorporates the other behaviorally-related function of hormones mentioned briefly above: that of hormones and an individual's *stimulus quality*. Many organism–environment interactions are social and, therefore, include other dynamic individuals. In these social interactions, the characteristics of each individual affects the behavior of the other; each individual serves as a stimulus to the other. An individual's quality or effectiveness as a stimulus is affected both by its behavioral reactions and by its hormonal state. Therefore, as an individual's behavioral reactions and hormonal state change as a function of its experiences in a situation, its stimulus quality should also change. Thus, the model presented in Figure 1-2 summarizes a dynamic relationship between hormones, behavior, and the environment, wherein the hormonal state of an individual affects both its behavior and its stimulus quality; and when the individual's hormonal state changes, so does its behavior and its quality as a stimulus.

The view summarized in this model articulates some common beliefs or hypotheses about hormone–behavior interactions—including statements about the long-chain relationship between hormones and behavior and about the mediation of those relationships—that will be examined in detail in later chapters. Some of the relational hypotheses are (1) that both the early hormonal state and the baseline hormonal state contributes to the determination of how intensely and in what form an individual will respond when stimulated; (2) that one of the functions of the hormonal responses to experience or behavioral action is to feed back and modify both the ongoing behavior of the individual in the situation and its reactions in future similar situations; and (3) that another function of such responses is to modify the individual's stimulus quality so that other individuals' reactions to it will be modified. Mediational hypotheses include the suggestions that (1) hormones can affect behavior through many mediating mechanisms, including hormonal effects on sensory receptor areas, on the general metabolic state, and on the brain; and (2) that the effects on endocrine function of having certain experiences or engaging in specific behaviors are mediated by changes in brain functioning. It should be pointed out that, in the case of the first mediating hypothesis, although hormones can affect behavior through multiple mediating mechanisms, behavioral action ultimately depends on neural activity. Therefore, even if the primary site of hormone action is not the brain (for example, if hormones are altering the general metabolic state), those nonneural actions must be integrated by the brain before behavior will be affected. This primacy of neural action for behavioral reactions explains why in the model presented in Figure 1-2 the box labeled "general metabolic state" and, of course, that labeled "receptors" are not *directly* connected to the behavioral and hormonal responses; they are only connected to these responses through "central neural processing."

The model presented in Figure 1-2 and the hypotheses it incorporates are the framework around which the rest of this book is organized. The discussions in each chapter begin with the effects of hormones on behavior and then turn to questions of the mediation of those hormonal effects. Then, the hormonal responses to experience are discussed, and the possible presence of long-chain hormone–behavior interactions is considered. It should be noted, however, that the model presented here is a generalization describing all possible relationships. We would not necessarily expect all relationships expressed in this model to be appropriate for all specific cases of hormones and behaviors. Therefore, rather than reevaluate the model as a whole for each behavior in each chapter, the adequacy of the model as a generalization will be considered only in Chapter 9.

TECHNIQUES OF STUDY

The models of the complex interaction between hormones and behavior just discussed were not derived from studies concerned with the total interaction between endocrine function and behavior, but from studies concerned with specific aspects or subunits of that relationship. For example, some studies have focused only on the effects of the baseline hormonal state on behavioral responses, others have studied the hormonal responses to experiences or behaving, and still others have attempted to study long-chain hormone–behavior interactions. Each class has used experimental designs and techniques particular to the kinds of questions asked. Before proceeding to a consideration of the data from these studies, it might be useful to review in a general way the types of experimental techniques used.

Identifying Hormone–Behavior Relationships

The goal of most studies in behavioral endocrinology is to analyze the causal relationships between certain aspects of endocrine function and the form and intensity of particular classes of behavioral responses. The first logical step in studying these relationships is to establish that a relationship exists at all. Establishing the existence of a relationship between a hormonal state and a behavior pattern can be accomplished in at least two ways. First, one can capitalize on natural changes in circulating hormone levels to show that levels of responding covary with or are correlated with natural changes in such levels. For example, it is well known that sexual receptivity varies with the stages of the reproductive cycle in the females of many species. Because the ovarian hormones vary with the reproductive cycle, there also is a correlation between changes in circulating (endogenous) ovarian hormone levels and levels of sexual receptivity.

Second, one can measure circulating hormone levels and observe a particular pattern of behaving or a particular behavioral trait at the same time. For example, in attempting to determine whether there is a relationship between aggressiveness and circulating androgen levels, one could measure androgen levels as individuals are engaged in an aggressive encounter. If more aggressive individuals exhibit higher (or lower) androgen levels than less aggressive individuals, it can be concluded that there is a correlation between androgen levels and levels of aggressiveness.

These types of correlational studies, however, only establish that a relationship exists between hormone levels and levels of behavioral responding. They do not reveal any causality in that relationship. For example, it cannot be determined from these types of studies whether the differences in androgen levels cause the differences in aggressiveness, whether the differences in aggressiveness cause the differences in androgen levels, or whether they are only "accidentally" related, through a third mechanism that affects them both. In order to determine the causality in correlational relationships it is necessary to conduct experimental studies, manipulating the level of one factor or variable while studying the effects of that manipulation on the other factor.

The Baseline Hormonal State and Initial Levels of Responding

Most studies of the effects of hormones on behavior have employed experimental designs where the baseline hormonal state is manipulated first, and then the effects of that manipulation on the individual's reactions to exciting stimuli are studied. Significantly, most have only studied initial responses to exciting stimuli, thereby avoiding the potential confound of changes in hormonal states as a function of initial experiences, a problem to be discussed in more detail below.

The first step in determining that a hormone affects a behavior might be to decrease the level of that particular hormone in the circulation and study the effects of this manipulation on responding. For example, if one wanted to determine whether the androgens affect male sexual behavior, one might begin by removing the animal's testes and seeing the effects of this operation on its reproductive behavior patterns. However, most endocrine glands secrete more than one hormone and removing any gland has profound effects on the state of the other endocrine glands and their secretions. Therefore, in order to demonstrate the dependence of a behavior on a particular hormone, one must be able to show that after decreasing the level of a hormone, one can restore levels of responding to normal by providing "replacement therapy" with that hormone. To extend our example, one might treat the castrated animal with injected (exogenous) androgens and observe whether there is a restoration of the behavior. If so, it would appear that the presence of the androgens is necessary for the normal expression of male sexual behavior.

Having established that a hormone is necessary for a particular behavior, one might ask whether varying the levels of that hormone within normal ranges leads to variations in the level of responding. Thus, one would seek the "dose–response relationship" between levels of the hormone and levels of responding. In our example, such a relationship might be established simply by injecting the animal with different dosages of an androgen and then studying its reproductive behavior. This method, however, is not the technique of choice. Injected hormones interact with endogenous secretions through the intricate feedback loops that control the activity of most endocrine glands. Therefore, it would be at least necessary to remove endogenous androgens from the circulation so that the experimenter could, in fact, *control* the circulating levels of these hormones experimentally. Thus, the design of a study intended to determine the effects of androgens on male sexual behavior might involve treating castrated, adrenalectomized animals with a range of dosages of an androgen and then studying the individual's sexual responses. Both operations would be necessary, because androgens are produced both in the testes and in the adrenals.

The Early Hormonal Environment and Adult Behavior Patterns

As discussed above, the early hormonal environment is important in the determination of adult behavior patterns. In some species, the prenatal (before birth) hormonal environment is more important for behavioral development than the postnatal environment, whereas in other species either both periods or just the postnatal period are important. Which period(s) is important often depends on the developmental level of the young at birth. For example, in humans, other primates, and guinea pigs, the young are born relatively mature, and the prenatal hormonal environment appears to be more important than the postnatal environment. On the other hand, in rats and mice, the young are born relatively immature, and both pre- and postnatal periods are important.

There are at least two kinds of experimental manipulations that can be used to determine the role of the early hormonal state in determining adult behavior. One is to raise the levels of these hormones, and a second is to lower particular hormone levels during early critical periods. Each of these kinds of manipulations can be made either prenatally or postnatally. In making prenatal manipulations, one can either treat the mother during pregnancy (thereby affecting the fetus by modifying the levels of hormones in the common circulation that the fetus shares with the mother) or treat the young directly. Raising prenatal hormone levels is relatively simple. In viviparous species (such as mammals) one often can simply inject the mother with the hormone being studied, and it will pass to the young. In oviparous species (such as birds) one can inject the test hormone directly into the egg (Adkins, 1975).

Lowering prenatal hormone levels is somewhat more complex. One might be able to lower prenatal hormone levels by removing the mother's endocrine glands that secrete the test hormone. In this way, unless the fetus produces sufficient amounts of the hormone to support both the mother and the fetus, the fetus's circulating hormone levels will drop. An alternative technique is to inject the mother (or the egg) with a chemical substance that reduces or blocks the secretion or action of the critical hormone. For example, the anti-androgen cyproterone acetate can be injected into the mother, resulting in a decrease in the functional activity of the fetus's circulating androgens (Ward & Renz, 1972). It should be noted that in modifying the mother's hormonal characteristics in order to change those of the fetus, one should be careful to determine first whether the substance to be used will pass from the mother to the young; that is, whether the substance passes the "placental barrier." For example, in manipulating prenatal pituitary-adrenal hormone levels, one should be aware that although corticosterone does pass the placental barrier, ACTH probably does not (Paul & D'Angelo, 1972).

In manipulating the postnatal hormonal state, raising postnatal hormone levels generally is accomplished by injecting the newborn with the test hormone. Often, a single treatment is effective, although some must be repeated. Lowering postnatal hormone levels can be accomplished in two ways. If one is a skilled surgeon, one can remove the neonate's critical glands. For example, to study the effects of reducing postnatal androgen levels on the adult sexual behavior of male rats, one can remove their testes during the postnatal period (e.g., Beach & Holz, 1946; Hart, 1968). The second technique is to inject the neonate with an "anti-hormone" that will block the secretion or action of the natural substance. As an example of this technique, Brain, Evans, and Poole (1974) studied the effects of reducing postnatal androgen levels on adult aggressive responding by injecting the neonates with a single dose of the anti-androgen cyproterone acetate during the postnatal period.

Some relatively recent studies have suggested that one can also manipulate the postnatal hormonal environment through "behavioral" techniques, e.g., by handling the neonate. It has been known for some time that handling an animal early in life affects its emotional reactions as an adult. It now seems likely that the effects of early handling on adult emotionality are mediated by postnatal pituitary-adrenocortical activity changes (Ader, 1975). Thus, there may be a behavioral means (handling) of modifying the postnatal hormonal environment.

An additional technique used to determine the relationships between the early hormonal environment and adult behavior patterns is to study the effects of naturally occurring endocrine abnormalities or endocrinopathies. For example, Money and Ehrhardt (1972) reported the results of many studies of human sex-hormone abnormalities during early developmental periods. Some subjects suffered from disorders leading to increases in androgen levels during early developmental stages, such as those observed in some female children of mothers with androgen secreting tumors, and others suffered from abnormally reduced early hormone levels. In many cases, Money and Ehrhardt reported evidence of marked changes in both physical characteristics and behavior.

Measuring the Hormonal Responses
to Stimulation or to Behaving

In order to determine the hormonal responses to having a particular experience or to engaging in a specific behavior, one need only collect a blood or urine sample from the subject during or following the experience or act. In most studies, urinary or plasma levels of either the hormones of interest or the products of the metabolism of these hormones are determined. In some cases, single measurements are made immediately following exposure to critical stimuli or engaging in particular behaviors, whereas in others, repeated measurements are made to determine the long-term responses to experience.

There are some methodological problems inherent in repeated sampling for long-term response measurements. For example, taking blood from an artery or a vein is quite stressful to the individual, and, therefore, the individual's hormone levels might reflect the stresses of repeated sampling more than an actual response to the experience being studied. Investigators have been able to circumvent this problem somewhat by inserting indwelling tubes or catheters into blood vessels so that blood samples can be collected with a minimum of disturbance to the individual.

Mason's (1968) elegant series of studies on the endocrine responses in the rhesus monkey to avoidance situations was designed to determine the hormonal responses to behaving or experience. In these studies, the investigators were interested in providing an "endocrine screen" or the total pattern of endocrine responses to avoidance situations. Mason and his colleagues maintained monkeys on a shock-avoidance schedule for 72 hours. Throughout this period, urine and blood samples were collected and analyzed for levels of a wide range of hormones and their metabolites. By using this type of design, Mason's group was able to determine the pattern of endocrine responses over time to this type of stressful experience.

Assessing the Role of Neural Mediators

Most behavioral endocrinologists agree that many of the effects of hormones on behavior are mediated by their effects on the state of the central nervous system circuits involved in the perception of critical stimuli and the integration of behavioral responses. Establishing that a particular brain site mediates the effects of a hormone on a behavior can be accomplished in a variety of ways. Although one could begin with any of the following steps, the sequence below represents one systematic approach that has been used.

First, one should establish which brain areas are important to which behaviors. This can be accomplished in a variety of ways, and the physiological psychology literature is filled with studies directed toward this end. However, two kinds of studies have been used most frequently to establish neural mediating areas for hormonal effects: lesion studies and stimulation studies. In a typical lesion study, one removes different parts of the brain and studies the resultant effects on behavior. If a lesion in a particular area alters the pattern of responding, it would appear that that area is somehow related to the normal expression of that behavior. In stimulation studies, one applies electrical stimulation to different brain sites and observes the behavioral effects. Again, if stimulating a particular site alters the pattern of responding, one might conclude that that neural area is somehow related to that behavior. Ideally, the two types of studies yield complimentary results. For example, lesions of the preoptic-hypothalamic area of the brain depress sexual responding in the males of many species, and stimulating these areas leads to increased sexual performance, at least in rats (Bermant & Davidson, 1974).

After establishing that a particular brain site is important in the control of a particular pattern of behavior, the next step might be to establish whether that area is sensitive to or affected by changes in the levels of the hormone in question. One technique for determination of hormone-sensitive brain sites is the measurement of the relative affinity or attraction of particular areas of the brain for particular hormones. In these studies, radiolabeled (radioactive) hormones are injected systemically, and then the relative concentrations of the radiolabeled substance in different brain areas are measured. An area that concentrates the hormone is considered to be particularly sensitive to or have a great affinity for that hormone. Of course, just because a brain site is sensitive to a hormone does not necessarily mean that that site is where the hormone acts to affect behavior.

One next might determine whether a particular hormone modifies the activity of the "critical" brain sites. This can be accomplished by injecting the test hormone either systemically or directly into the brain area and measuring whether there are changes in the electrical activity of that brain site. For example, if one wishes to determine whether androgens affect the activity of the preoptic area, one might increase systemic androgen levels and determine whether the electrical activity in the preoptic area is altered. Alternatively, one could inject androgens directly into the preoptic area and simultaneously record the local activity of that brain area. If such treatments do not affect the activity of the brain area, it is unlikely that that area is involved in the mediation of the effects of the test hormone on behavior.

Once it has been established that a particular brain site is important in the control of a behavior and that that brain site is sensitive to and affected by a hormone that affects that behavior, one can turn to a direct test of whether that hormone affects that behavior by modifying the state of that particular brain site. This determination typically is carried out by first removing the hormone from the circulation by removing its source (the gland that secretes it), and then replacing the hormone only in the brain site in question. If local application into a brain area is sufficient to counteract the effects of removing a hormone from the total circulation, one can conclude that only the neural actions of that hormone are necessary for the normal display of the behavior being studied. For example, having established that the preoptic area is important to the display of male sexual behavior, and having established that the activity of the preoptic area is affected by the androgens, one can ask whether the androgens affect male sexual behavior because they modify the state of the preoptic area. If local application of an androgen into the preoptic area counteracts the effects of castration on sexual behavior, it can be concluded that only the neural action of this androgen is necessary for the normal display of male sexual responses. This kind of study does not, of course, limit the number of sites at which androgens can be working, but it does indicate one site where such hormones do work. Most investigators believe that the brain is organized into circuits, rather than discrete centers, and, therefore, hormones might be able to exert their effects at any point in a circuit.

In the same way that direct implantation of hormones into "critical" brain sites is the most direct test of whether the brain mediates hormonal effects on behavior in adulthood, the same technique can be used to establish that early hormonal effects on adult responding are mediated by local effects of these hormones on the infant's brain. For example, Nadler (1968, 1973) administered testosterone directly into the hypothalamus of infant female rats. This treatment produces the same masculinizing effects on adult sexual behavior as do systemic injections of this androgen.

Most behavioral endocrinologists also believe that the central nervous system mediates the effects of experience or behaving on endocrine function. Demonstration of the role of the brain as mediator of the effects of experience on endocrine function has been more difficult than demonstrating its role as mediator of hormonal effects on behavior. One cannot inject an experience into restricted brain sites and study resultant effects on hormone secretion in the same way that one can inject hormones into the brain and study behavioral effects. Therefore, much of the belief that the brain mediates experiential effects on endocrine function is based on commonalities between those brain sites whose activity is affected by experience and those sites which affect endocrine function. An example of this kind of analysis was provided before for the case of agonistic experiences.

One can, however, disrupt the functioning of some parts of the brain and then study the effects of this modification on the hormonal responses to experience. If altering the functioning of a particular brain site changes the form or intensity of the hormonal responses to experience, it would then appear that that brain site is involved in the mediation of the effects of that experience on endocrine function. For example, Endröczi and Nyákás (1971) studied the role of the septum in the effects of conflict on corticosterone secretion. They placed a lesion in the septum and found that the corticosterone responses to conflict were exaggerated, thus suggesting that the septum is important in the mediation of the effects of conflict on adrenocortical functioning. This kind of study does not, of course, tell us specifically whether the lesion alters the hormonal responses to experience because that brain site is important in the accurate perception of the stimulus situation or because that brain site is critical to adrenocortical functioning in general. It does show in a general way, however, that this brain site is important to the display of normal endocrine responses to experience.

Studying Long-Chain Hormone–Behavior Interactions

Although most theoretical models of hormone–behavior interactions have included the proposition that the relationships among the environment, endocrine function, and behavior are continuous and dynamic, relatively few investigators have examined hormone–behavior interactions in their dynamic forms. Those who have focused on long-chain hormone–behavior interactions have used two techniques. One involves what might be called "partialling" of the chain, and the other involves disrupting one part of the chain and observing the effects of this disruption on the rest of the sequence. Lehrman's classic work on the reproductive behavior of the ring dove is the most complete analysis of long-chain hormone–behavior interactions; the technique of partialling the chain was used. Lehrman and colleagues conducted an elaborate series of studies which, first, articulated both the sequence of behaviors occurring during courtship and egg incubation and the environmental stimuli that elicit or potentiate each stage in the behavioral sequence. They then analyzed both the hormonal factors on which each of the behaviors depends and the hormonal changes that occur following each stage in the "stimulus-behavior-stimulus-behavior" chain. As a part of this analysis they even were able to determine which hormonal changes were elicited by external stimuli and which were elicited by engaging in specific behaviors. Through this type of detailed analysis of each step in the total sequence of environmental-behavioral-hormonal events they were able to show that engaging in courtship behaviors (which depends at least partly on hormonal factors) causes certain hormonal secretions that facilitate the building of nests. Building of nests causes the secretion of other hormonal factors, which induce the birds to sit on eggs. Sitting on eggs induces the secretion of another hormone which maintains brooding behavior and readies the birds to feed the young when they hatch (see Lehrman, 1965, for a detailed account of this work).

Nock and Leshner (1976) used the second technique, disruption of the chain, to study a long-chain hormone–behavior interaction that occurs in competitive situations. Their studies were a test of the hypothesis that although an animal's baseline hormonal state may determine the form and intensity of its initial behavioral responses, the animal's experiences in the agonistic situation lead to changes in its hormonal state that then feed back and can lead to changes in its pattern of agonistic responding. This hypothesis suggests a long-chain interaction involving an animal's baseline hormonal state, its initial responses and experiences, a change in its hormonal state caused by those experiences, and, then, a change in its behavior caused by the change in its hormonal state. In order to test this hypothesis, Nock and Leshner disrupted the chain by preventing the hormonal responses to the experience of defeat. They controlled the animal's hormone levels throughout the encounter at a fixed level. Therefore, if the hypothesis were true, preventing hormonal change in response to defeat should have prevented or altered the behavioral changes that ordinarily accompany this experience. Significantly, disrupting the chain by preventing the hormonal responses to defeat both delayed and decreased the changes in behavior that ordinarily accompany this experience, thereby establishing a causal connection between the hormonal responses to defeat and the behavioral changes that accompany and follow this experience.

A *Potential Problem in Interpreting Studies of Hormone–Behavior Interactions*

The existence of both behavioral effects of the baseline hormonal state and feedback effects of the hormonal responses to experience on ongoing and subsequent behavioral responses may pose a problem in interpreting the results of traditional studies of hormones and behavior. This problem stems from the fact that the frequently used techniques of removing a gland and treating with a fixed hormone dosage actually result in modifications of both the baseline hormonal state and the hormonal responses to experience. For example, if we castrate a rat and then treat it with a fixed dosage of testosterone we really are doing two things: First, we are modifying its baseline hormonal state, because the hormonal manipulations are made prior to exposing the animal to critical stimuli. But, second, we also are controlling its androgen responses to those stimuli; no gland is there to produce the hormonal response. Therefore, the results of this kind of study could present a serious problem in interpretation: Do they reflect the effects of the baseline hormonal state on behavior or the effects of modifying the hormonal responses to experience, with their feedback effects on behavioral responses?

Can one know whether an observed effect is a result of altering the baseline hormonal state or a result of altering the hormonal responses to experience? There are at least two possible solutions to this problem. First, one can rely on standard correlational studies to determine whether there are relationships between the baseline hormonal state and the behavior in question, or between the magnitude of the hormonal response and the level of responding, or both. If one discovers a correlation between endogenous changes in hormone levels and levels of the behavior, then it is probable that there is a relationship between the baseline hormonal state and the behavior. In the case of sexual behavior, we shall see (Chapter 5) that there are dramatic correlations between endogenous changes in gonadal hormone levels across the estrous cycle and levels of sexual responding in female animals. Thus, it is likely that experimental manipulations that produce similar hormonal changes and alter responding in the predicted way are in fact telling us about the effects of the baseline hormonal state; we know from the correlational studies that there is some relationship.

On the other hand, if there is no correlation between normal endogenous hormonal changes and changes in the behavior, then it would seem unlikely that experimental studies are telling us about the effects of the baseline hormonal state. For example, in the case of avoidance responding (Chapter 7), no clear correlations between endogenous hormone level changes and levels of avoidance responding have been identified. Thus, it may be that the baseline hormonal state is not involved in the control of this behavior. On the other hand, there are strong correlations between the magnitude of the hormonal responses to stress and the level of avoidance responding. Therefore, experimental manipulations made prior to avoidance training may affect avoidance responding because they modify the hormonal responses to this experience (with their feedback effects on behavior), rather than because they alter the baseline hormonal state.

A second possible means for separating the effects of the baseline hormonal state from the feedback effects of the hormonal responses to experience would be to rely on correlational studies examining hormone–behavior relationships over time. One can "map" the time courses of hormonal and behavioral changes. Then, if a behavioral event occurs before the hormonal change, it would be impossible to argue that the hormonal change plays a role in controlling the behavior. Alternatively, if the behavioral event occurs only after the hormonal change, one would have to look for potential feedback effects whereby the hormonal change might in some way be responsible for the change in behavior.

This potential interpretive problem is dealt with in the following discussions by, as much as possible, considering correlational studies first. In this way, we can have some idea about whether or not the baseline hormonal state might be involved in the control of a behavior before attempting to interpret accurately the relevant experimental studies. Unfortunately, there have been only very few correlational studies examining the time courses of behavioral and hormonal events in any detail, and, therefore, that kind of interpretive aid is not readily available.

SUMMARY AND COMMENT

The purpose of this chapter was to provide an introduction to some of the major theoretical and technical issues in behavioral endocrinology. We have reviewed how hormones might be related to behavior and some theoretical models which have been proposed to describe this complex relationship. In discussing techniques of study, we have surveyed some of the experimental designs used to determine hormonal effects on behavior, the relationship between the early hormonal environment and adult behavior patterns, the hormonal responses to experience or behaving, the role of the central nervous system as mediator of hormone–behavior interactions, and the long-chain interrelationship between hormones and behavior in its dynamic form.

The remainder of the book is devoted to a general review of the literature. Many of the issues raised in this introductory chapter will be discussed in more detail, and the theoretical issues raised here will be reevaluated in Chapter 9. The reviews that follow are not intended to be complete; references to more complete reviews will be provided in each chapter. Rather, these reviews are intended to provide the reader with an overview of what is known about the relationship between endocrine function and each of the classes of behavior or experience. Chapter 2 considers the relationship between hormones and the class of behaviors whose major function appears to be maintaining the internal economy of the organism, the regulatory behaviors. Chapters 3 and 4 treat the role of hormones in social behaviors, Chapters 5 and 6 are concerned with reproductive behaviors, and Chapters 7 and 8 are concerned with the relationship of hormones to emotion, emotionality, and mood.

REFERENCES

Ader, R.   Early experience and hormones: emotional behavior and adrenocortical hormones. In B. E. Eleftheriou & R. L. Sprott (Eds.), *Hormonal Correlates of Behavior, Vol. 1.* New York: Plenum Press, 1975, pp. 7-33.

Adkins, E. K.   Hormonal basis of sexual differentiation in the Japanese quail. *Journal of Comparative and Physiological Psychology*, 1975, 89, 61-71.

Antelman, S. M. & Brown, T. S.   Hippocampal lesions and shuttlebox avoidance behavior: a fear hypothesis. *Physiology and Behavior*, 1972, 9, 15-20.

Balász, R., Potel, A. J. & Hajós, F.   Factors affecting the biochemical maturation of the brain: effects of hormones during early life. *Psychoneuroendocrinology*, 1975, 1, 25-36.

Beach, F. A.   *Hormones and Behavior.* New York: Hoeber, 1948.

Beach, F. A.   Retrospect and prospect. In F. A. Beach (Ed.), *Sex and Behavior.* New York: Wiley, 1965.

Beach, F. A.   Behavioral endocrinology and the study of reproduction. *Biology of Reproduction*, 1974, 10, 2-18.
Beach, F. A.   Behavioral endocrinology: an emerging discipline. *American Scientist*, 1975, 63, 178-187.
Beach, F. A. & Holz, A. M.   Mating behavior in male rats castrated at various ages and injected with androgen. *Journal of Experimental Zoology*, 1946, 101, 91-142.
Bermant, G. & Davidson, J. M.   *Biological Bases of Sexual Behavior.* New York: Harper and Row, 1974.
Brain, P. F., Evans, C. M. & Poole, A. E.   Studies on the effects of cyproterone acetate administered in adulthood or in early life on subsequent endocrine function and agonistic behavior in male albino laboratory mice. *Journal of Endocrinology*, 1974, 61, xlv.
Davenport, J. W. & Dorcey, T. P.   Hypothyroidism: learning deficit induced in rats by early exposure to thiouracil. *Hormones and Behavior*, 1972, 3, 97-112.
Davidson, J. M.   Hormones and reproductive behavior. In S. Levine (Ed.), *Hormones and Behavior*. New York: Academic Press, 1972, pp. 63-134.
Dunlap, J. L., Preis, L. K. & Gerall, A. H.   Compensatory ovarian hypertrophy as a function of age and neonatal androgenization. *Endocrinology*, 1972, 90, 1309-1314.
Eleftheriou, B. E.   Effects of aggression and defeat on brain macromolecules. In B. E. Eleftheriou & J. P. Scott (Eds.), *Physiology of Aggression and Defeat*. New York: Plenum Press, 1971, pp. 65-90.
Eleftheriou, B. E. & Church, R. L.   Brain 5-hydroxytryptophan decarboxylase in mice after exposure to aggression and defeat. *Physiology and Behavior*, 1968, 3, 323-325.
Eleftheriou, B. E. & Sprott, R. L.   *Hormonal Correlates of Behavior.* New York: Plenum Press, 1975.
Endröczi, E. & Nyákás, C.   Effect of septal lesion on exploratory activity, passive avoidance learning, and pituitary-adrenal function in the rat. *Acta Physiologica Academiae Scientiarum Hungaricae*, 1971, 39, 351-360.
Goy, R. W., Bridson, W. E. & Young, W. C.   Period of maximal susceptibility of the prenatal female guinea pig to masculinizing actions of testosterone propionate. *Journal of Comparative and Physiological Psychology*, 1964, 57, 166-174.
Goy, R. W. & Goldfoot, D. A.   Hormonal influences on sexually dimorphic behavior. In *Handbook of Physiology—Endocrinology II, Part I*. Washington: American Physiological Society, 1973, pp. 169-186.
Hart, B. L.   Neonatal castration: influence on neural organization of sexual reflexes in male rats. *Science*, 1968, 160, 1135-1136.

Horn, G.   Physiological and psychological aspects of selective percep-tion. In D. S. Lehrman, R. A. Hinde & E. Shaw (Eds.), *Advances in the Study of Behavior, Vol. I.* New York: Academic Press, 1965, pp. 155-215.

Joffe, J. M., Milkovic, K. & Levine, S.   Effects of changes in maternal pituitary-adrenal function on behavior of rat offspring. *Physiology and Behavior,* 1972, 8, 425-430.

Kamel, F., Mock, E. J., Wright, W. W. & Frankel, A. I.   Alterations in plasma concentrations of testosterone, L.H., and prolactin associated with mating in the male rat. *Hormones and Behavior,* 1975, 6, 277-288.

Komisaruk, B. R., Adler, N. T. & Hutchinson, J.   Genital sensory field: enlargement by estrogen treatment in female rats. *Science,* 1972, 178, 1295-1298.

Kow, L. M. & Pfaff, D. W.   Effects of estrogen treatment on the size of the receptive field and response threshold of pudendal nerve in the female rat. *Neuroendocrinology,* 1974, 13, 299-313.

Lehrman, D. S.   Interaction between internal and external environ-ment in the regulation of the reproductive cycle of the ring dove. In F. A. Beach (Ed.), *Sex and Behavior.* New York: Wiley, 1965, pp. 355-380.

LeMagnen, J.   Les phenoménes olfactosexuals chez le rat blanc. *Ar-chives of the Science of Physiology,* 1952, 6, 295-331.

Leshner, A. I.   A model of hormones and agonistic behavior. *Physiol-ogy and Behavior,* 1975, 15, 225-235.

Leshner, A. I. & Walker, W. A.   Dietary self-selection, activity, and carcass composition of rats fed thiouracil. *Physiology and Behavior,* 1973, 10, 373-378.

Levine, S. (Ed.), *Hormones and Behavior.* New York: Academic Press, 1972.

Levine, S. & Mullins, R. F.   Hormonal influences on brain organiza-tion in infant rats. *Science,* 1966, 152, 1585-1592.

Lisk, R. D.   Hormonal regulation of sexual behavior in poluestrus mammals common to the laboratory. In *Handbook of Physiology, Sec-tion 7, Vol. 2.* Washington: American Physiological Society, 1973, 223-260.

Lissák, K. (Ed.),   *Hormones and Brain Function.* New York: Plenum Press, 1973.

Marañon, G.   Contribution á l'étude de l'action émotive de l'adréna-line. *Revue Francaise d'Endocrinologie,* 1924, 2, 301-325.

Mason, J. W.   Organization of the multiple endocrine response to avoidance in the monkey. *Psychosomatic Medicine,* 1968, 30, 774-790.

McEwen, B. S., Pfaff, D. W. & Zigmond, R. E.   Factors influencing sex hormone uptake by rat brain regions. II. Effects of neonatal treatment and hypophysectomy on testosterone uptake. *Brain Research,* 1970, 21, 17-28.

Modigh, K. Effects of isolation and fighting in mice on the rate of synthesis of noradrenalin, dopamine, and 5-hydroxytriptamine in the brain. *Psychopharmacologia,* 1973, 33, 1-17.

Money, J. & Ehrhardt, A. A. *Man & Woman, Boy & Girl.* Baltimore: Johns Hopkins Press, 1972.

Nadler, R. D. Masculinization of female rats by intracranial implantation of androgens in infancy. *Journal of Comparative and Physiological Psychology,* 1968, 66, 157-167.

Nadler, R. D. Further evidence on the intra-hypothalamic locus for androgenization of female rats. *Neuroendocrinology,* 1973, 12, 110-119.

Nock, B. L. & Leshner, A. I. Hormonal mediation of the effects of defeat on agonistic responding in mice. *Physiology and Behavior,* 1976, 17, 111-119.

Nyákás, C. & Endröczi, E. Effect of neonatal corticosterone administration on behavioral and pituitary-adrenocortical responses in the rat. *Acta Physiologica Academiae Scientiarum Hungaricae,* 1972, 42, 231-241.

Paul, D. H. & D'Angelo, S. A. Dexamethasone and corticosterone administration to pregnant rats: effects on pituitary-adrenocortical function in the newborn. *Proceedings of the Society for Experimental Biology and Medicine,* 1972, 140, 1360-1364.

Phoenix, C. H., Goy, R. W., Gerall, A. A. & Young, W. C. Organizing action of prenatally administered testosterone propionate in the tissues mediating mating behavior in the female guinea pig. *Endocrinology,* 1959, 65, 369-387.

Ryzhenkov, V. E. Brain monoaminergic mechanisms and hypothalamic-pituitary-adrenal activity. In K. Lissák (Ed.), *Hormones and Brain Function.* New York: Plenum Press, 1973, pp. 285-286.

Sawyer, C. H. & Gorski, R. A. (Eds.), *Steroid Hormones and Brain Function.* Berkeley: University of California Press, 1971.

Strand, F. L., Stoboy, H. & Cayer, A. A possible direct action of ACTH on nerve and muscle. *Neuroendocrinology,* 1974, 13, 1-20.

Turner, C. F. & Bagnara, J. T. *General Endocrinology,* 5th ed. Philadelphia: W. B. Saunders, 1971.

Vernikos-Danellis, J. Effects of hormones on the central nervous system. In S. Levine (Ed.), *Hormones and Behavior,* New York: Academic Press, 1972, pp. 11-62.

Ward, I. L. & Renz, F. J. Consequences of perinatal hormone manipulation on the adult sexual behavior of female rats. *Journal of Comparative and Physiological Psychology,* 1972, 78, 349-355.

Welch, A. S. & Welch, B. L. Isolation, reactivity and aggression: evidence for an involvement of brain catecholamines and serotonin. In B. E. Eleftheriou & J. P. Scott (Eds.), *Physiology of Aggression and Defeat.* New York: Plenum Press, 1971, pp. 91-142.

Welch, B. L. & Welch, A. S.　Sustained effects of brief daily stress (fighting) upon brain and adrenal catecholamines and adrenal, spleen, and heart weights of mice. *Proceedings of the National Academy of Sciences,* 1969, 63, 100-107.

Whalen, R. K. (Ed.), *Hormones and Behavior.* Toronto: Van Nostrand, 1967.

Young, W. C.　The hormones and mating behavior. In W. C. Young (Ed.), *Sex and Internal Secretions.* Baltimore: Williams & Wilkins, 1961, pp. 1173-1239.

Chapter 2

SOME REGULATORY
BEHAVIORS

The term *regulatory behaviors* refers to a fairly broad class of behaviors whose primary functions appear to be the maintenance of physiological or metabolic constancies in the body. Many of these behaviors seem both to affect and to be affected by the individual's hormonal state. In this chapter we shall review some of the relationships between endocrine function and eating, dietary self-selection, and running activity—the regulatory behaviors to which behavioral endocrinologists have devoted most attention. The discussions that follow are summaries of what is known in this area. The reader interested in more detail might consult the more comprehensive reviews by Panksepp (1975), Wade (1972, 1976), and Woods, Decke, and Vasselli (1974).

Why should endocrine function and the regulatory behaviors be related? The concept "regulatory behavior" implies that a particular type of behavioral response is involved in the regulation or maintenance of some physiological characteristic at an optimal or "set-point" level, much as in any homeostatic system. In the case of the behaviors to be considered here, the critical parameter seems most often to be related to the levels of the body tissue stores that are important both to growth and to the availability of energy. The levels of the body tissue stores are dependent on intermediary metabolic processes, such as protein, fat, and carbohydrate metabolisms, and, of course, these processes are intimately related to levels of endocrine activity. Because changes in hormonal states produce dramatic changes in intermediary metabolic reactions and because the regulatory behaviors respond to changes in metabolic states (and, in turn, feed back and affect those states), it seems reasonable that the regulatory behaviors also should be related to endocrine activity.

Hormones seem to affect the regulatory behaviors in two ways. One is by producing metabolic changes which cause deviations from the set-point or optimum for the critical characteristic or parameter. The second mechanism involves actually altering or re-setting the optimal level or set-point. In the first case, hormonal changes alter the existing or current level of the critical parameter, creating a deviation from the set-point that must be corrected. The level of the regulatory behavior then changes in order to correct that deviation. In this way, behavior can serve as a regulatory mechanism that compensates for deviations from metabolic set-points. An example is provided by the case of sodium consumption. Adrenalectomized rats suffer sodium deficiencies because they cannot retain sodium in the absence of the mineralocorticoids. They respond to this deficiency by increasing their dietary intake of sodium, thereby returning the endogenous level of this mineral toward the optimum (Clark & Clausen, 1943).

In the second case, hormones appear to actually shift the set-point or optimal level for the critical parameter, rather than simply cause deviations from the existing set-point. Then, changes in the level of the regulatory behavior aid in the achievement of the new set-point level. For example, some investigators believe that eating can serve as a regulatory behavior that facilitates the maintenance of body weight or body fat stores at optimal levels. If an individual is below the set-point for body weight, it will increase its food intake until the set-point is achieved. If, however, the individual is above the set-point level for body weight, it will decrease its food intake until body weight returns to that optimal level (e.g., Kennedy, 1966; Mayer 1955). Some hormones, such as the estrogens, may affect eating by modifying or shifting the set-point level for body weight or body fat. When ovariectomized rats are injected with estrogens, their food intake decreases until they become lean, and when estrogen treatment is discontinued, their food intake increases until body weight returns to pretreatment levels. This type of finding has been interpreted as showing that estrogen treatment lowers the set-point for body weight, and that the resultant changes in food intake represent a mechanism for achieving the newly established optimal body weight level (Wade, 1972, 1976).

In addition to affecting the regulatory behaviors, hormones may be involved in the mediation of behavioral effects on metabolic states. Engaging in regulatory behaviors often leads to changes in endocrine function, and these changes in hormonal states could be responsible for the effects of those behaviors on the levels of metabolic stores. For example, engaging in running wheel activity leads to decreases in body fat levels. Running in activity wheels also leads to increases in the secretion of the glucocorticoids from the adrenal cortex. Importantly, injecting glucocorticoids into non-running animals can lead to the same changes in body fat levels as does running, suggesting that the glucocorticoid response to engaging in exercise might be involved in the mediation of the effects of that behavior on body fat levels (Leshner, 1971).

The fact that hormones both affect regulatory behaviors and might mediate the effects of regulatory behaviors on critical parameters suggests that there could be long-chain hormone–behavior interactions in the case of these behaviors, similar to those discussed in a general way in Chapter 1. This possibility will be considered in more detail as we review the relevant literature. Before turning to that review, it might be useful to note that the majority of studies examining hormones and regulatory behaviors have used only rodents as subjects and, therefore, the generality of the relationships to be discussed here may be somewhat limited. We shall discuss that generality to some degree as we proceed.

FOOD INTAKE

There is little question that eating can function as a regulatory behavior. This behavior is the primary mechanism for the intake of both calories and the nutrients that are necessary to sustain life. However, total food intake and the selection of specific nutrients have been studied separately, and, therefore, these behaviors will be considered separately in this chapter.

Theories of the regulatory nature of feeding have focused on both the "short-term" and the "long-term" control of food intake. When considering the short-term control of food intake, one is interested in the stimuli involved in the initiation or termination of feeding episodes. On the other hand, when considering the long-term control of food intake, one is interested in the factors that control the amount of food eaten over time or over many meals. Most traditional views of the short-term regulation of food intake have proposed what might be called "depletion-repletion" models of food intake. They suggest that eating is initiated in response to a depletion or reduction in the circulating level of a critical metabolite, such as blood sugar, and that eating terminates with the repletion of that metabolite (e.g., Mayer, 1955). Some recent evidence, however, has suggested that the traditional depletion-repletion view may be inappropriate for the short-term control of feeding, and that other influences, e.g., ecological factors, may be controlling the initiation and/or termination of feeding episodes (Collier, Hirsch & Hamlin, 1972; Hirsch, 1973). It is not within the realm of our discussion to decide among these views of the short-term control of feeding. However, the reader should keep in mind that the issue is unsettled.

In contrast to their views of the short-term situation, most theorists seem to agree that in a long-term sense, feeding is a regulatory behavior directed toward the control of some parameter related to body weight or body composition. Most mammalian species seem to have set-points around which body weight and composition are regulated (body weight and composition levels are relatively constant over time), and deviations from these set-points seem to be the factors determining the amount of food eaten over time (Kennedy, 1966; Nisbett, 1972; Wade, 1972, 1976). Of course, although these theorists speak about "body weight regulation" and "body weight set-points," animals do not have scales in their feet, and most investigators agree that it is not body weight per se that is being regulated. Rather, it probably is some other characteristic on which body weight depends, such as body fat stores, that is the critical parameter. The term "body weight regulation" will be used here because of convention, and the reader is asked to keep in mind that this term usually means body weight and/or composition regulation and that studies of body weight regulation alone carry the assumption that some other parameter is really being studied, the level of which is reflected in body weight.

It is unlikely that hormones stimulate food intake directly. Rather, they more likely affect eating either by modifying the states of those cues that do signal the need to eat, or they affect the neural mechanisms that are responsible for the control of eating and the amount of food consumed (Panksepp, 1975). Moreover, some hormones may serve primarily in the mediation of the effects of eating on body tissue stores, rather than in affecting eating characteristics. These potential roles and mechanisms will be considered for each hormone system separately.

The Gonadal Hormones

There are marked gender differences in both food intake and body weight and composition: the males of most species both weigh more and eat more than their female counterparts. These sex differences appear to be at least partly a result of sex differences in gonadal hormone secretions, and a great amount of attention has been directed toward the role of the gonadal hormones, particularly the ovarian hormones, in the control of food intake.

Although castrating male rats leads to only a relatively slight reduction in both body weight and food intake, ovariectomizing female rats leads to marked increases in both of these parameters. In fact, ovariectomized females consume about the same amount of food as do intact male rats, and, although the body weight levels of ovariectomized females still are below those of males, both groups exhibit the same carcass tissue proportions. Table 2-1 presents the results of a study examining the effects of gonadectomy on body weight and composition in adult male and female rats (from Leshner & Collier, 1973). Note that although the body compositions of intact male and female rats are quite different, the body composition proportions of ovariectomized females are quite similar to those of males.

These kinds of findings have led to the suggestion that the ovarian hormones exert inhibitory influences on food intake and body weight, and that the presence of the female sex hormones can partly account for the observed gender differences in food intake and body weight and composition (e.g., Wade, 1976). Further support for this position comes from studies showing that hormone treatments during early developmental stages that "mas-

Table 2-1
The Effects of Gonadectomy on Body Weight and Composition

Group	Body Weight (g)	Water (%)	Fat (%)	Protein (%)
Intact males	324.5	60.7	15.8	12.8
Castrated males	316.7	58.8	18.2	12.7
Intact females	204.8	63.7	10.7	14.1
Ovariect. females	251.4	59.9	16.1	13.6

culinize" females morphologically also lead to adult body weight and food intake levels that are quite similar to those of genetic males (Bell & Zucker, 1971; Slob & van der Werff ten Bosch, 1975).

There is substantial evidence to suggest that the most important ovarian hormones in the control of food intake and body weight are the estrogens. In many female mammals, there is a dramatic reduction in both body weight and food intake around the time of ovulation. This periovulatory decrease in food intake and body weight has been observed in the females of species as diverse as rats, pigs, goats, sheep, and monkeys (Baile & Forbes, 1974; Czaja, 1975; Tarttelin & Gorski, 1971). Figure 2-1 presents an example of food intake levels across the estrous cycle in the rat, and demonstrates the magnitude of the periovulatory decrease in the amount of food consumed. In addition, around the time of ovulation, there is a marked rise in the circulating level of the estrogens. Therefore, there is an inverse correlation between circulating estrogen levels and food intake. This correlation led many investigators to begin to examine in detail the role of the ovarian hormones in the estrous cycle variations in food intake.

As discussed before, removing the ovarian hormones by ovariectomy leads to an increase in body weight and food intake. However, the increase in food intake is only transitory; food intake returns to more normal levels as body weight reaches a higher plateau (Mook et al., 1972). Moreover, treating ovariectomized rats with estrogens returns their food intake to lower levels and seems to lower the level at which body weight is regulated (Dubuc, 1974; Wade, 1975). The other major class of ovarian hormones, the progestogens, does not seem to affect either food intake or body weight in ovariectomized rats, although it can block the restorative effects of estrogen treatment (Wade, 1975).

These findings show that changes in estrogen levels can alter both body weight and food intake levels, and they suggest that the periovulatory decrease in these parameters probably is a result

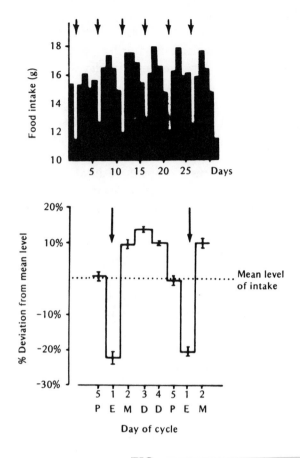

FIG. 2-1

Cyclic fluctuations in actual food intake of one rat (upper figure) correlated with its vaginal cycle. Vertical arrows indicate vaginal estrus. The lower figure presents the average cycle as determined by the percent deviation from the mean level of food intake during 21 estrous cycles in 7 rats. Abbreviations: D, diestrus; E, estrus; M, metestrus; and P, proestrus (from Tarttelin & Gorski, *Physiology and Behavior*, 1971, 7, 848; by permission of Pergamon Press).

of the increased estrogen levels characteristic of this period. Significantly, estrogens affect food intake in rats that are at fairly high body weight levels, but these hormones do not affect eating in lean rats (Zucker, 1972). This finding suggests that estrogen's effects on food intake may be secondary to its effects on body weight; that is, estrogen depression of food intake may represent an attempt to achieve an estrogen-induced lowered set-point for body weight. If the animal already is lean, estrogen will not reduce the body weight set-point further, and food intake will not be decreased. However, if the animal is heavy, estrogen does lower the set-point for body weight, and food intake does decrease until that new set-point is reached. Conversely, ovariectomy raises the body weight set-point, and food intake increases; but it increases only until the new body weight level is reached. According to this interpretation, eating is a regulatory behavior involved in the achievement and maintenance of the set-point for body weight, and the estrogens affect food intake because they alter the set-point for body weight. The interested reader is referred to the excellent reviews by Wade (1972, 1976) for a more detailed discussion of this argument.

It should be noted that the ovarian hormones are not always effective in modifying food intake and body weight. Specifically, manipulations of the levels of the ovarian hormones do not begin to affect food intake and body weight until puberty has been reached. Ovariectomy will not increase food intake and body weight and estrogen treatment will not decrease these characteristics until the animal achieves this developmental stage. It could be that the mechanisms that mediate gonadal hormone effects have not matured and are not responsive to changes in ovarian hormone levels until the time of puberty. Or, it could be that some other characteristic of the prepubertal animal, such as the high level of growth hormone, masks the effects of the ovarian hormones on food intake and body weight (Ross & Zucker, 1974; Wade & Zucker, 1970a). The latter possibility will be discussed in more detail when the role of growth hormone in food intake is considered.

How do the ovarian hormones exert their effects on food intake and body weight? The most probable explanation seems to be that the ovarian hormones affect eating by modifying the states of the central neural circuits that exert primary control over food intake and body weight. Although there are many brain sites that are important in the control of food intake and weight, the ventromedial hypothalamus (VMH) has been implicated as the primary site for the mediation of the effects of estrogen on food intake. This brain site appears to be an important part of the neural circuit that controls body weight and composition, and appears quite important in the neural control of food intake (e.g., Kennedy, 1969).

Implanting estradiol benzoate directly into the VMH is effective in counteracting the stimulatory effects of ovariectomy on food intake and body weight, whereas estrogen implants into other hypothalamic areas are much less effective (Beatty, O'Briant & Vilberg, 1974; Wade & Zucker, 1970b). However, although the VMH may be the most potent site where brain implants of estrogens can affect food intake and body weight, it probably is not the only site. Ovariectomy and estrogen treatment still affect body weight and food intake in rats with lesions in the VMH, suggesting that the estrogens can affect food intake in other sites as well (King & Cox, 1973).

The progestogens may also affect food intake by acting on the brain. Although progesterone implants into the VMH do not affect feeding in ovariectomized (heavy) rats, progesterone implants into the dorsomedial hypothalamus will stimulate feeding in adrenalectomized-ovariectomized (lean) animals (Jankowiak & Stern, 1974). In addition, in sheep, progesterone implants into the lateral ventricles of the brain block the depressive effects of estrogen on food intake (Forbes, 1974). This finding reinforces the suggestion that progesterone blocks the depressive effects of estrogens on food intake.

The Pancreatic Hormones

Both pancreatic hormones, insulin and glucagon, have been shown to have marked effects on food intake, and their effects generally are opposite: Insulin treatment leads to an increase in food intake in most species (sheep are one exception), whereas glucagon treatment leads to a decrease in food intake (at least in rats and humans) (Baile & Forbes, 1974; Hoebel & Teitelbaum, 1966; Schulman et al., 1957; Stunkard, Van Itallie & Reis, 1955; Woods, Decke & Vasselli, 1974). The effects of insulin on food intake have been studied extensively, although relatively little experimental attention has been directed toward the details of the effects of glucagon.

Insulin treatments lead to an increase in food intake and body weight, and cessation of insulin treatment is followed by a decline in both of these measures until the individual achieves its pretreatment body weight level, at which point food intake returns to normal (Hoebel & Teitelbaum, 1966; Mandell, 1971). Although insulin has a wide range of metabolic effects, most investigators seem to believe that it affects food intake by decreasing carbohydrate availability and utilization.

Insulin treatment leads to a decrease in blood sugar levels, and it does this in a dose-response fashion: progressively increasing insulin dosages lead to progressive decreases in blood sugar levels. However, it does not affect food intake in this same type of dose-dependent way. There appears to be a threshold or minimum insulin dosage needed to induce excess eating, and larger dosages do not seem to lead to greater increases in food intake (Booth & Pitt, 1968). Thus, insulin's effects are not really determining; they are "all-or-none."

Although insulin does not affect feeding in the same dose-dependent way that it affects blood sugar levels, blood sugar levels and feeding do appear to be related in insulin-treated animals. If one provides large amounts of glucose at the same time that insulin is injected, the induction of eating is delayed. This delay in the insulin induction of eating may occur because the glucose treatment temporarily counteracts the effects of insulin on blood sugar levels (Booth & Pitt, 1968). In this way, insulin would be seen as affecting eating because it causes a decrease in blood sugar levels.

The relationship between carbohydrate levels and the insulin induction of feeding may be mediated by the neural circuits that control feeding. Many theorists (e.g., Mayer, 1955) have argued that although food intake may not be dependent on *circulating* glucose levels, eating may be initiated in response to a decrease in the availability and utilization of glucose in the brain. Significantly, changes in insulin levels do seem to affect the sensitivity of some brain sites to glucose. For example, the VMH of animals with low insulin levels appears relatively insensitive to glucose, and the sensitivity of this area is restored if insulin is administered (Debons, Krimsky & From, 1970; Debons et al., 1969). However, this brain site does not appear essential to insulin's effects on feeding, because lesions of the VMH do not prevent the insulin induction of food intake (York & Bray, 1972).

It also has been suggested that insulin may exert its action on food intake through modifying the functioning of the lateral hypothalamus, and this brain site may be necessary for the induction of eating by insulin. Some studies (e.g., Epstein & Teitelbaum, 1967; Wayner, Cott, Millner & Tartaglione, 1971) have found that lesions of the lateral hypothalamus prevent the increase in food intake that normally accompanies insulin treatment, although other studies (e.g., Stricker, Friedman & Zigmond, 1975) have found that lateral hypothalamic lesions do not affect insulin's actions on food intake. However, insulin treatment does not appear to affect the excitability of the lateral hypothalamus: Low dosages of insulin do not alter the amount of electrical stimulation needed to elicit eating from the lateral hypothalamus (Berthoud & Baettig, 1974).

This brief discussion of the effects of insulin on food intake may leave the reader with a feeling of uneasiness, but the mechanisms of insulin's actions on food intake are not clearly understood. Unfortunately, this kind of ambiguity surrounds many other relationships between hormones and behavior, and underscores the need for more concentrated research in this field.

The Thyroid and Adrenocortical Hormones

Relatively little attention has been directed toward the role of the thyroid and adrenocortical hormones in food intake, but some information has been collected. Thyroidectomy reduces food intake, and replacement therapy with thyroxine restores the food intake of thyroidectomized rats. Furthermore, creating hyperthyroidism by injecting intact rats with thyroxine stimulates food intake (Soulairac, 1967; Warkentin, Warkentin & Ivey, 1943). These actions of the thyroid hormones could possibly reflect some change in the neural circuits that control food intake, although it seems more likely that the very broad metabolic effects of the thyroid hormones are at least somehow involved in the effects of these hormones on food intake.

In rats, adrenalectomy reduces food intake, and replacement therapy with glucocorticoids restores it to normal levels (Leshner, 1971). Treatment of intact rats with glucocorticoids, however, seems to have a bimodal effect on food intake: low dosages of corticosterone stimulate feeding, whereas high dosages decrease food intake (Panksepp, 1975; Van Putten, Van Bekkum & Querido, 1953).

Panksepp (1975) has suggested that such effects reflect different mechanisms of action: low dosages of corticosterone may stimulate food intake because they also stimulate insulin release (an insulin rebound to the hyperglycemia produced by corticoid treatment), whereas high dosages depress food intake because they produce such extreme hyperglycemia. Similarly, adrenalectomy might affect food intake through its effects on carbohydrate metabolism, but it also could decrease food intake as a side effect of the general debilitation that results from removing this gland.

Hypophysectomy and Growth Hormone

The pituitary is often called the "master gland" because in many ways it controls the functioning of the rest of the endocrine system. Because of such broad influence, pituitary activity should affect food intake, if only because its secretions affect other hormones that can modify food intake. It is known that hypophysectomy reduces food intake, and that replacement therapy with some pituitary hormones, such as growth hormone, can at least partially restore the food intake of hypophysectomized animals (Panksepp, 1975). However, relatively little experimental attention has been directed toward the role of the pituitary hormones per se in the control of feeding.

The pituitary has been studied most extensively as a potential mediator of some central neural effects on feeding and body composition. Because the activity of the anterior pituitary is dependent on the secretion of both releasing and inhibiting factors from the area of the basal hypothalamus, some investigators have questioned whether the effects of VMH lesions on food intake and body weight might be mediated by changes produced by these lesions in the release of the anterior pituitary hormones. The findings of the earliest studies were mostly negative. It has generally been found that hypophysectomy does not prevent the stimulatory effects of VMH lesions on either food intake or body weight (Han, 1968; Kennedy, 1969), although hypophysectomy does delay the onset of hyperphagia following these lesions (Cox, Kakolewski & Valenstein, 1968). These studies, however, only examined whether or not an intact pituitary is necessary for VMH lesion effects. It seems more likely that these brain lesions would produce changes in the ratio or relationship among the pituitary hormones, rather than deplete them totally. Therefore, the ratio among pituitary hormones might be what is critical in the mediation of neural effects on food intake and body weight.

Woods, Decke, and Vasselli (1974) have proposed a theory implicating growth hormone, in combination with insulin, in the mechanism by which eating is related to body weight or composition regulation. According to this theory, the body weight set-point is determined by the insulin/growth hormone ratio. If there is a change in this ratio, food intake is altered until the body weight-ratio relationship is corrected. For example, Woods and his colleagues suggest that lesions of the VMH increase the insulin/growth hormone ratio, and, then, the set-point for body weight is raised. Food intake then increases until the new body weight set-point is achieved. Alternatively, lesions of the lateral hypothalamus produce a decrease in the insulin/growth hormone ratio, the set-point for body weight is lowered, and food intake decreases until this new set-point is achieved. However, this theory is based primarily on indirect evidence, and an evaluation of its accuracy will have to await further direct empirical tests.

Growth hormone has also been implicated in the nonresponsiveness of prepubertal female rats to estrogen, discussed earlier. The reader may recall that estrogen treatment does not decrease food intake in prepubertal rats, although it does decrease feeding in adult females (e.g., Wade & Zucker, 1970a). But, if prepubertal female rats are hypophysectomized, they do exhibit decreased feeding following estrogen treatment. This finding suggests that some pituitary factor present during the prepubertal period counteracts or masks the depressive effects of estrogen on feeding (Wade & Zucker, 1970a). As support for this hypothesis, it has been found that if prepubertal hypophysectomized rats (who now are responsive to the depressive effects of estrogen) are treated with growth hormone, they again become unresponsive to estrogen. This finding suggests that the high levels of growth hormone characteristic of early development are the critical factors masking the depressive effects of estrogen on food intake (Wade, 1974).

The Intestinal Hormones

As food passes through the stomach and enters the small intestine, the latter begins to secrete hormone-like substances, secretin and cholecystokinin. Some recent evidence has suggested that the release of at least one of these hormones, cholecystokinin, may be involved in the mechanisms of satiety (the termination of eating).

Gibbs, Young, and Smith (1973a) first found that fasted rats, given the opportunity to eat, stop eating when injected with cholecystokinin (but not secretin). The authors then showed that cholecystokinin prevents eating even when rats are fitted with gastric fistulas and food cannot enter the small intestine (Gibbs, Young & Smith, 1973b). Thus, food entering the intestine is not necessary for satiety if cholecystokinin is present.

In a third paper, Antin et al. (1975) reported the results of a series of studies examining the behavior patterns of rats treated with cholecystokinin. In these studies, they found that although other means of stopping eating, such as quinine treatment, simply produce a cessation of eating, cholecystokinin treatment elicits the complete pattern of satiety behaviors: The rat stops eating, then grooms, explores, and rests. Thus, this preliminary evidence suggests that the intestinal hormone cholecystokinin may provide a satiety cue.

This possible role for the intestinal hormone responses to food consumption may be an example of a long-chain hormone–behavior interaction. That is, the hormonal responses to engaging in the behavior (eating) seem to feed back and affect that behavior in progress. Thus, we see both hormonal effects on feeding (as in the cases of the hormones discussed earlier in this section) and feedback effects of the hormonal responses to eating on ongoing feeding responses.

Comment: Food Intake

In this section we have discussed many cases where hormones affect behavior and one case where the hormonal responses to food consumption might be feeding back and modifying ongoing behavioral responses. It might be useful to emphasize again that although many hormones can affect food intake, such effects may be exerted in different ways. Specifically, in some cases, such as that of the estrogens, hormonal effects on feeding appear to be a result of the effects of these hormones directly on the circuits in the brain that control eating. In other cases, however, such as that of the thyroid hormones and the glucocorticoids, hormonal effects on feeding appear to be the result of altering general metabolic states. Even though such metabolic changes must be sensed by the brain in order to be expressed as changes in behavior, the mechanism of hormone action is via the general metabolic state, not directly via the brain circuits that control the behavior.

DIETARY SELF-SELECTION

Nutritional intake really includes more than just total food intake. Animals living in the wild rarely encounter a foodstuff that provides all of the needed nutrients. Therefore, in order to meet all their nutritional requirements, animals must select their foods from a variety of sources. Some experimental attention has been directed to the selection of foods by laboratory animals, and most studies conducted to date have shown that laboratory animals (and, interestingly, infant but not adult humans) are quite capable of selecting adequate diets from a fairly wide range of sources.

Nutritional requirements can be modified in many ways, including changes induced by altered environmental conditions and by changes in the animal's physiological state. No matter how nutritional requirements are altered, this change should be reflected in modications of dietary selection patterns. Modifying an individual's hormonal state seems to alter its nutritional requirements, and this change can be brought about in different ways. Some hormonal manipulations may change dietary self-selection patterns because they modify the set-point level for body weight and/or composition. Others produce metabolic changes that either cause demands for or produce intolerance of specific nutrients. The probable modes of action of specific hormonal changes will be considered as we review the relationship between specific hormones and dietary self-selection patterns.

The Gonadal Hormones

In contrast to the large number of studies examining the relationships between the gonadal hormones and total food intake, relatively few have considered how the gonadal hormones might affect dietary self-selection patterns. Those studies that have been conducted have focused primarily on the relationship of the ovarian hormones to self-selection patterns.

In general, males select a greater proportion of their diets as protein than do females, and this gender difference in selection patterns seems to be at least indirectly related to gonadal hormone levels. Removing the gonadal hormones from the circulation by gonadectomy seems to have long-lasting effects on dietary self-selection patterns. Although castrating male rats produces only a slight increase in the percentage of the diet selected as protein, ovariectomizing females leads to a marked increase in percentage protein intake. In fact, ovariectomized females select the same dietary proportions as males (Leshner & Collier, 1973).

Both the gender difference in dietary self-selection by intact animals and the effects of ovariectomy on the dietary self-selection patterns of females seem to be related to the effects of the gonadal hormones on the body weight or composition set-point. Ovariectomized female rats not only select the same dietary proportions as males, their carcass tissue proportions are also the same as those of males (Table 2-1). Therefore, it may be that ovariectomy produces females who select the same dietary proportions as males because this operation readjusts the body composition set-point at a level equal to that of males. In this way, dietary self-selection is seen as one of the mechanisms for achieving and maintaining that new set-point level most efficiently (Leshner & Collier, 1973).

In intact females, the ovarian hormones undergo many kinds of natural variations, and some of these changes seem correlated with changes in dietary self-selection patterns. The relatively short-term changes in the levels of the ovarian hormones across the estrous cycle do not appear to affect the proportions of nutrients selected by female rats. However, as the levels of these hormones remain changed over longer time periods, there are changes in self-selection patterns. For example, as pregnancy progresses, the intakes of dietary protein and fat increase, and this altered self-selection pattern persists throughout lactation. On the other hand, carbohydrate intake remains stable throughout pregnancy and lactation (Leshner, Siegel & Collier, 1972; Richter & Barelare, 1938). But, this selective increase in protein and fat intake during pregnancy and lactation may not be related *directly* to changes in hormone levels, because pregnant and lactating rats need extra protein to support the development of the fetus and young, probably independently of concomitant changes in hormone levels.

Insulin

Early studies showed that total pancreatectomy leads to a decrease in carbohydrate intake, and that insulin treatment leads to a selective increase in the intake of this nutrient (Richter, 1942). More recent studies, however, have found that insulin leads to increases in both protein and carbohydrate intake (Mandell, 1971). This discrepancy about the effects of insulin may reflect differences in dosages used or differences in the means of studying self-selection patterns; this kind of contradictory evidence emphasizes the need for additional study.

By what mechanism does insulin affect dietary self-selection patterns? As discussed before, insulin has rather broad effects on metabolic processes, and this pancreatic hormone could affect any parameter related to food intake because of any of these metabolic actions. However, one study by Mandell (1971) has suggested that insulin may affect dietary self-selection patterns (and perhaps food intake in general) by raising the set-point for body weight or composition, rather than by producing changes in the levels of circulating metabolites. In Mandell's study, insulin injections led to increases in body weight and food intake, as would be expected, and the increase in food intake was accomplished by increasing both protein and carbohydrate intakes. This increase in food intake was maintained as long as insulin injections were continued. When insulin treatment was discontinued, food intake decreased below pretreatment levels, and remained reduced until body weight returned to the level of controls. This post-treatment reduction in food intake was accomplished almost completely by a selective decrease in carbohydrate intake. Figure 2-2 shows the pattern of protein and carbohydrate intakes following withdrawal of insulin treatment. Mandell interpreted her findings as suggesting that total food intake increases during insulin treatment because the set-point level for body weight or composition is elevated. The intake of all nutrients is increased in order to maximize weight gain. When insulin treatment is discontinued, the set-point level for body weight returns to the level of untreated controls, and the animal reduces its food intake until that level is reached. Mandell argued that the animals selectively decrease carbohydrate intake because this is the most effective way of losing weight without suffering protein depletion.

The Adrenocortical Hormones

The adrenocortical steroids exert two kinds of effects on dietary self-selection patterns, and both seem to be related to the major metabolic actions of these hormones. The first is related to the

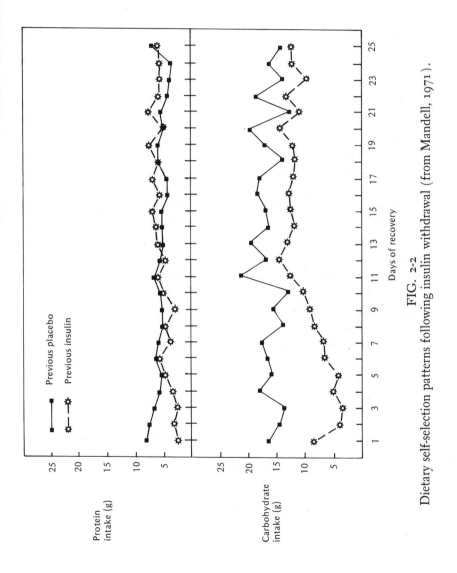

FIG. 2-2

Dietary self-selection patterns following insulin withdrawal (from Mandell, 1971).

mineralocorticoid actions of the corticosteroids. In many species, such as mice and rats, removing the adrenal glands leads to an increase in the dietary intake of sodium (Clark & Clausen, 1943; Richter, 1941). In fact, in those species that respond to adrenalectomy by increasing sodium intake, there is no need to provide any additional treatment in order to guarantee survival. However, there are other species, such as the hamster and the gerbil, in which there is no compensatory increase in sodium intake following adrenalectomy (Cullen & Scarborough, 1970; Zucker, Wade & Ziegler, 1972), and in these species, mineralocorticoid therapy is needed.

In those species that do respond to adrenalectomy with increased sodium consumption, replacement therapy with mineralocorticoids, such as desoxycorticosterone (DOC), returns the sodium intake of adrenalectomized animals to normal levels (Richter, 1941). These findings, therefore, suggest that withdrawal of the mineralocorticoids following adrenalectomy leads to sodium depletion, which, in turn, is compensated for by an increase in the dietary intake of substances containing sodium.

There is one seemingly inconsistent aspect of this relationship between the mineralocorticoids and sodium intake. Treatment of intact rats with mineralocorticoids leads to an increase in sodium intake (Rice & Richter, 1943; Weisinger & Woods, 1971), a phenomenon contrary to expectations based on the depressive effects of the mineralocorticoids on sodium intake in adrenalectomized rats. This strange effect is not clearly understood at present, although it does not seem to reflect some sodium depleting action of the mineralocorticoids in intact animals, because these hormones do increase the retention of sodium.

The second type of effect of adrenocortical hormone manipulations on dietary self-selection also seems to be related to the metabolic actions of the glucocorticoids. However, the results of studies considering the effects of adrenalectomy on protein and carbohydrate intakes (the nutrients one would expect to be related to glucocorticoid action) have yielded conflicting results. Some studies (Clark & Clausen, 1943) have found no effect of adrenalectomy on the intake of either protein or carbohydrate, others (Richter, 1941; Soulairac, 1967) have found adrenalectomy to reduce carbohydrate intake but not protein intake, whereas still others (Lát, 1967; Leshner, 1972) have found adrenalectomy to decrease protein intake but not carbohydrate intake. Leshner (1972) suggested that a decrease in protein intake is the most probable change to be expected following adrenalectomy, because this operation produces a major deficit in gluconeogenesis (the conversion of protein to carbohydrates). This deficit might result in adrenalectomized animals being unable to utilize dietary proteins completely. If this is so, then adrenalectomized rats should avoid these nutrients. Moreover, in most studies animals have been maintained on salt solutions in order to counteract the mineralocorticoid deficiency that accompanies this operation, and this type of treatment has been shown to counteract the effects of adrenalectomy on the intestinal absorption of carbohydrates. Therefore, adrenalectomized rats maintained on salt solutions should not suffer from too great an inability to utilize dietary carbohydrates, and they should not avoid this nutrient. Of course, final resolution of the contradictory findings on protein and carbohydrate intakes after adrenalectomy will have to await further experimentation.

The Thyroid Hormones

Only a few studies have examined the effects of thyroid hormone manipulations on dietary self-selection patterns, and their findings have been quite consistent. Inducing hypothyroidism by either thyroidectomy or thiouracil treatment leads to a selective reduction in the intake of carbohydrates (Leshner & Walker, 1973; Soulairac, 1967). This relationship between carbohydrate intake levels and thyroid hormone levels probably reflects the metabolic effects of the thyroid hormones on energy availability and utilization.

Comment: Dietary Self-Selection

As in the discussion of food intake, we have seen many cases where modifications in hormonal states result in modifications of dietary selection patterns, and, as in the case of total food intake, these hormonal effects seem to be exerted in a variety of ways. Some hormonal changes seem to affect dietary self-selection patterns by altering the general metabolic state. Such general metabolic effects either create the need for specific nutrients, such as in mineralocorticoid effects on sodium consumption, or alter the ability of the animal to utilize nutrients, as in the case of glucocorticoid effects. On the other hand, there also are cases, such as that of insulin, where hormonal modifications might be affecting dietary selection patterns because these hormonal changes alter the set-points around which body composition is regulated. These kinds of distinctions have not been studied extensively in the self-selection of nutrients, but they raise some interesting questions for future investigations.

RUNNING ACTIVITY

Everyone who has had a pet mouse or hamster has noticed that it exhibits what may seem superficially to be a useless behavior: it will run for hours in a little wheel without getting anywhere. Some common thoughts about why the animal runs in the wheel include (1) that the animal is bored and running provides distraction, (2) that the animal is running in order to find something missing from its environment (Wald & Jaksson, 1944), or (3) that the animal is exercising in order to keep its muscles toned in the restricted environment of its home cage. Much recent evidence has suggested that running in activity wheels really is a regulatory behavior, and that its energy-expending characteristics make it an efficient mechanism for controlling body weight or composition. Many investigators (e.g., Collier, 1969; Leshner, 1971; Wade,

1976) have argued that animals engage in this type of exercise in order to achieve or maintain the set-point levels for body weight and/or composition.

There are basically three ways in which hormones could be related to the regulatory aspects of voluntary exercise. First, hormones could affect levels of running by modifying the set-points for body weight or composition. If the set-point is raised, running decreases; if the set-point is lowered, running levels increase.

Hormones also could affect running activity more indirectly, through their general metabolic effects. Changes in hormonal states lead to marked changes in both body weight and body composition, and as those values deviate from the set-point, activity levels should change. Therefore, hormones could affect activity levels by causing deviations from the regulatory set-points.

Third, there is some preliminary evidence that the adrenocortical hormones may be involved in the maintenance of running. There is a marked rise in glucocorticoid levels during and following bouts of exercise, which may feed back and signal to the animal how much it has exercised (Leshner & Walker, unpublished). This possibility will be discussed in more detail when we consider the adrenocortical hormones and activity.

The Gonadal Hormones

In the same way that there are gender differences in total food intake and dietary selection patterns, there are marked gender differences in running activity patterns. The hormonal factors controlling running differ for males and females, and, therefore, the two sexes will be considered separately here.

THE FEMALE There is a pronounced estrous-cycle rhythm in running activity levels in female rats (Fig. 2-3), and, as in the case of food intake, this rhythm seems related to estrous-cycle variations in estrogen levels. Ovariectomy decreases running in female rats by abolishing the estrous peaks, and estrogen replacement therapy in-

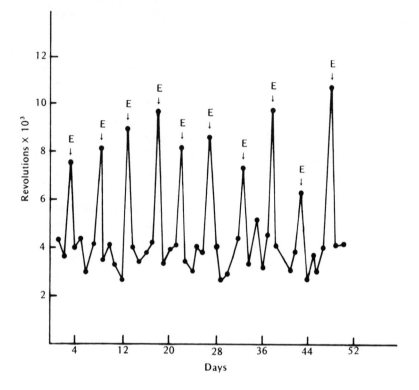

FIG. 2-3

Estrous cycle variation in running activity levels (E indicates estrous day) (from Stern, *Physiology and Behavior*, 1970, 5, 1278, by permission of Pergamon Press).

creases the overall activity levels of ovariectomized females (Gerall, Napoli & Cooper, 1973; Stern & Zwick, 1972). Progesterone, on the other hand, has no effect on running activity in ovariectomized rats, although it does decrease running in intact rats (perhaps because this hormone treatment makes the rats pseudopregnant). Interestingly, progesterone treatment will decrease running in ovariectomized rats treated with estrogen. This finding suggests that progesterone may be capable of counteracting the stimulatory actions of the estrogens (Rodier, 1971). Thus, because estrogen stimulates running, and because estrogens are high around the time of estrus, it seems most likely that the periovulatory increase in estrogen levels is responsible for the estrous increase in running.

It has been argued (e.g., Wade, 1972) that, as in the case of food intake, estrogens affect running because they produce changes in the set-point for body weight or composition. Because running activity is an efficient mechanism for reducing body weight and body fat, as the estrogens lower the body weight or composition set-point, running levels should increase. However, there also is some evidence suggesting that estrogen effects on running activity are distinct from the effects of these hormones on the body weight set-point. For example, although, as discussed above, estrogen effects on food intake are dependent on the rat's body weight at the time of hormone treatment (recall that estrogen does not affect food intake in lean rats), estrogen stimulates running no matter what the animal's weight (Gentry, Wade & Roy, 1976). Thus, estrogen effects on activity may be independent of the effects of this class of hormone on body weight regulation.

Two lines of evidence suggest that estrogen effects on running activity are mediated through changes in central neural activity. First, early hormonal manipulations can exert temporally distant effects on adult activity levels, and, as discussed before, early hormonal effects on regulatory behaviors probably are mediated by the relatively permanent changes that these manipulations cause in neural activity. Neonatal androgen treatment decreases the magnitude of the estrous peaks in running activity in adulthood (Gerall, 1967). In addition, neonatal androgenization seems to decrease adult running by decreasing the adult female's sensitivity to the stimulatory effects of estrogen on activity (Gerall, Stone & Hitt, 1972). These findings suggest that early hormonal manipulations may affect adult running wheel activity patterns by altering the brain's sensitivity to estrogens circulating in adulthood. As a caution in interpreting these findings, however, it should be noted that neonatally androgenized females do not respond in adulthood in exactly the same way as do males (Gentry & Wade, 1976). Thus, the early hormonal environment does not totally determine adult activity patterns.

Second, estrogens can stimulate running when injected only into the brain. Estrogen will stimulate running when injected in many hypothalamic sites in both intact and ovariectomized females. However, estrogen implants into the VMH do not seem to affect activity, although they do depress feeding (Colvin & Sawyer, 1969; Wade & Zucker, 1970b). This difference between feeding and activity shows that although these behaviors do covary, they may be controlled quite differently.

THE MALE Much less experimental attention has been directed toward the hormonal basis of running activity in males than in females. It is known that castration reduces activity and that replacement therapy with testosterone will restore the activity levels of castrates to normal. This finding suggests that testosterone has a stimulatory effect on running in males, since its removal leads to decreased running.

A recent study by Roy and Wade (1975) has suggested that testosterone may stimulate running in the male because it is converted (aromatized) to estrogens. Roy and Wade treated castrated males with either testosterone, dihydrotestosterone (a metabolite of testosterone that cannot be converted to estrogen), or estradiol. They found that both testosterone and estradiol restored activity in castrates but that dihydrotestosterone was without effect. Because testosterone can be aromatized to estrogens naturally, they suggested that testosterone stimulates running in male rats because it is converted to estrogen, not because of some androgenic property. If this is the case, then, castration would reduce running levels because it leads to withdrawal of the substance (testosterone) from which the estrogens would be produced.

The Glucocorticoids

Because the adrenocortical hormones have such profound effects on intermediary metabolism, it is not surprising that the glucocorticoids can affect running activity. Adrenalectomy virtually abolishes running in rats, and replacement therapy with moderate dosages of corticosterone restores the activity levels of adrenalectomized rats to normal (Leshner, 1971). However, as in the case of food intake discussed before, treatment of intact rats with glucocorticoids appears to have a bimodal effect on running activity: treatment with low dosages stimulates running, whereas treatment with high dosages decreases running levels (Beatty, Scouten & Beatty, 1971; Kendall, 1970; Leshner, 1971).

Why does adrenalectomy abolish running wheel activity? Withdrawal of the glucocorticoids leads to many changes in intermediary metabolism, including a depression of body fat levels. In fact, adrenalectomizing rats leads to the same decrease in percentage fat levels as does running. Because the opportunity to exercise appears to lower the set-point for body fat levels—at least such levels are lower in exercising rats—and because adrenalectomized rats who already are at that set-point do not run, Leshner (1971) proposed that adrenalectomized rats do not run in activity wheels because they do not need to; they already have achieved the optimum set-point for body fat.

How can one account for the bimodal effect of corticosterone on running in intact rats? Not only do changes in glucocorticoid levels affect activity levels, but running in activity wheels also seems to modify adrenocortical hormone levels: Rats running in activity wheels exhibit increased levels of the glucocorticoids. Perhaps significantly, rats not given the opportunity to exercise respond to corticosterone treatment with a depression in fat levels equal to that caused by running. Therefore, the increases in glucocorticoid levels that accompany running may be one of the mechanisms by which exercise affects body fat levels (Leshner, 1971).

This dual relationship between the glucocorticoids and running activity (the glucocorticoids affect activity levels and running affects glucocorticoid levels) may help account for the bimodal effect of corticosterone on running wheel activity in intact rats. Figure 2-4 presents the results of a study examining the dose-response relationship between corticosterone dosages and running activity levels in intact and adrenalectomized rats. Note that in adrenalectomized rats, increasing corticosterone dosages increases running levels, even above the level of placebo-treated intact rats. On the other hand, in intact animals, increasing dosages of corticosterone lead to greater increases in activity levels until a fairly high dosage is reached, at which point activity levels begin to decline (Leshner & Walker, unpublished). Combining these findings with the finding that running itself can increase corticosterone levels, it seems reasonable to suggest that the following sequence of events normally occurs: (1) The rat begins to run in the wheel, and (2) corticosterone levels begin to rise. (3) This increase in corticosterone levels leads to an increase in activity levels, which (4) leads to a further increase in corticosterone levels. (5) When corticosterone reaches a very high level, running activity then begins to decline. It seems as if the corticosterone responses to activity might be able to feed back and serve as a cue regulating the amount of running. Slight increases in corticosterone levels stimulate motor activity, but, when corticosterone levels become very high, they decrease running. This suggestion, of course, requires experimental verification, but it may be an example of a long-chain hormone–behavior interaction, where the hormonal responses to engaging in a behavior feed back and affect the continuing display of that behavior.

The Thyroid Hormones

Relatively little attention has been directed toward the role of the thyroid hormones in running activity. It is known that inducing hypothyroidism by either thyroidectomy or thiouracil treatment leads to decreases in activity levels in direct proportion to the

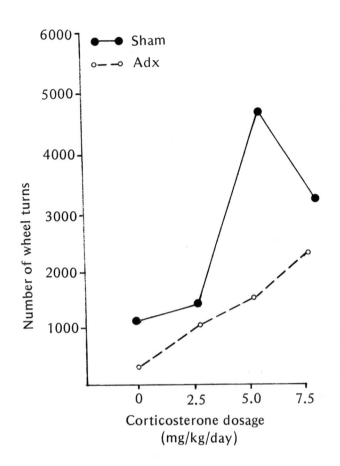

FIG. 2-4
The effects of corticosterone on running activity in intact (Sham) and adrenalectomized (Adx) rats (from Leshner & Walker, unpublished).

degree of hypothyroidism induced, a dose-response relationship. In addition, feeding hypothyroid rats thyroid powder restores their activity levels to that of euthyroid rats (Richter, 1933; Stern, 1970).

These effects appear to be related to the general metabolic action of the thyroid hormones. Inducing hypothyroidism leads to a decrease in body fat levels in nonexercising animals, but does not affect the fat levels of rats given the opportunity to run. Therefore, it seems that hypothyroid animals that exercise achieve the same body fat level as do euthyroid animals, although the hypothyroid animals run less. It seems likely that they run less because they are closer to the optimum level for body fat to begin with than are euthyroid animals, and, therefore, they do not need to run as much to reach the target level for body fat (Leshner & Walker, 1973).

SUMMARY AND COMMENT

The discussion in this chapter has suggested that hormones can affect regulatory behaviors in at least two ways: (1) By altering the general metabolic state, thereby causing deviations from the set-points for critical parameters toward which a regulatory behavior is directed; the level of the behavior then is changed in order to correct that deviation. (2) By changing or resetting the level of the set-point itself. In this case, the existing level of the parameter is not changed by the hormone, but the level differs from the new set-point. The level of the behavior then changes in order to achieve the new set-point.

The net effect of both mechanisms on regulatory behaviors is the same. In both cases, the behavior changes because the existing level of the critical parameter deviates from the set-point level. However, in the first case the hormone has caused a deviation from the existing set-point by altering the general metabolic state, whereas in the second case the hormone has altered the target level to be achieved (the set-point has been shifted), not the individual's general metabolic state.

This chapter has reviewed the relationship between endocrine function and three regulatory behaviors related to energy balance: eating, dietary self-selection, and running activity. For each behavior, hormone systems were considered separately. However, the reader should keep in mind that these systems do not in fact operate independently of each other. Unfortunately, very little experimental attention has been directed toward the interaction among different endocrine factors in their relationships to these behaviors.

In addition, although we have considered the regulatory behaviors separately, it is important to remember that no individual really lives in such a vacuum that it engages in one behavior exclusively. The regulatory behaviors can and do interact to determine the state of energy balance and to regulate critical parameters at their set-point levels. For example, when the body weight or composition set-point is lowered by estrogen during the periovulatory period, food intake decreases (reducing nutritional intake), and running activity increases (increasing energy expenditure). The combined effects of these behavioral changes provide a more efficient means of achieving the new set-point than would altering either behavior alone (Wade, 1976).

Hormones also seem to be involved in the mechanisms by which some behaviors exert their regulatory actions. Engaging in those behaviors or altering their levels produces changes in endocrine function which then lead to changes in metabolic states. Again, the combined endocrine effects of engaging in multiple regulatory behaviors would be more efficient than any single endocrine change, and many behaviors may act together to produce a composite of endocrine changes that is most efficient in altering metabolic states.

The fact that hormones both affect and are affected by regulatory behaviors suggests that long-chain hormone–behavior interactions could operate here. Although very little experimental attention has been devoted to this question directly, we have seen some preliminary evidence suggesting that these kinds of relationships do exist. One case discussed involves the potential role of the intestinal hormone cholecystokinin in the termination of feeding episodes. A second case involves a potential feedback effect of the glucocorticoid responses to running activity. Of course, there are many other possible long-chain hormone–behavior interactions that could exist, but these have not been studied explicitly.

REFERENCES

Antin, J., Gibbs, J., Holt, J., Young, R. C. & Smith, G. P.   Cholecystokinin elicits the complete behavioral sequence of satiety in rats. *Journal of Comparative and Physiological Psychology*, 1975, 89, 784-790.

Baile, C. A. & Forbes, J. M.   Control of feed intake and regulation of energy balance in ruminants. *Physiological Reviews*, 1974, 54, 160-214.

Beatty, W. W., O'Briant, D. A. & Vilberg, T. R.   Suppression of feeding by intrahypothalamic implants of estradiol in male and female rats. *Bulletin of the Psychonomic Society*, 1974, 3, 273-274.

Beatty, W. W., Scouten, C. W. & Beatty, P. A.   Differential effects of dexamethasone and body weight loss on two measures of activity. *Physiology and Behavior*, 1971, 7, 869-871.

Bell, D. D. & Zucker, I.   Sex differences in body weight and eating: organization and activation by gonadal hormones in the rat. *Physiology and Behavior*, 1971, 7, 27-34.

Berthoud, H. R. & Baettig, K.   Effects of insulin and 2-deoxy-d-glucose on plasma glucose levels and lateral hypothalamic eating threshold in the rats. *Physiology and Behavior*, 1974, 12, 547-556.

Booth, D. A. & Pitt, M. E.   The role of glucose in insulin-induced feeding and drinking. *Physiology and Behavior*, 1968, 3, 447-453.

Clark, W. G. & Clausen, D. F.   Dietary "self-selection" and appetite of untreated and treated adrenalectomized rats. *American Journal of Physiology*, 1943, 139, 70-79.

Collier, G.   Body weight loss as a measure of motivation in hunger and thirst. *Annals of the New York Academy of Sciences*, 1969, 157, 594-609.

Collier, G., Hirsch, E. & Hamlin, P. H.   The ecological determinants of reinforcement in the rat. *Physiology and Behavior*, 1972, 9, 705-716.

Colvin, G. B. & Sawyer, C. H.   Induction of running activity by intracerebral implants of estrogen in ovariectomized rats. *Neuroendocrinology*, 1969, 4, 309-320.

Cox, V. C., Kakolewski, J. W. & Valenstein, E. S.   Effects of ventromedial hypothalamic damage in hypophysectomized rats. *Journal of Comparative and Physiological Psychology*, 1968, 65, 145-148.

Cullen, J. W. & Scarborough, D. E.   Behavioral and hormonal prophylaxis in the adrenalectomized gerbil (*Meriones unguculatus*). *Hormones and Behavior*, 1970, 1, 203-210.

Czaja, J. A.   Food rejection by female Rhesus monkeys during the menstrual cycle and early pregnancy. *Physiology and Behavior*, 1975, 14, 579-587.

Debons, A. F., Krimsky, I., & From, A.   A direct action of insulin on the hypothalamic satiety center. *American Journal of Physiology*, 1970, 219, 938-943.

Debons, A. F., Krimsky, I., From, A. & Clouten, R. J.   Rapid effects of insulin on the hypothalamic satiety center. *American Journal of Physiology*, 1969, 217, 1114-1118.

Dubuc, P. V.   Effects of estradiol implants on body weight regulation in castrated and intact female rats. *Endocrinology*, 1974, 95, 1733-1736.

Epstein, A. N. & Teitelbaum, P.   Specific loss of the hypoglycemic control of feeding in recovered lateral rats. *American Journal of Physiology*, 1967, 213, 1159-1167.

Forbes, J. M.   Feeding in sheep modified by intraventricular estradiol and progesterone. *Physiology and Behavior*, 1974, 12, 741-747.

Gentry, R. T. & Wade, G. N.   Sex differences in sensitivity of food intake, body weight and running wheel activity to ovarian steroids in rats. *Journal of Comparative and Physiological Psychology*, 1976, 90, 747-754.

Gentry, R. T., Wade, G. N. & Roy, E. J.   Individual differences in estradiol-induced behaviors and in neural ^{3}H-estradiol uptake in rats. *Physiology and Behavior*, 1976, 17, 195-200.

Gerall, A. A.   Effects of early postnatal androgen and estrogen injections on the estrous activity cycles and mating behavior of rats. *Anatomical Record*, 1967, 157, 97-104.

Gerall, A. A., Stone, L. S. & Hitt, J. C.   Neonatal androgen depresses female responsiveness to estrogen. *Physiology and Behavior*, 1972, 8, 17-20.

Gerall, A. A., Napoli, A. M. & Cooper, U. C.   Daily and hourly estrous running in intact, spayed and estrone implanted rats. *Physiology and Behavior*, 1973, 10, 225-229.

Gibbs, J., Young, R. C. & Smith, G. P.   Cholecystokinin decreases food intake in rats. *Journal of Comparative and Physiological Psychology*, 1973, 84, 488-495. (a)

Gibbs, J., Young, R. C. & Smith, G. P.   Cholecystokinin elicits satiety in rats with open gastric fistulas. *Nature*, 1973, 245, 323-325. (b)

Han, P. W.   Obesity in force-fed, hypophysectomized rats bearing hypothalamic lesions. *Proceedings of the Society for Experimental Biology and Medicine*, 1968, 127, 1057-1060.

Hirsch, E.   Some determinants of intake and patterns of feeding in the guinea pig. *Physiology and Behavior*, 1973, 11, 687-704.

Hoebel, B. G. & Teitelbaum, P.   Weight regulation in normal and hypothalamic hyperphagic rats. *Journal of Comparative and Physiological Psychology*, 1966, 61, 189-193.

Jankowiak, R. & Stern, J. J.   Food intake and body weight modifications following medial hypothalamic hormone implants in female rats. *Physiology and Behavior*, 1974, 12, 875-879.

Kendall, J. W.   Dexamethasone stimulation of running activity in the male rat. *Hormones and Behavior*, 1970, 1, 327-336.

Kennedy, G. C.   Food intake, energy balance and growth. *British Medical Bulletin*, 1966, 22, 216-220.

Kennedy, G. C.   Interactions between feeding behavior and hormones during growth. *Annals of the New York Academy of Sciences*, 1969, 157, 1049-1061.

King, J. M. & Cox, V. C.   The effects of estrogen on food intake and body weight following ventromedial hypothalamic lesions. *Physiological Psychology*, 1973, 1, 261-264.

Lát, J.   Self-selection of dietary components. In *Handbook of Physiology, Sect. 6: Alimentary Canal, Vol. 1 Food and Water Intake.* Washington: American Physiological Society, 1967, pp. 367-386.

Leshner, A. I.   The adrenals and the regulatory nature of running wheel activity. *Physiology and Behavior*, 1971, 6, 551-558.

Leshner, A. I.   The effects of adrenalectomy on protein-carbohydrate choice. *Psychonomic Science*, 1972, 27, 289-290.

Leshner, A. I. & Collier, G.   The effects of gonadectomy on the sex differences in dietary self-selection patterns and carcass compositions of rats. *Physiology and Behavior*, 1973, 11, 671-676.

Leshner, A. I., Siegel, H. I. & Collier, G.   Dietary self-selection by pregnant and lactating rats. *Physiology and Behavior*, 1972, 8, 151-154.

Leshner, A. I. & Walker, W. A.   Dietary self-selection, activity and carcass composition of rats fed thiouracil. *Physiology and Behavior*, 1973, 10, 373-378.

Mandell, D.   The effects of insulin on dietary self-selection. Unpublished Master's Thesis, Bucknell University, 1971.

Mayer, J.   Regulation of energy intake and the body weight: the glucostatic theory and the lipostatic hypothesis. *Annals of the New York Academy of Science*, 1955, 63, 15-42.

Mook, D. G., Kenney, N. J., Roberts, S., Nussbaum, A. I. & Rodier, W. I.   Ovarian-adrenal interactions in regulation of body weight by female rats. *Journal of Comparative and Physiological Psychology*, 1972, 81, 198-211.

Nisbett, R. E. Hunger, obesity and the ventromedial hypothalamus. *Psychological Review*, 1972, 79, 433-453.

Panksepp, J. Hormonal control of feeding behavior and energy balance. In B. E. Eleftheriou & R. L. Sprott (Eds.), *Hormonal Correlates of Behavior*, Vol. 2. New York: Plenum Press, 1975, pp. 657-695.

Rice, K. & Richter, C. P. Increased sodium chloride and water intake of normal rats treated with desoxycorticosterone acetate. *Endocrinology*, 1943, 33, 106-115.

Richter, C. P. The role played by the thyroid gland in the production of gross bodily activity. *Endocrinology*, 1933, 17, 73-87.

Richter, C. P. Decreased carbohydrate appetite of adrenalectomized rats. *Proceedings of the Society for Experimental Biology and Medicine*, 1941, 48, 577-579.

Richter, C. P. Increased dextrose appetite of normal rats treated with insulin. *American Journal of Physiology*, 1942, 135, 781-787.

Richter, C. P. & Barelare, B. Nutritional requirements of pregnant and lactating rats studied by the self-selection method. *Endocrinology*, 1941, 28, 179-192.

Rodier, W. I. Progesterone-estrogen interactions in the control of activity-wheel running in the female rat. *Journal of Comparative and Physiological Psychology*, 1971, 74, 465-474.

Ross, G. E. & Zucker, I. Progesterone and the ovarian-adrenal modulation of energy balance in rats. *Hormones and Behavior*, 1974, 5, 43-62.

Roy, E. J. & Wade, G. N. Role of estrogens in androgen-induced spontaneous activity in male rats. *Journal of Comparative and Physiological Psychology*, 1975, 89, 573-579.

Schulman, J. L., Carleton, J. L., Whitney, G. & Whitehorn, C. Effect of glucagon on food intake and body weight in man. *Journal of Applied Physiology*, 1957, 11, 419-421.

Slob, A. K. & van der Werff ten Bosch, J. J. Sex differences in body growth in the rat. *Physiology and Behavior*, 1975, 14, 353-398.

Soulairac, A. Control of carbohydrate intake. In *Handbook of Physiology, Section 6: Alimentary Canal, Vol. 1. Food and Water Intake.* Washington: American Physiological Society, 1967, pp. 387-398.

Stern, J. J. The effects of thyroidectomy on the wheel running activity of female rats. *Physiology and Behavior*, 1970, 5, 1277-1279.

Stern, J. J. & Zwick, G. Hormonal control of spontaneous activity during the estrus cycle of the rat. *Psychological Reports*, 1972, 30, 983-988.

Stricker, E. M., Friedman, M. I. & Zigmond, M. J. Glucoregulatory feeding by rats after intraventricular 6-hydroxy-dopamine or lateral hypothalamic lesions. *Science*, 1975, 189, 895-897.

Stunkard, A. J., Van Itallie, T. B. & Reis, B. B. The mechanism of satiety: effect of glucagon on gastric hunger contractions in man. *Proceedings of the Society for Experimental Biology and Medicine*, 1955, 89, 258-261.

Tarttelin, M. F. & Gorski, R. A. Variations in food and water intake in the normal and acyclic female rat. *Physiology and Behavior*, 1971, 7, 847-852.

Van Putten, L. M., van Bekkum, D. W. & Querido, A. Influence of cortisone and ACTH on appetite. *Acta Endocrinologica*, 1953, 12, 159-166.

Wade, G. N. Gonadal hormones and behavioral regulation of body weight. *Physiology and Behavior*, 1972, 8, 523-534.

Wade, G. N. Interaction between estradiol-17B and growth hormone in control of food intake in weanling rats. *Journal of Comparative and Physiological Psychology*, 1974, 86, 359-362.

Wade, G. N. Some effects of ovarian hormones on food intake and body weight in female rats. *Journal of Comparative and Physiological Psychology*, 1975, 88, 183-193.

Wade, G. N. Sex hormones, regulatory behaviors and body weight. In J. S. Rosenblatt, R. A. Hinde, E. Shaw & C. G. Beer (Eds.), *Advances in the Study of Behavior*, Vol. 6. New York: Academic Press, 1976, pp. 201-279.

Wade, G. N. & Zucker, I. Development of hormonal control over food intake and body weight in female rats. *Journal of Comparative and Physiological Psychology*, 1970, 70, 213-220. (a)

Wade, G. N. & Zucker, I. Modulation of food intake and locomotor activity in female rats by diencephalic hormone implants. *Journal of Comparative and Physiological Psychology*, 1970, 72, 328-336. (b)

Wald, G. & Jackson, B. Activity and nutritional deprivation. *Proceedings of the National Academy of Sciences*, 1944, 30, 255-263.

Warkentin, J., Warkentin, L. & Ivey, A. C. The effect of experimental thyroid abnormalities on appetite. *American Journal of Physiology*, 1943, 139, 139-146.

Wayner, M. J., Cott, A., Millner, J. & Tartaglione, R. Loss of 2-deoxy-D-glucose induced eating in recovered lateral rats. *Physiology and Behavior*, 1971, 7, 881-884.

Weisinger, R. S. & Woods, S. C. Aldosterone-elicited sodium appetite. *Endocrinology*, 1971, 89, 538-544.

Woods, S. C., Decke, E. & Vasselli, J. R. Metabolic hormones and regulation of body weight. *Psychological Review*, 1974, 81, 26-43.

York, D. A. & Bray, G. A. Dependence of hypothalamic obesity on insulin, the pituitary and the adrenal gland. *Endocrinology*, 1972, 90, 885-894.

Zucker, I.   Body weight and age as factors determining estrogen responesiveness in the rat feeding systems. *Behavioral Biology*, 1972, 7, 527-542.

Zucker, I., Wade, G. N. & Ziegler, R.   Sexual and hormonal influences on eating, taste preferences and body weight of hamsters. *Physiology and Behavior*, 1972, 8, 101-111.

Chapter 3

AGONISTIC BEHAVIOR

The *agonistic behaviors* include the aggressive, submissive, and defensive reactions that occur in competitive situations. In this discussion, *aggression* is considered to be any action by which one individual either causes or threatens to cause physical injury to another. This definition is designed to include both injurious forms of aggression, such as attacking and fighting, and noninjurious forms of aggression, such as ritualized threats and displays. In turn, *submissive* or *defensive behaviors* include the wide range of behavior patterns such as flight, passivity, avoidance, and the stereotyped postures exhibited by defeated or subordinate individuals (see Leshner, 1975).

Agonistic responses can be seen in a variety of settings, and it has been argued that the responses exhibited in different kinds of situations really constitute distinct categories of behavior that are only superficially related. Moyer (1968) has suggested that there are seven major types of circumstances that can elicit agonistic reactions, and that the behaviors occurring in these different situations can be distinguished on the bases of the stimuli that elicit them, their response topographies, and the physiological factors that affect them. We shall use Moyer's classification here, and we shall discuss three classes of responses: *intermale* agonistic behaviors, *irritable* agonistic reactions, and *predatory* agonistic behaviors. These are the categories whose relationships to endocrine function have received the most attention. It should be noted, however, that these three classes of agonistic reactions have not received equal amounts of attention. Much more is known about the relationship between endocrine function and intermale agonistic responding than is known about endocrine function and the other two classes of reactions. Therefore, our discussion will be weighted heavily in the direction of the first class of responses. Another category of agonistic responses, maternal aggression, will be discussed in Chapter 6.

Although most studies have examined the relationship between hormones and agonistic behavior directly, some have used a more indirect approach, examining the relationship between hormones and the outcome of agonistic interactions, dominance/subordinance relationships. The relationship between hormones and dominance will be considered in a separate section following the discussion of intermale agonistic behavior, the type of responses to which dominance seems most closely related.

The subject of hormones and human aggression is discussed in a separate section at the end of this chapter because human aggression has been studied in ways that are quite different from the ways in which agonistic responding has been studied in nonhuman animals. Furthermore, human aggression has not been categorized in the same way that forms of animal aggression have. These kinds of differences emphasize the need for caution in attempting to generalize from studies of nonhuman animals to the human case.

The literature on hormones and agonistic behavior is vast, and we shall not attempt to provide a comprehensive review of that literature here. The interested reader is referred to the more comprehensive reviews by Conner (1972), Floody and Pfaff (1974), Edwards and Rowe (1975), and Leshner (1975).

INTERMALE AGONISTIC BEHAVIOR

The term *intermale agonistic behavior* refers to the group of aggressive and submissive or defensive reactions that occur when two unfamiliar members of the same species meet. This term is somewhat misleading, because there are many cases of females exhibiting similar types of agonistic responses under similar circumstances. But, the term "intermale" has been used extensively, and it will be used here in keeping with convention. It should be noted, however, that the review that follows will not be limited to the case of agonistic interactions between males.

Studies of hormones and intermale agonistic behavior have focused on three subunits of that total relationship: (1) the effects of hormones on agonistic responding, (2) the effects of agonistic experiences on endocrine function, and (3) the role of hormones in the mediation of the effects of agonistic experiences on ongoing agonistic responses. These subrelationships will be considered separately, and their interactions will be discussed as we proceed in this chapter.

Hormonal Effects on Agonistic Responding

Most experimental studies concerned with the effects of hormones on intermale agonistic behaviors have examined the relationship between what we have called the baseline hormonal state and the levels of these responses. These studies have either examined or manipulated the individual's hormonal state before the animal is exposed to agonistic stimuli. Primary attention has been directed to the effects of two groups of hormones, the androgens and the hormones of the pituitary-adrenocortical axis, and these two groups will be considered separately here. In addition, the two components of agonistic responding, aggression and submission, have been studied separately, and will be so considered here.

THE ANDROGENS AND AGGRESSION There are three lines of correlational evidence suggesting that the androgens are related to levels of aggressiveness. First, there are seasonal variations in levels of aggressiveness, and these changes coincide with seasonal variations in testosterone levels: as testosterone levels rise during the breeding season, so do levels of aggression. This kind of correlation between aggressiveness and androgen levels has been observed in species as diverse as birds, rodents, and primates (Crook & Butterfield, 1968; Healey, 1967; Sadleir, 1965; Wilson & Boelkins, 1970). Second, in male mice, aggressiveness first is exhibited at the time of puberty, when testosterone levels are rising (Brian & Nowell, 1969a; McKinney & Desjardins, 1973). In fact, treating juvenile male mice with androgens increases their aggressiveness (Levy & King, 1953; Svare & Gandelman, 1975). Third, there is some evidence of a correlation between adult baseline androgen levels and levels of aggressiveness, at least in mice and rhesus monkeys (Brain & Nowell, 1969b; Lagerspetz, Tirri & Lagerspetz, 1968; Rose, Holaday & Bernstein, 1971). Curiously, although there appears to be a correlation between androgen levels and aggressiveness in the rhesus monkey, there appears to be no such correlation in the Japanese snow monkey, which also is a member of the genus *Macaca* (Eaton & Resko, 1974). Thus, there are three lines of evidence demonstrating that there is some relationship between androgen levels and levels of aggressiveness, two showing that changes in androgen levels are correlated with changes in levels of aggressiveness and one showing a correlation between baseline or resting androgen levels and levels of this behavior.

Experimental studies have shown that the androgens are important to the display of aggression in many species, thereby demonstrating some causality in the correlation discussed above. Castration can lead to a decrease in aggressiveness, and replacement therapy with moderate dosages of the androgens can restore the aggressiveness of castrates (Beeman, 1947; Tollman & King, 1956; Ulrich, 1938). A thorough dissection of the correlation discussed above would require a study of the potential dose-response relationship between androgen dosages and levels of aggressiveness, but, surprisingly, this obvious study has never been conducted. What is known is that there appears to be a threshold androgen dosage needed to induce fighting in castrates; that is, as testosterone dosages are increased, more and more mice will fight (Fig. 3-1) (Edwards, 1969). However, no study to date has systematically compared levels of aggressiveness, such as how much or how intensely an animal attacks, in individuals treated with different androgen dosages.

It also is interesting to note that treatment of castrated mice with very high androgen dosages does not restore their aggressive-

FIG. 3-1
The percentage of castrated males fighting at each dosage level (modified from Edwards, *Physiology and Behavior*, 1969, 4, 336, by permission of Pergamon Press).

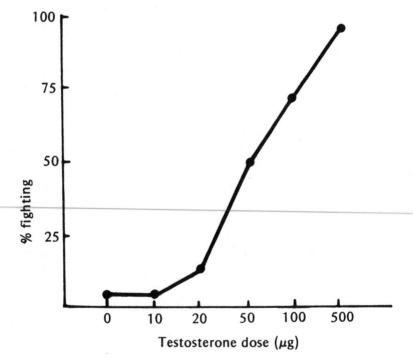

ness (Bevan, Bevan & Williams, 1958; Bevan et al., 1957). This finding, when combined with the results of studies of the effects of castration, suggests that there may be a bimodal relationship between androgen levels and levels of aggressiveness: both very low and very high androgen levels lead to decreased aggressiveness. Of course, the studies showing the ineffectiveness of high androgen dosages in restoring the aggressiveness of castrated mice have used extremely high dosages, and, therefore, the observed effects may represent a pharmacological rather than a physiological phenomenon.

There also is some evidence that raising the androgen levels of intact mice can alter their aggressiveness. Injecting relatively non-aggressive mice with testosterone has been reported to increase their aggressiveness (Banarjee, 1971). In addition, exposing male mice to a female in estrus increases their aggressiveness (Taylor, 1975), and this effect may be mediated by changes in androgen levels. Exposure to an estrous female can lead to increases in androgen levels (Kamel et al., 1975), and, therefore, the effects of contact with these females on aggressiveness may be a result of the concomitant increase in androgen levels.

GENDER DIFFERENCES IN AGGRESSIVENESS The males of most mammalian species are more aggressive than the females (Gray, 1971; Seward, 1945), and this gender difference in aggressiveness seems to be related both to the early hormonal environment and to the adult hormonal condition. Androgen treatment during early developmental stages predisposes female rodents and primates to be aggressive if androgen treatment is reapplied in adulthood (Eaton, Goy & Phoenix, 1973; Edwards, 1968). In addition, male mice castrated on postnatal Day 1 usually will not exhibit aggression in adulthood. Thus, androgenic hormones present during early critical periods seem to predispose mice to be aggressive in adulthood, so long as androgen is present at that time. This stimulation of adult aggressiveness by androgenic hormones early in development seems to be the result of a sensitization of the individual to circulating androgens in adulthood. Nonandrogenized female mice and neonatally castrated male mice require massive dosages of androgen provided for long time periods in adulthood before these animals will fight, whereas androgenized females and intact males need much less androgen in adulthood to activate aggressive responses (Brain & Evans, 1975; Svare, Davis & Gandelman, 1974; Vom Saal, Gandelman & Svare, 1976; Vom Saal, Svare & Gandelman, 1976).

Although males typically are more aggressive than females (the hamster is one exception), many female mammals do exhibit aggression, which may depend on the activity of the ovarian hormones. For example, there are cyclical changes in aggressiveness accompanying the menstrual cycle in the rhesus monkey, and manipulations of the female rhesus ovarian hormone state seem to affect the amount of aggression displayed (Michael, 1971; Michael & Zumpe, 1970).

In the golden hamster, the female is quite a bit more aggressive than the male and will attack both males and females (Payne & Swanson, 1971, 1972a). Although the male hamster's aggressiveness clearly appears to be under the same kind of androgenic control as that of other rodents (Payne & Swanson, 1972a; Vandenbergh, 1971), the effects of hormones on aggression in the female hamster are not yet clear. Some studies have suggested that the female hamster's hormonal state does not affect her level of aggressiveness (Floody & Pfaff, 1974; Vandenbergh, 1971), whereas other studies have suggested that the ovarian hormones are important. Both Kislak and Beach (1955) and Payne and Swanson (1972b) have reported that ovariectomy decreases the aggressiveness of female hamsters. However, one of those studies found that estrogen, but not progesterone, could increase the aggressiveness of ovariectomized hamsters (Kislak & Beach, 1955), whereas the other study found that progesterone but not estrogen could increase the aggressiveness of these animals (Payne & Swanson, 1972b). These differences may result from methodological differences between studies, but, clearly, additional research is needed to clarify the role of hormonal factors in the control of aggression in female hamsters.

THE PITUITARY-ADRENAL HORMONES AND AGGRESSION Although classically the androgens were considered the only hormones important to the control of aggression, some more recent studies have implicated the hormones of the pituitary-adrenocortical axis in the determination of levels of aggressiveness. It should be noted at the outset that the effects of pituitary-adrenocortical manipulations on aggression are not so dramatic as those of androgen manipulations, and that the effects of the pituitary-adrenal hormones are not always consistent across both strains of animals and methods of testing (Burge & Edwards, 1971; Bronson & Desjardins, 1971).

There is some evidence from correlational studies that levels of pituitary-adrenal activity are related to levels of aggressiveness. For example, in rhesus monkeys, highly aggressive animals have higher circulating levels of the 17-hydroxycorticosteroids than less aggressive monkeys (Levine et al., 1970). In addition, members of a more aggressive strain of mice have been shown to have heavier adrenal glands than members of a less aggressive strain (Lagerspetz, Tirri & Lagerspetz, 1968).

Turning to experimental studies, removing the glucocorticoids from the circulation by adrenalectomy leads to a decrease in aggressiveness (Brain, Nowell & Wouters, 1971; Harding & Leshner, 1972; Sigg, 1969), and replacement therapy with corticosterone can restore the aggressiveness of adrenalectomized mice (Candland & Leshner, 1974). Treatment of intact mice with moderate dosages of the glucocorticoids seems to stimulate aggressiveness (Kostowski, Rewerski & Piechocki, 1970), whereas treatment with high glucocorticoid dosages decreases their aggressiveness (Candland & Leshner, 1974). In addition, injecting nonaggressive mice with glucocorticoids can increase their aggressiveness (Banarjee, 1971).

Because a change in adrenocortical activity always is accompanied by a change in the pituitary secretion of adrenocorticotropic hormone (ACTH), and because ACTH has been shown to have extra-adrenal effects on other behaviors (see Chapter 7), interest developed in the question of whether there is a direct relationship between ACTH levels and levels of aggressiveness. Treatment with ACTH over long time periods decreases aggressiveness in mice (Brain, Nowell & Wouters, 1971; Leshner et al., 1973), and the decrease appears to be independent of the effects of this pituitary peptide on either adrenocortical or gonadal activity (recall that ACTH treatment can depress the gonadal secretion of the androgens). ACTH will reduce the aggressiveness of mice even if they have adequate amounts of testosterone and if they cannot respond to the ACTH treatment with increases in corticosterone levels (Leshner et al., 1973).

This effect of ACTH on aggressiveness also can account for the observed effects of adrenalectomy. Adrenalectomy is accompanied by a sustained rise in ACTH levels which may be responsible for the depressive effects of this operation on aggressiveness. Thus, it is likely that manipulations that alter the levels of both ACTH and the glucocorticoids, such as adrenalectomy or ACTH treatment, affect aggressiveness because they modify ACTH levels; the changes in glucocorticoid levels are irrelevant.

ACTH may have different effects on aggressiveness when it is administered over only a very short period of time: short-term ACTH treatment appears to increase rather than decrease aggressiveness (Brain & Evans, 1973). In contrast to the long-term effects just discussed, the short-term excitatory effect appears to be a result of the effects of ACTH on corticosterone secretion. Short-term ACTH treatment increases the aggressiveness of mice that can respond to this peptide with an increase in corticosterone secretion (intact mice), but ACTH treatment does not affect the aggressiveness of mice with controlled corticosterone levels. Therefore, the increase in corticosterone levels that normally accompanies ACTH treatment is necessary for this pituitary peptide to exert its stimulatory effects (Leshner & Walker, 1972).

In summary, a long-lasting increase in pituitary-adrenal activity leads to a decrease in aggressiveness in mice, which appears to be a result of an extra-adrenal action of ACTH. On the other hand, a short-term increase in such activity leads to an increase in aggressiveness, probably because of the actions of the glucocorticoids.

HORMONES AND SUBMISSION During an agonistic encounter, one individual typically remains the aggressor, and the other individual becomes less and less aggressive and more and more submissive as it is defeated. Although many studies have examined the effects of hormones on aggressive responding, relatively little experimental attention has been directed toward the role of hormones in submissiveness. Some studies, however, have begun to examine the role of endocrine factors in characteristics related to submission, and these studies have focused on the hormones of the pituitary-adrenocortical axis and on the androgens.

No correlational studies have examined specifically the relationship between hormonal states and submissiveness. However, those studies which have shown correlations between either glucocorticoid or androgen levels and aggressiveness may also be showing correlations (the reverse) between these hormones and nonaggressiveness. Because submissive animals do not attack, one could argue that these studies have shown correlations between hormone levels and one element of submissiveness, nonaggressiveness.

Many theorists believe that submissive behaviors are avoidance responses, and that they serve primarily either to inhibit attack by the aggressor or to enable the defeated animal to escape from the attacker (Lorenz, 1966; Scott, 1946, 1967). Therefore, some studies have begun to examine the role of hormones in the avoidance component of submissive responding, which has been called "avoidance-of-attack." These studies have used a passive avoidance task where the aversive stimulus is attack by a trained fighter (see also Chapter 7). By studying how many trials it takes the test animal to learn to avoid the trained fighter, and by studying how well the animal retains the passive avoidance response once it has been learned, one can examine an animal's readiness or tendencies to avoid attack.

Both decreasing and increasing pituitary-adrenocortical activity for long time periods lead to an increase in the tendency to avoid attack (Leshner, Moyer & Walker, 1975). Interestingly, this bimodal relationship between pituitary-adrenal activity and avoidance-of-attack is opposite to that observed for these hormones and aggressiveness, where both decreases (as are induced by hypophysectomy) and increases (as are induced by ACTH treatment) in pituitary-adrenal activity lead to decreases in aggressiveness. However, the critical pituitary-adrenal hormones in the cases of aggression and avoidance-of-attack appear to be different. As discussed above, in the case of aggression, ACTH appears to be the critical hormone; it affects aggressiveness independently of its effects on glucocorticoid levels. On the other hand, in the case of avoidance-of-attack, the critical hormone appears to be corticosterone. Corticosterone treatment alone is sufficient to restore the avoidance behavior of hypophysectomized mice to normal levels, and ACTH only affects the avoidance tendencies of mice that are able to respond to this treatment with increases in corticosterone levels; mice with controlled corticosterone levels are unresponsive to ACTH treatment (Moyer & Leshner, 1976). Then, because in intact animals ACTH and corticoid levels ordinarily covary, changes in pituitary-adrenal activity affect both aggressiveness and avoidance tendencies, and they do so in opposite ways. However, as mentioned, the two behaviors are controlled by different hormones.

The suggestion that increases in pituitary-adrenal activity increase the tendency to avoid attack and, therefore, perhaps submissiveness is supported by the findings of a study by Brain and Poole (1974). They found that ACTH treatment decreases the likelihood that an animal will fight back if attacked, and this treatment decreases the latency for a test mouse to be defeated by a trained fighter mouse.

Turning to the androgens, although manipulations of adult androgen levels have dramatic effects on aggressiveness, these kinds of manipulations appear to have no effect on the tendency to avoid attack (Fig. 3-2). Neither castration nor treatment of castrated mice with testosterone affects the number of trials needed to learn to avoid attack or how well the response is retained (Leshner & Moyer, 1975). These findings provide preliminary evidence that the level of the androgens is irrelevant to the tendency to avoid attack and, therefore, perhaps to submissiveness. As in the case of the pituitary-adrenocortical hormones, this interpretation is supported by the findings of a study examining the tendency of androgen-manipulated animals to fight back when attacked. Barfield, Busch, and Wallen (1972) reported that although castrated rats will not initiate attacks, they will fight back if they are attacked. Therefore, manipulating androgen levels does not affect another behavioral characteristic of submissive animals, the tendency to fight back if attacked.

In summary, both decreases and increases in pituitary-adrenocortical activity lead to increases in the tendency to avoid attack and a decrease in fighting back when attacked, both of which are characteristics of submissive animals. On the other hand, manipulating androgen levels has no effect on either of these behavioral characteristics, suggesting that the level of the androgens is irrelevant to submissiveness.

COMMENT: HORMONAL EFFECTS ON AGONISTIC RESPONDING The findings discussed in this section show that the hormonal bases of the two components of intermale agonistic responding are different. Whereas the androgens appear to be quite important to aggression, they appear irrelevant to submissiveness. In addition, although generally the pituitary-adrenal hormones affect both

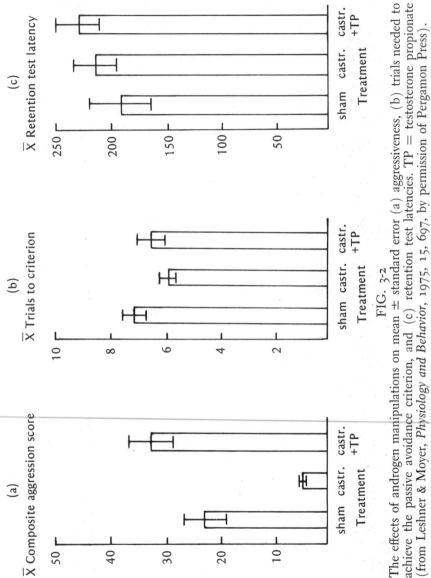

FIG. 3-2

The effects of androgen manipulations on mean ± standard error (a) aggressiveness, (b) trials needed to achieve the passive avoidance criterion, and (c) retention test latencies. TP = testosterone propionate (from Leshner & Moyer, *Physiology and Behavior*, 1975, 15, 697, by permission of Pergamon Press).

aggressiveness and submissiveness, the critical pituitary-adrenal hormones are different in the two cases. ACTH seems to be the critical pituitary-adrenal hormone in the case of aggression, whereas the glucocorticoids appear to be critical in the control of submission.

These differences in hormonal effects on aggression and submission have important implications for the behavioral study of agonistic responding. Investigators interested in this class of behaviors often seem to assume that aggressiveness and submissiveness are opposite ends of a single continuum; that is, that as an animal becomes less aggressive it automatically becomes more submissive, and the reverse. However, the findings discussed in this section show that aggressiveness and submissiveness can be manipulated separately. For example, a castrated mouse might be less aggressive but it is not necessarily more submissive than an intact animal. Thus, although aggressiveness and submissiveness may ordinarily vary in opposite ways, they are not opposite extremes of a single process; they can be manipulated separately and, therefore, are separable components of agonistic responding (see Leshner & Moyer, 1975).

MEDIATION OF HORMONAL EFFECTS ON AGONISTIC RESPONDING How do hormones exert their effects on agonistic responding? The findings reviewed here show that an animal's baseline hormonal state prior to exposure to agonistic stimuli affects both the form and intensity of its agonistic responses to those stimuli. For example, animals with high levels of pituitary-adrenocortical activity react relatively nonaggressively to and quite readily avoid other potentially aggressive members of the same species. An important remaining question concerns the mediation of these hormonal effects.

As discussed in Chapter 1, there are many ways that hormones might affect behavior: by altering general metabolic states, by altering the state of the sensory receptors that receive information about critical stimuli, or by altering the state of the neural mechanisms that are responsible for the interpretation of stimuli and the coordination of responses. In the case of agonistic behavior, it seems most likely that hormones affect responding by modifying the state of critical brain circuits. Moyer (1971) has suggested that the androgens affect aggressiveness by sensitizing critical neural circuits to certain kinds of stimuli. Leshner (1975) expanded this argument somewhat by suggesting that the same hormonal manipulations can affect both aggressive and submissive components of agonistic responding by sensitizing certain neural circuits and desensitizing others. For example, increases in pituitary-adrenocortical activity might make an animal less aggressive and more readily submissive because these hormonal changes sensitize the neural circuits controlling submissiveness and desensitize the circuits controlling aggressiveness. This kind of interpretation seems plausible, since the neural mechanisms that control aggressive and avoidance responses appear to be different (Endröczi & Koranyi, 1969), and specific hormones do affect different brain sites differently. However, these propositions remain primarily speculative; there have been relatively few experimental studies dealing directly with the mediation of hormonal effects on agonistic responding.

Some preliminary evidence does support the view that hormonal effects on agonistic responding are neurally mediated. Implants of testosterone into the septal area of the brain restore the aggressiveness of castrated mice (Owen, Peters & Bronson, 1974), and implants of testosterone into the preoptic area can restore the aggressiveness of castrated ring doves (Barfield, 1971). Thus, androgen treatments limited to the brain can counteract the effects of decreasing androgen levels in the general circulation. Although there have been no direct tests of whether hormone implants into the brain can affect submissive responses, it is clear that hormones can affect other kinds of avoidance responses, such as shock-mediated responses, through directly modifying the state of specific neural circuits (Endröczi, 1972).

Effects of Experience on Endocrine Function

Not only do hormones affect agonistic behavior, but experiences in agonistic situations appear to have marked effects on both pituitary-adrenocortical and pituitary-gonadal function. Following competition, defeated animals show increased levels of adrenocortical activity, whereas victorious animals seem unaffected (Archer, 1970; Bronson & Eleftheriou, 1964, 1965a). In fact, the mere threat of defeat is sufficient to induce increases in adrenocortical activity in previously defeated mice (Bronson & Eleftheriou, 1965b). The effects of exposure to different numbers of defeats on plasma corticosterone levels are shown in Figure 3-3.

FIG. 3-3

Plasma corticosterone levels after 0, 1, 2, 4, or 8 exposures per day to trained fighters or empty cages for one week (modified from Bronson & Eleftheriou, *General and Comparative Endocrinology*, 1964, 4, 11, by permission of Academic Press).

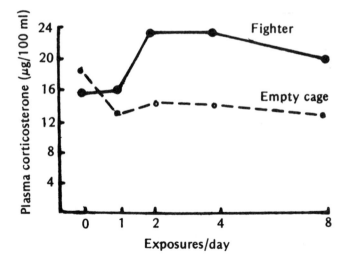

On the other hand, the effects of fighting on pituitary-gonadal function are less clear than those on pituitary-adrenocortical activity. For example, although Vale and his colleagues (Vale, Lee & Ray, 1970; Vale, Vale & Harley, 1971) found no direct effects of fighting or defeat on testicular function in mice, Bronson and Desjardins (1971) found that defeat, but not victory, depresses gonadal activity in these rodents.

Fighting also affects gonadotropin levels, and the nature of the animal's agonistic experiences determines the form and duration of its gonadotropin responses to competition. Fighting leads to decreased serum levels of both luteinizing hormone (LH) and follicle stimulating hormone (FSH), and the magnitude of this depression of gonadotropin levels is greater in defeated than in victorious mice (Bronson, Stetson & Stiff, 1973). The temporal characteristics of the gonadotropin responses to competition also are different for defeated and victorious mice: FSH levels remain depressed longer following fighting in defeated mice than in victorious mice. However, LH levels remain depressed for long post-experience time periods, and the outcome of the fight does not influence the rate of return of LH levels toward normal levels (Bronson, 1973).

How do these agonistic experiences lead to changes in endocrine function? As discussed in Chapter 1, the peripheral receptors that receive information from the external environment are not directly connected to the endocrine glands, and experience surely is not integrated in the endocrine system. Therefore, it is likely that the effects of victory or defeat are mediated through the nervous system, which both is sensitive to the state of the peripheral receptors and integrates the functioning of the endocrine system. Agonistic experiences produce dramatic changes in the state of the central nervous system circuits which control endocrine function. Defeat has a significant effect on protein synthesis in the brain (Eleftheriou, 1971) and alters the state of the brain neurotransmitter systems. Daily fighting experiences lead to increases in central catecholamine and serotonin levels, and these increases are more pronounced in some brain areas than in others (Eleftheriou & Church, 1968a, 1968b; Welch & Welch, 1971). This altered neurotransmitter activity in particular brain circuits, such as the limbic circuits, should be reflected in altered activity levels of both the pituitary-adrenocortical and pituitary-gonadal axes, since these endocrine subsystems are under the control of the same brain areas (e.g., Ryzhenkov, 1973; Sawyer & Gorski, 1971; Taylor, Matheson & Dafny, 1971).

Hormonal Mediation of the Effects of Defeat on Agonistic Response Patterns

The reader may have noticed that there is a striking similarity between the effects of defeat on endocrine function and those endocrine manipulations that are most effective in modifying initial levels of agonistic responding in naive animals. First, defeated mice exhibit increased levels of pituitary-adrenocortical activity and, probably, decreased levels of gonadal activity. Second, naive animals with experimentally-induced increases in pituitary-adrenal activity and decreases in gonadal activity are less aggressive and more submissive than normal animals. Interestingly, defeat leads to the same behavioral characteristics, nonaggressiveness and submissiveness, as do these hormonal manipulations. On the basis of this similarity, it has been suggested that the behavioral responses to defeat, nonaggressiveness and submissiveness, are in part caused by the hormonal responses to this experience; that is, that there is a long-chain hormone–behavior interaction whereby the hormonal responses to defeat feed back and modify ongoing agonistic responses (Leshner, 1975).

Nock and Leshner (1976) tested this hypothesis directly by preventing the hormonal responses to defeat (by controlling hormone levels) and observing the pattern of agonistic responding throughout an encounter. These hormonal responses were prevented by hypophysectomizing the mice and treating them with fixed replacement dosages of ACTH and testosterone prior to and during the encounter. Thus, if the hormonal responses to defeat are important to the behavioral responses to this experience, preventing those hormonal changes should prevent or at least decrease the behavioral changes that normally accompany defeat.

Nock and Leshner found that animals that could not react hormonally to defeat fought longer and took longer to become submissive than did normal animals. In addition, the animals with controlled hormone levels became nonaggressive and submissive later in the encounter than did noncontrolled animals (Fig. 3-4). Thus, preventing the hormonal responses to defeat delayed and decreased

FIG. 3-4
Mean number of (a) attacks and (b) submissive postures in each half of an agonistic encounter. (Groups: CH-V = controlled-hormone, victorious; CH-D = controlled-hormone, defeated; SH-V = intact, victorious; SH-D = intact, defeated) (modified from Nock & Leshner, *Physiology and Behavior*, 1976, 17, 113, by permission of Pergamon Press).

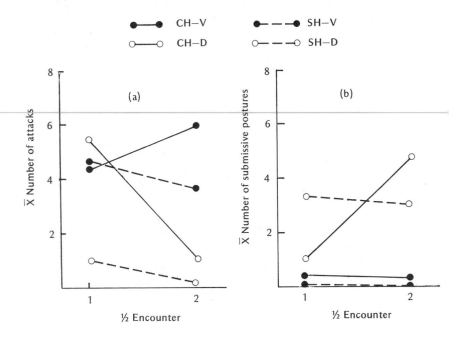

the behavioral changes that ordinarily accompany this experience. Because preventing these hormonal responses altered the pattern of agonistic responding of defeated mice, Nock and Leshner concluded that the hormonal responses to defeat ordinarily feed back and facilitate the expression of nonaggressive, submissive behaviors following this experience.

DOMINANCE RELATIONSHIPS

The studies just discussed have examined agonistic responding directly, either by observing whether an individual fights or submits or by studying how much it fights or submits. An alternative measure of aggressiveness that has frequently been used is more indirect: studying the outcome of agonistic interactions, or dominance/subordinance relationships. Most theorists agree that dominance status can reflect levels of aggressiveness, as long as the definition of aggression includes the ritualized threats that many animals use in place of actual attacks. This belief is based on the high correlations between levels of aggressiveness and the attainment of dominance (who wins or loses) and between an individual's already-achieved status (the dominance position it maintains) and its level of aggressiveness (Buirski et al., 1973; Ginsburg & Allee, 1942; Scott, 1944). Furthermore, both the attainment and maintenance of dominance status seem to be dependent on the display of agonistic behaviors. Therefore, studies of the relationship between endocrine function and dominance also are examining, at least indirectly, the relationship between endocrine function and agonistic responding.

Many studies have examined the correlation between dominance status and endocrine activity levels, and the hormones of both the pituitary-adrenal and pituitary-gonadal axes seem to be related to dominance rank. In general, subordinate animals exhibit higher levels of adrenocortical activity than do dominant animals. This increase has been observed in species as diverse as mice (Louch &

Higginbotham, 1967; Southwick & Bland, 1959), rats (Popova & Naumenko, 1972), wolf cubs (Fox & Andrews, 1973), and rhesus monkeys (Sassenrath, 1970). It has been suggested that subordinate animals have higher levels of pituitary-adrenal activity because they are constantly exposed to the stresses of being defeated or the threat of defeat.

The relationship between pituitary-gonadal activity and dominance is the reverse of that for pituitary-adrenal activity: dominant animals appear to have higher levels of gonadal activity than subordinates (e.g., Bronson & Marsden, 1973 for mice; Rose, Holaday & Bernstein, 1971 for rhesus monkeys). Figure 3-5 shows the mean testosterone levels of rhesus monkeys of different ranks. Interestingly, at least in the rhesus monkey, as an animal achieves a high

FIG. 3-5
Mean ± standard errors for each quartile of the dominance rank order. The most dominant animals, rank order 1-8, had significantly higher testosterone concentrations than those in the lower quartiles (reprinted from Rose et al., *Nature*, Vol. 231, 367, 1971).

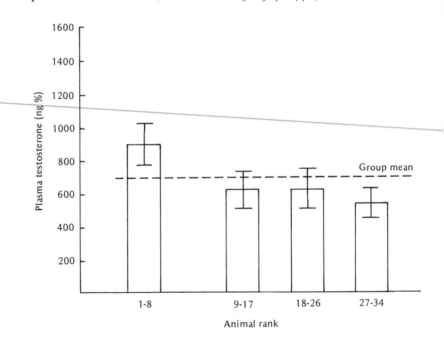

dominance position, its testosterone levels rise. As its dominance status is reduced, testosterone levels decline. This finding suggests that androgen levels may represent a response to or a characteristic of being in a particular dominance position, thereby suggesting some causality in the correlation between androgen levels and dominance status: an animal's rank may determine its androgen levels (Rose, Gordon & Bernstein, 1972). This proposition is consistent with the results of those studies of the hormonal responses to competition which showed that defeat (which would lead to a reduction in rank) leads to a decrease in pituitary-gonadal activity (see above).

In light of our earlier discussions, where we saw that androgen levels affect levels of aggressiveness, the findings of these correlational studies may seem surprising because they suggest that dominance status determines androgen levels, rather than vice versa. But, experimental studies also have demonstrated the importance of the androgenic hormones in the maintenance of dominance status. Castration of a dominant animal will lead to a reduction in status in mice (Lee & Naranjo, 1972), chickens (Guhl, 1964), and some primates (e.g., Clark & Birch, 1945). Interestingly, once an animal has been relegated to a low rank, raising androgen levels will not raise the individual's rank (Guhl, 1964; Lee & Naranjo, 1972; Mirsky, 1955). This lack of effect on subordinate animals has been attributed to the powerful effects of social experiences which, in the case of subordinance, seem prepotent over any potential effects of hormonal manipulations (Guhl, 1964).

These findings about hormones and dominance are basically consistent with the findings discussed before about hormones and intermale agonistic behavior. There appear to be significant correlations between endocrine activity and dominance status, and these correlations are similar in form to those between endocrine activity and direct measures of agonistic responding. That is, there have been reports of a correlation between levels of aggressiveness and levels of androgen activity, and dominant (aggressive) animals seem to have higher androgen levels than subordinate (less aggressive and submissive) animals. In addition, defeated animals exhibit high levels of pituitary-adrenocortical activity, as do subordinate animals. Finally, experimental manipulations show that at least androgenic manipulations can lead to changes in dominance status, and these effects are similar to the effects of those manipulations on aggressiveness.

The findings discussed in this section raise the possibility of there being a long-chain hormone–behavior interaction operating in the case of androgen levels and dominance. Recall that the correlational studies discussed here suggest that the rank an animal holds can determine its androgen levels, and that experimental studies also have suggested that an animal's androgen levels can affect its dominance status. These two relationships could be connected in important ways. Specifically, it could be that an animal's initial androgen levels first contribute to the determination of the rank the animal will achieve. Then, if the animal's rank later decreases (for whatever reason) its androgen levels will fall. That fall in androgen levels might then feed back and lower the animal's level of aggressiveness, which, in turn, would contribute to keeping that individual at a low rank. Of course, this kind of hypothesis is speculative, and its evaluation would have to await direct experimental tests.

IRRITABLE AGGRESSION

When animals are in pairs or larger groups, they seem to respond to environmental irritations with the display of aggression toward other group members. Moyer (1968) has labeled this type of aggression *irritable aggression*. Because it usually is studied using shock as the irritating stimulus, it is often referred to as *shock-elicited aggression*.

There are some similarities and some dissimilarities between the relationship of endocrine function and irritable aggression and that of endocrine function and intermale aggression. As in the case of intermale aggression, there is a gender difference in shock-elicited aggressiveness: males exhibit more aggression following irritation than females. In addition, this gender difference appears to be at least in part androgen dependent. Castrating adult male rats reduces the amount of aggression displayed, and replacement therapy with testosterone restores aggressiveness to the level of controls (Hutchinson, Ulrich & Azrin, 1965; Milligan, Powell & Borasio, 1973). In addition, neonatal castration of male rats leads to adult levels of shock-elicited aggression equal to those of females (Conner & Levine, 1969). Thus, in the same way that the presence or absence of the androgens may be responsible for the gender differences in intermale aggressiveness, they may be responsible for the gender differences in irritable aggression.

However, the pituitary-adrenal hormones do not appear to be involved in the control of irritable aggression, as they are in the case of intermale aggression. Although there are marked increases in pituitary-adrenocortical activity following fighting in the shock-elicited situation (Conner, Vernikos-Danellis & Levine, 1971), manipulating pituitary-adrenal activity levels does not affect the amount of aggression displayed. Implants of cortisol into the median eminence, which decrease circulating levels of the pituitary-adrenal hormones, have no effect on the amount of aggression elicited by shocking the animals (Erskine & Levine, 1973).

PREDATORY AGGRESSION

The attacking of prey may be viewed as an example of aggression (Moyer, 1968), and some laboratory studies have begun to examine the role of endocrine factors in the control of what is called *predatory aggression*. One problem with these studies is that the animals used as stimuli do not represent prey that the test animal, usually the laboratory rat, would encounter naturally. Typical stimulus prey used in these laboratory studies include mice and frogs.

Castration in adulthood has no effect on either mouse-killing or frog-killing (Bernard, 1974; Karli, 1958). On the other hand, removing the androgens during the neonatal period by castration does reduce mouse-killing in adult rats (Baenninger, 1974). These findings suggest that predatory aggression is not dependent on androgens circulating in adulthood, but that the neural "organization" of critical circuits for the control of this behavior is dependent on the presence of androgens early in life.

HUMAN AGGRESSION

The studies discussed so far all were conducted with nonhuman subjects. Human agonistic behavior often appears to be different in form from that of other animals, and there have been many controversies about what does and does not constitute an agonistic response in humans. In addition, human agonistic behaviors have not been categorized as extensively as have those of nonhuman animals. Therefore, a direct comparison of the role of hormones in animal and human agonistic responses is not yet possible.

The few studies that have been conducted with human subjects have focused on the relationship between androgen levels and various behaviors labeled as aggression, and the findings of these studies have not been consistent. Persky, Smith, and Basu (1971) first examined the correlations between testosterone production rates and a range of measures of aggressiveness in three groups of human subjects: young men, older men, and psychiatric patients. They found relatively few significant correlations among their measures, but they did find a significant correlation in young men between testosterone production rates and levels of hostility as measured by the Buss-Durkee Hostility Inventory (Fig. 3-6). Curiously, there was no correlation between these same measures in

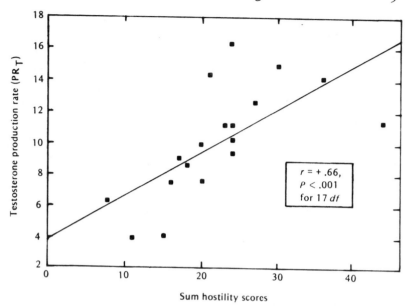

FIG. 3-6
Testosterone production rate as a function of hostility score on the
Buss-Durkee Hostility Inventory for 18 young men (modified from
Persky, Smith & Basu, *Psychosomatic Medicine*, 1971, 33, 270, by
permission of the American Psychosomatic Society)

older men. On the other hand, Doering et al. (1974) attempted
to replicate this study using repeated measures of both testosterone
levels and hostility. Although they did find some within-subject
correlations between testosterone levels and levels of aggression,
they found no consistent relationship in groups.

Kreuz and Rose (1972) examined the correlations between testosterone levels and three measures of aggressiveness in male prison
inmates. They found no correlations between plasma testosterone
levels and measures of aggressiveness taken while the subjects were
in prison. However, they did find a significant negative correlation
between age at first conviction for an aggressive act and plasma

testosterone levels: the earlier an inmate had been convicted for the first time, the higher his testosterone levels at the time of the study. But, since those inmates who had been convicted earlier had been in prison for a longer time, it is possible that the observed correlation really is between length of imprisonment and testosterone levels, and does not reflect a static characteristic of inmates imprisoned earlier.

In another study of prison inmates, Ehrenkranz, Bliss, and Sheard (1974) did find a relationship between aggressiveness and androgen levels. They found that inmates rated as quite aggressive had significantly higher plasma testosterone levels than inmates ranked as nonaggressive.

One should be cautious, however, in interpreting the results of these studies of prison inmates, because many people believe that all inmates are relatively more aggressive than noninmates. Therefore, the results of these types of studies may not be generalizable to the general population.

For obvious ethical reasons, there have been no systematic experimental studies of the relationship between hormones and aggression in humans. However, the clinical literature is filled with reports of the effects of reducing androgen levels either by castration or by treatment with anti-androgens for sex-related crimes (see also Chapter 5). As would be expected, habitual sex offenders show great "improvement" or remission of their symptoms following reductions in androgen levels. But, it is unclear whether such "improvements" are due to direct effects on aggression or whether they are due to effects on sexual motivation (see reviews in Kling, 1975; Money et al., 1975).

SUMMARY AND COMMENT

Most studies of endocrine function and agonistic behavior have focused on what have been called intermale agonistic responses.

These studies have shown that: (1) The baseline hormonal state contributes to the determination of the form and intensity of the individual's initial responses to agonistic stimuli. Under one hormonal condition, the individual reacts quite aggressively and is not readily submissive. Under another hormonal condition, the individual will react nonaggressively and be readily submissive. These hormonal effects on intermale agonistic responding probably are mediated by the central nervous system circuits that are responsible for the control of agonistic behaviors. (2) Experiences in agonistic situations lead to changes in endocrine function, and the form of those experiences seems to determine the form of the hormonal change: defeated and victorious animals exhibit different hormonal responses to competition. (3) The hormonal responses to competition seem to feed back and facilitate the behavioral changes that accompany different agonistic experiences, since preventing the hormonal responses (at least to defeat) alters the pattern of changes in agonistic responding that normally accompany this experience. Therefore, there appears to be a long-chain hormone–behavior interaction between endocrine function and agonistic behavior: An animal's baseline hormonal state first affects the form and intensity of its initial responses to agonistic stimuli. The individual's initial experiences and behavioral responses then lead to changes in its hormonal state. Then, these changes in its hormonal state feed back and modify its pattern of agonistic responding, etc.

Relatively little experimental attention has been directed toward the role of endocrine factors in the control of other types of agonistic responses. The few studies that have been conducted suggest that (1) as in intermale aggression, the level of the androgens is important in the determination of the intensity of irritable aggressive responses. (2) Unlike intermale aggression, in irritable aggression the level of the pituitary-adrenal hormones is unimportant. (3) On the other hand, adult hormone levels, at least those of the androgens, seem unimportant to predatory aggression, although the early hormonal environment does seem to play a role in the determination of adult responses.

Some preliminary evidence suggests that hormones may be related to the amount of aggression displayed by humans as well as animals. There have been a few correlational studies showing a relationship between androgen levels and levels of aggressiveness, and some clinical studies have suggested that altering androgen levels might modify some types of aggressive responses. However, the results of studies of human subjects have not been consistent, and, therefore, any decisions about the role of hormones in human agonistic responding should await additional evidence.

REFERENCES

Archer, J.   Effects of aggressive behavior on the adrenal cortex in male laboratory mice. *Journal of Mammology*, 1970, 51, 327-333.

Baenninger, R.   Effects of day 1 castration on aggressive behavior of rats. *Bulletin of the Psychonomic Society*, 1974, 3, 189-190.

Banarjee, U.   The influence of some hormones and drugs on isolation-induced aggression in male mice. *Communications in Behavioral Biology*, 1971, 6, 163-170.

Barfield, R. J.   Activation of sexual and aggressive behavior by androgen implanted into the male ring dove brain. *Endocrinology*, 1971, 89, 1470-1476.

Barfield, R. J., Busch, D. E. & Wallen, K.   Gonadal influences on agonistic behavior in the male domestic rat. *Hormones and Behavior*, 1972, 3, 247-259.

Beeman, E. A.   The effect of male hormone on aggressive behavior in mice. *Physiological Zoology*, 1947, 20, 373-405.

Bernard, B. K.   Frog killing (ranacide) in the male rat: lack of effect of hormonal manipulations. *Physiology and Behavior*, 1974, 12, 405-408.

Bevan, J. M., Bevan, W. & Williams, B. F.   Spontaneous aggressiveness in young castrate C3H mice treated with three dose levels of testosterone. *Physiological Zoology*, 1958, 31, 284-288.

Bevan, W., Levy, G. W., Whitehouse, J. M. & Bevan, J. M.   Spontaneous aggressiveness in two strains of mice castrated and treated with one of three androgens. *Physiological Zoology*, 1957, 30, 341-349.

Brain, P. F. & Evans, C. M.   Some recent studies on the effects of corticotrophin on agonistic behaviour in the house mouse and the golden hamster. *Journal of Endocrinology*, 1973, 57, xxxix-xl.

Brain, P. F. & Evans, C. M. Attempts to influence fighting and threat behavior in adult isolated female CFW mice in standard opponent aggression tests using injected and subcutaneously implanted androgens. *Physiology and Behavior*, 1975, 14, 551-556.

Brain, P. F. & Nowell, N. W. Some endocrine and behavioral changes in the development of the albino laboratory mouse. *Communications in Behavioral Biology*, 1969, 4, 203-220. (a)

Brain, P. F. & Nowell, N. W. Some behavioral and endocrine relationships in adult male, laboratory mice subjected to open field and aggression tests. *Physiology and Behavior*, 1969, 4, 945-947. (b)

Brain, P. F., Nowell, N. W. & Wouters, A. Some relationships between adrenal function and the effectiveness of a period of isolation in inducing intermale aggression in albino mice. *Physiology and Behavior*, 1971, 6, 27-29.

Brain, P. F. & Poole, A. E. The role of endocrines in isolation-induced intermale fighting in albino laboratory mice. I. Pituitary adrenocortical influences. *Aggressive Behavior*, 1974, 1, 39-69.

Bronson, F. H. Establishment of social rank among grouped male mice: relative effects on circulating FSH, LH and corticosterone. *Physiology and Behavior*, 1973, 10, 947-951.

Bronson, F. H. & Desjardins, C. Steroid hormones and aggressive behavior in mammals. In B. E. Eleftheriou & J. P. Scott (Eds.), *Physiology of Aggression and Defeat*. New York: Plenum Press, 1971, pp. 43-63.

Bronson, F. H. & Eleftheriou, B. E. Chronic physiological effects of fighting in mice. *General and Comparative Endocrinology*, 1964, 4, 9-14.

Bronson, F. H. & Eleftheriou, B. E. Relative effects of fighting on bound and unbound corticosterone in mice. *Proceedings of the Society for Experimental Biology and Medicine*, 1965, 118, 146-149. (a)

Bronson, F. H. & Eleftheriou, B. E. Adrenal response to fighting in mice: separation of physical and psychological causes. *Science*, 1965, 147, 627-628. (b)

Bronson, F. H. & Marsden, H. M. The preputial gland as an indicator of social dominance in male mice. *Behavioral Biology*, 1973, 9, 625-628.

Bronson, F. H., Stetson, M. H. & Stiff, M. E. Serum FSH and LH in male mice following aggressive and nonaggressive interactions. *Physiology and Behavior*, 1973, 10, 369-372.

Buirski, P., Kellerman, H. M., Plutchik, R., Weininger, R. & Buirski, N. A field study of emotions, dominance and social behavior in a group of baboons (*Papio anubis*). *Primates*, 1973, 14, 67-78.

Burge, K. G. & Edwards, D. A.   The adrenal gland and the pre- and post-castrational aggressive behavior of male mice. *Physiology and Behavior*, 1971, 7, 885-888.

Candland, D. K. & Leshner, A. I.   A model of agonistic behavior: endocrine and autonomic correlates. In L. V. DiCara (Ed.), *Limbic and Autonomic Nervous Systems Research*. New York: Plenum Press, 1974, pp. 137-163.

Clark, G. & Birch, H. G.   Hormonal modifications of social behavior. I. The effects of sex-hormone administration on the social status of a male castrate chimpanzee. *Psychosomatic Medicine* 1945, 7, 321-329.

Conner, R. L.   Hormones, biogenic amines and aggression. In S. Levine (Ed.), *Hormones and Behavior*. New York: Academic Press, 1972, pp. 209-233.

Conner, R. L. & Levine, S.   Hormonal influences on aggressive behavior. In S. Garattini and E. B. Sigg (Eds.), *Aggressive Behavior*. New York: Wiley, 1969, pp. 150-163.

Conner, R. L., Vernikos-Danellis, J. & Levine, S.   Stress, fighting and neuroendocrine function. *Nature*, 1971, 234, 564-566.

Crook, J. H. & Butterfield, P. A.   Effects of testosterone propionate and luteinizing hormone on agonistic and nest building behavior of *Quela quela*. *Animal Behavior*, 1968, 16, 370-384.

Doering, C. H., Brodie, H. K. H., Kraemer, H., Becker, H. & Hamburg, D. A.   Plasma testosterone levels and psychologic measures in men over a 2-month period. In R. C. Friedman, R. M. Richart, and R. L. vande Wiele (Eds.), *Sex Differences in Behavior*. New York: Wiley, 1974, pp. 413-431.

Eaton, G. G., Goy, R. W. & Phoenix, C. H.   Effects of testosterone treatment in adulthood on sexual behavior of female pseudohermaphrodite rhesus monkeys. *Nature*, 1973, 242, 119-120.

Eaton, G. G. & Resko, J. A.   Plasma testosterone and male dominance in a Japanese macaque (*Macaca fuscata*) troop compared with repeated measures of testosterone in laboratory males. *Hormones and Behavior*, 1974, 5, 251-259.

Edwards, D. A.   Mice: fighting by neonatally androgenized females. *Science*, 1968, 16, 1027-1028.

Edwards, D. A.   Early androgen stimulation and aggressive behavior in male and female mice. *Physiology and Behavior*, 1969, 4, 333-338.

Edwards, D. A. & Rowe, F. A.   Neural and endocrine control of aggressive behavior. In B. E. Eleftheriou and R. L. Sprott (Eds.), *Hormonal Correlates of Behavior, Vol. 1*. New York: Plenum Press, 1975, pp. 275-303.

Ehrenkranz, J., Bliss, E. & Sheard, M. H.   Plasma testosterone: correlation with aggressive behavior and social dominance in men. *Psychosomatic Medicine*, 1974, 36, 469-475.

Eleftheriou, B. E.   Effects of aggression and defeat on brain macro-molecules. In B. E. Eleftheriou and J. P. Scott (Eds.), *Physiology of Aggression and Defeat.* New York: Plenum Press, 1971, pp. 65-90.

Eleftheriou, B. E. & Church, R. L.   Brain 5-hydroxytryptophan de-carboxylase in mice after exposure to aggression and defeat. *Physiology and Behavior,* 1968, 3, 323-325. (a)

Eleftheriou, B. E. & Church, R. L.   Brain levels of serotonin and norepinephrine in mice after exposure to aggression and defeat. *Physiology and Behavior,* 1968, 3, 977-980. (b)

Endröczi, E.   *Limbic System, Learning and Pituitary-Adrenal Function.* Budapest: Akademiai Kiado, 1972.

Endröczi, E. & Koranyi, L.   Integration of emotional reactions in the brain stem, diencephalic and limbic system. In S. Garattini and E. B. Sigg (Eds.), *Aggressive Behavior.* New York: Wiley, 1969, pp. 132-140.

Erskine, M. S. & Levine, S.   Suppression of pituitary-adrenal activity and shock-induced fighting in rats. *Physiology and Behavior,* 1973, 11, 787-790.

Floody, O. R. & Pfaff, D. W.   Steroid hormones and aggressive behavior: approaches to the study of hormone sensitive brain mechanisms for behavior. *Research Publications of the Association for Research in Nervous and Mental Disease,* 1974, 52, 149-185.

Fox, M. W. & Andrews, R. V.   Physiological and biochemical correlates of individual differences in behavior of wolf cubs. *Behavior,* 1973, 46, 129-139.

Ginsburg, B. & Allee, W. C.   Some effects of conditioning on social dominance and subordination in inbred strains of mice. *Physiological Zoology,* 1942, 15, 485-506.

Gray, J. A.   Sex differences in emotional behavior in mammals including man: endocrine bases. *Acta Psychologica,* 1971, 35, 29-46.

Guhl, A. M.   Psychophysical interrelations in the social behavior of chickens. *Psychological Bulletin,* 1964, 61, 277-285.

Harding, C. F. & Leshner, A. I.   The effects of adrenalectomy on the aggressiveness of differently housed mice. *Physiology and Behavior,* 1972, 8, 437-440.

Healey, M. C.   Aggression and self-regulation of population size in deermice. *Ecology,* 1967, 48, 377-392.

Hutchison, R. R., Ulrich, R. E. & Azrin, N. H.   Effects of age and related factors on the pain-aggression reaction. *Journal of Comparative and Physiological Psychology,* 1965, 59, 365-369.

Kamel, F., Mock, E. J., Wright, W. W. & Frankel, A. I.   Alterations in plasma concentrations of testosterone, LH, and prolactin associated with mating in the male rat. *Hormones and Behavior,* 1975, 6, 2772-2788.

Karli, P.   Hormones steroides et comportment d'aggression inter-specific rat-souris. *Journal of Physiology and General Pathology*, 1958, 50, 346-357.

Kislak, J. W. & Beach, F. A.   Inhibition of aggressiveness by ovarian hormones. *Endocrinology*, 1955, 56, 684-692.

Kling, A.   Testosterone and aggressive behavior in man and non-human primates. In B. E. Eleftheriou and R. L. Sprott (Eds.), *Hormonal Correlates of Behavior*, Vol. 1. New York: Plenum Press, 1975, pp. 305-323.

Kostowski, W., Rewerski, W. & Piechocki, T.   Effects of some steroids on aggressive behavior in mice and rats. *Neuroendocrinology*, 1970, 6, 311-318.

Kreuz, L. E. & Rose, R. M.   Assessment of aggressive behavior and plasma testosterone in a young criminal population. *Psychosomatic Medicine*, 1972, 34, 321-332.

Lagerspetz, K. Y. H., Tirri, R. & Lagerspetz, K. M. J.   Neurochemical and endocrinological studies of mice selectively bred for aggressiveness. *Scandinavian Journal of Psychology*, 1968, 9, 157-160.

Lee, C. T. & Naranjo, N.   Effects of castration and androgen on the social dominance of BALB/cJ mice. *Physiological Psychology*, 1974, 2, 93-98.

Leshner, A. I.   A model of hormones and agonistic behavior. *Physiology and Behavior*, 1975, 15, 225-235.

Leshner, A. I. & Moyer, J. A.   Androgens and agonistic behavior in mice: relevance to aggression and irrelevance to avoidance-of-attack. *Physiology and Behavior*, 1975, 15, 695-699.

Leshner, A. I., Moyer, J. A. & Walker, W. A.   Pituitary-adrenocortical activity and avoidance-of-attack in mice. *Physiology and Behavior*, 1975, 15, 689-693.

Leshner, A. I., Walker, W. A., Johnson, A. E., Kelling, J. S., Kreisler, S. J. & Svare, B. B.   Pituitary adrenocortical activity and intermale aggressiveness in isolated mice. *Physiology and Behavior*, 1973, 11, 705-711.

Leshner, A. I. & Walker, W. A.   The adrenals and intermale aggression. Paper presented at the meeting of the Psychonomic Society, St. Louis, 1972.

Levine, M. D., Gordon, T. P., Peterson, R. H. & Rose, R. M.   Urinary 17-OHCS response of high- and low-aggressive rhesus monkeys to shock avoidance. *Physiology and Behavior*, 1970, 5, 919-924.

Levy, J. V. & King, J. A.   The effects of testosterone propionate on fighting behavior in young male C57BL/10 mice. *Anatomical Record*, 1953, 117, 562-563.

Lorenz, K.   *On Aggression*. New York: Bantam Books, 1966.

Louch, C. D. & Higginbotham, M. The relation between social rank and plasma corticosterone levels in mice. *General and Comparative Endocrinology*, 1967, 8, 441-444.

McKinney, T. D. & Desjardins, C. Postnatal development of the testis, fighting behavior and fertility in house mice. *Biology of Reproduction*, 1973, 9, 279-294.

Michael, R. P. Hormonal factors and aggressive behavior in the rhesus monkey. In *Proceedings of the International Society for Psychoneuroendocrinology*. Basel: S. Karger, 1971, pp. 412-423.

Michael, R. P. & Zumpe, D. Aggression and gonadal hormones in captive rhesus monkeys (*Macaca mulatta*). *Animal Behavior*, 1970, 18, 1-10.

Milligan, W. L., Powell, D. A. & Borasio, G. Sexual variables and shock-elicited aggression. *Journal of Comparative and Physiological Psychology*, 1973, 83, 441-450.

Mirsky, A. F. The influence of sex hormones on social behavior in monkeys. *Journal of Comparative and Physiological Psychology*, 1955, 48, 327-335.

Money, J., Wiedeking, C., Walker, P., Migeon, C., Meyer, W. & Borgaonkar, D. 47,SYY and 46,SY male with antisocial and/or sex-offending behavior: antiandrogen therapy plus counseling. *Psychoneuroendocrinology*, 1975, 1, 165-178.

Moyer, J. A. & Leshner, A. I. Pituitary-adrenal effects on avoidance-of-attack in mice: separation of the effects of ACTH and corticosterone. *Physiology and Behavior*, 1976, 17, 297-301.

Moyer, K. E. Kinds of aggression and their physiological basis. *Communications in Behavioral Biology*, 1968, 2, 65-87.

Moyer, K. E. *The Physiology of Hostility*. Chicago: Markham, 1971.

Nock, B. L. & Leshner, A. I. Hormonal mediation of the effects of defeat on agonistic responding in mice. *Physiology and Behavior*, 1976, 17, 111-119.

Owen, K., Peters, P. J. & Bronson, F. H. Effects of intracranial implants of testosterone propionate on intermale aggression in the castrated male mouse. *Hormones and Behavior*, 1974, 5, 83-92.

Payne, A. P. & Swanson, H. H. The effect of castration and ovarian implantation on aggressive behavior of male hamsters. *Journal of Endocrinology*, 1971, 51, 217-218.

Payne, A. P. & Swanson, H. H. The effect of sex hormones on the agonistic behavior of the male golden hamster (*Mesocricetus auratus*). *Physiology and Behavior*, 1972, 8, 687-691. (a)

Payne, A. P. & Swanson, H. H. The effect of sex hormones on the aggressive behavior of the female golden hamster (*Mesocricetus auratus*, Waterhouse). *Animal Behavior*, 1972, 20, 782-787. (b)

Persky, H., Smith, K. D. & Basu, G. Relation of psychologic measures of aggression and hostility to testosterone production in man. *Psychosomatic Medicine*, 1971, 33, 265-277.

Popova, N. K. & Naumenko, E. V. Dominance relations and the pituitary-adrenal system in rats. *Animal Behavior*, 1972, 20, 108-111.

Rose, R. M., Gordon, T. P. & Bernstein, I. S. Plasma testosterone levels in the male rhesus: influences of sexual and social stimuli. *Science*, 1972, 178, 643-645.

Rose, R. M., Holaday, J. W. & Bernstein, I. S. Plasma testosterone, dominance rank and aggressive behavior. *Nature*, 1971, 231, 366-368.

Ryzhenkov, V. E. Brain monoaminergic mechanisms and hypothalamic-pituitary-adrenal activity. In K. Lissák (Ed.), *Hormones and Brain Function*. New York: Plenum Press, 1973, pp. 285-286.

Sadleir, R. M. F. S. The relationship between agonistic behavior and population changes in the deermouse, *Peromyscus maniculatus* (Wagner). *Journal of Animal Ecology*, 1965, 34, 331-352.

Sassenrath, E. N. Increased adrenal responsiveness related to social stress in rhesus monkeys. *Hormones and Behavior*, 1970, 1, 283-290.

Sawyer, C. H. & Gorski, R. A. (Eds.), *Steroid Hormones and Brain Function*. Berkeley: University of California Press, 1971.

Scott, J. P. An experimental test of the theory that social behavior determines social organization. *Science*, 1944, 99, 42-43.

Scott, J. P. Incomplete adjustment caused by frustration of untrained fighting mice. *Journal of Comparative Psychology*, 1946, 39, 379-390.

Scott, J. P. Discussion. In C. D. Clemente and D. B. Lindskey (Eds.), *Aggression and Defense*. Berkeley: University of California Press, 1967, pp. 45-51.

Seward, J. P. Aggressive behavior in the rat. I. General characteristics, age, and sex differences. *Journal of Comparative Psychology*, 1945, 38, 175-197.

Sigg, E. B. Relationship of aggressive behavior to adrenal and gonadal function in male mice. In S. Garattini and E. B. Sigg (Eds.), *Aggressive Behavior*. New York: Wiley, 1969, pp. 143-149.

Southwick, C. H. & Bland, V. P. Effect of population density on adrenal glands and reproductive organs of CFW mice. *American Journal of Physiology*, 1959, 197, 111-114.

Svare, B. B., Davis, P. G. & Gandelman, R. Fighting behavior in female mice following chronic androgen treatment during adulthood. *Physiology and Behavior*, 1974, 12, 399-403.

Svare, B. B. & Gandelman, R. Aggressive behavior of juvenile mice: influence of androgen and olfactory stimuli. *Developmental Psychobiology*, 1975, 8, 405-415.

Taylor, A. N., Matheson, G. K. & Dafney, N. Modification of the responsiveness of components of the limbic midbrain circuit by corticosteroids and ACTH. In C. H. Sawyer, and R. A. Gorski (Eds.), *Steroid Hormones and Brain Function.* Berkeley: University of California Press, 1971, pp. 67-78.

Taylor, G. T.   Male aggression in the presence of an estrous female. *Journal of Comparative and Physiological Psychology,* 1975, 89, 246-252.

Tollman, J. & King, J. A.   The effects of testosterone propionate on aggression in male and female C57BL/10 mice. *British Journal of Animal Behaviour,* 1956, 4, 147-149.

Ulrich, J.   The social hierarchy in albino mice. *Journal of Comparative Psychology,* 1938, 25, 373-413.

Vale, J. R., Lee, C. T. & Ray, D.   The effect of defeat upon the reproductive behavior and upon adrenal, testes and seminal vesicle weights of C57BL/6 mice. *Communications in Behavioral Biology,* 1970, 5, 225-236.

Vale, J. R., Vale, C. A. & Harley, J. P.   Interaction of genotype and population number with regard to aggressive behavior, social grooming, and adrenal and gonadal weight in male mice. *Communications in Behavioral Biology,* 1971, 6, 209-221.

Vandenbergh, J. G.   The effects of gonadal hormones on the aggressive behavior of adult golden hamsters (*Mesocricetus auratus*). *Animal Behavior,* 1971, 19, 589-594.

Vom Saal, F. S., Gandelman, R. & Svare, B.   Aggression in male and female mice: evidence for changed neural sensitivity to neonatal but not adult androgen. *Physiology and Behavior,* 1976, 17, 53-57.

Vom Saal, F. S., Svare, B. & Gandelman, R.   Time of neonatal androgen exposure influences length of testosterone treatment required to induce aggression in adult male and female mice. *Behavioral Biology,* 1976, 17, 391-397.

Welch, A. S. & Welch, B. L.   Isolation, reactivity and aggression: evidence for an involvement of brain catecholamines and serotonin. In B. E. Eleftheriou and J. P. Scott (Eds.), *Physiology of Aggression and Defeat.* New York: Plenum Press, 1971, pp. 91-142.

Wilson, A. P. & Boelkins, R. C.   Evidence for seasonal variation in aggressive behavior by *Macaca mulatta. Animal Behavior,* 1970, 18, 719-724.

Chapter 4

PHEROMONAL AND ULTRASONIC COMMUNICATION

The concept of stimulus quality was introduced in Chapter 1 to connote the effectiveness of an individual as a stimulus of another individual's behavior. In recent years, one element of an individual's stimulus quality has received a great amount of attention in relation to the functioning of the endocrine system. This aspect is related to the chemical signals or *pheromones* that individuals release into the external environment, affecting the behavior and/or physiological states of other individuals (Bruce, 1970; Gleason & Reynierse, 1969).

Much experimental and theoretical attention has been directed toward the functions of pheromones in communication among individuals, including both the behavioral and physiological responses to these signals. Many of the issues related to the functions of pheromones really are not within the realm of this book, and excellent reviews of that literature are available to the interested reader (e.g., Bronson, 1971; Bruce, 1970; Gleason & Reynierse, 1969; Vandenbergh, 1975). The focus in this chapter will be on the relationship between endocrine function and pheromonal communications, and the review that follows is organized around the functions and classes of pheromones.

Before proceeding too far, we should pause and mention that the term "pheromone" may not be totally appropriate when used in the context of communication through odorous signals in mammals. The concept of pheromones was originally used in the context of odorous communication among insects, and "pheromonal communication" often connotes some instinctual or reflexive response to those signals. It is nowhere near certain, however, that odorous signals as used by mammals would meet that requirement. It is quite possible that the meaning of odorous signals must be learned in mammals (e.g., Goldfoot et al., 1976), and, therefore, a label that connotes some innate responsiveness to those signals would be inappropriate. However, the term "pheromone" is the one used most often in describing communication through odor signals in mammals, and, therefore, it will be used here.

There appear to be two primary classes of pheromones, distinguishable by their types of effects. The first class includes the *releasing* or *signaling* pheromones, those that seem to cause either the initiation of particular behaviors or changes in the pattern of behaving. Among the signaling pheromones are those used in territorial marking, those eliciting or inhibiting agonistic responses, those serving for sexual recognition and attraction, and those sustaining contact between mothers and young.

The second class includes the *primer* pheromones, which induce changes in endocrine or neuroendocrine activity in the receiver. Most priming pheromonal effects are related to reproductive functioning and include effects on estrous cyclicity, the onset of puberty, and the maintenance of pregnancy.

The final section of this chapter considers a different, but perhaps related, mode of social communication that has been receiving increasing attention in the last few years. It involves the use of ultrasonic calls to relay information about sexual status, and recent studies have suggested that *ultrasonic calling* is affected by the endocrine statuses of both the communicator and the receiver. A brief review of this new and exciting literature will be provided at the end of this chapter.

Returning to pheromones, we might first ask whether there is a general relationship between endocrine function and pheromonal communication. It should be noted at the outset that, as in any communication system, effective pheromonal communication ultimately depends on both the sender and the receiver. It is likely that the endocrine states of both individuals are critical to accurate or effective communication. Therefore, one might ask questions both about the relationship between hormones and the emission of pheromones and about the relationship between hormones and the reception or perception of pheromonal signals.

In the case of the sender, hormones can affect both the production and the release of pheromones. It is clear that hormones can affect pheromonal production by modifying the state of the glands or organs where the pheromones are manufactured and released, because many of these glands depend on hormones for their integrity. However, it also seems likely that hormones affect pheromonal release through modifying the state of the neural circuits that control the behaviors necessary for the emission or effective placement of the pheromones. Examples of both modes of action are provided by the case of territorial marking in gerbils (see below), where hormones can affect the production of pheromones both at the level of the glands that produce the substances and by affecting the neural circuits that control the marking behavior necessary for the deposition of the pheromone (Thiessen, Yahr & Owen, 1973).

In the case of the receiver or responder, hormones seem to be related to pheromonal communication in the same ways that they are related to any other reaction to exciting stimuli (recall the discussion in Chapter 1): (1) The hormonal state of the individual can affect its responses to pheromonal stimuli, and (2) the reception or perception of pheromonal signals can lead to modifications in the individual's hormonal state. These possibilities will be considered in more detail as we progress.

SIGNALING PHEROMONES

The signaling pheromones are signs that communicate the state of one individual or its territory to other individuals. These pheromones originally were called "releasing" pheromones because their emission can elicit behavioral responses or changes in behavior from other individuals. However, not all pheromones that are signals seem to elicit behavioral change or action from the perceivers, and, as in the case of territorial marking, there need not be another individual present in order for the pheromone to be emitted. Therefore, Bronson (1971) suggested that the term "signaling" pheromone is more appropriate than "releasing" pheromone, arguing that these substances really are signals denoting the state of an individual. Whether or not another individual will respond depends on a number of perhaps extraneous factors, such as the hormonal state of the receiver, not on the state of the communicator.

Four signaling pheromones will be discussed here: those used in marking territories or home ranges, those effective in modifying reactions in agonistic situations, those serving for sex recognition and/or attraction, and the maternal pheromone, which seems to be an attractant for the young. Bronson (1971) has suggested that the same pheromone(s) may be operating in more than one of these cases (for example, the female's attractant pheromone and her aggression-inhibiting pheromone may be the same substance), but these classes of pheromones have been studied separately, and, therefore, they will be reviewed separately here.

Territorial Marking

Many mammalian species have specialized scent glands, and these animals seem to use the substances produced in these glands to mark their home ranges (Johnson, 1973; Thiessen et al., 1970). There has been a fairly extensive discussion in the literature about the functions of this marking behavior; some investigators believe that the marking indicates territorial claims, and others believe it serves other functions (Johnson, 1973). Whether or not marking really is "territorial" in all or most cases seems unresolved, and we shall refer to the marking of one's home range as "territorial marking" in keeping with tradition and for the sake of simplicity.

In most species, the males exhibit more marking than the females (Johnson, 1973; Turner, 1975), and the incidence of marking in both males and females appears to be dependent on the levels of sex hormones circulating in adulthood. In addition, some recent evidence suggests that the gender differences in adult marking levels is related to the early hormonal environment. Neonatal androgen treatment increases the marking level of female gerbils to the levels of males, and neonatal castration of male gerbils reduces their marking levels to that of females (Turner, 1975).

THE MALE There is some correlational evidence suggesting that the level of marking in male rodents is related to circulating androgen levels. First, in many species, territorial marking first appears at the time of puberty, when testosterone levels are rising (Johnson, 1973). Second, there are seasonal variations in levels of marking in some species, which coincide with seasonal variations in testosterone levels: when testosterone levels rise during the breeding season, so do marking levels (Johnson, 1973). Third, there appears to be a positive correlation between marking rates and dominance rank. Dominant hamsters and gerbils mark more than subordinates, and, as discussed in Chapter 3, there seems to be a correlation between dominance rank and androgen levels (Blum & Thiessen, 1971, for the gerbil; Drickamer, Vandenbergh & Colby, 1973, for the hamster). Finally, one study reported a positive correlation between marking levels and seminal vesicle weights, a measure often used as an index of androgen activity (Blum & Thiessen, 1971). Thus, although there have been no direct studies correlating circulating androgen levels and levels of territorial marking, there is some evidence that androgen levels and marking might be related.

The experimental evidence generally supports the belief that marking rates depend on circulating androgen levels. Castration reduces marking in gerbils, rats, and cats (Price 1975; Hart, 1974; Thiessen, Friend & Lindzey, 1968), although it does not seem to affect marking in male hamsters and dogs (Hart, 1974; Whitsett, 1975). In addition, in those species where castration does reduce marking, replacement therapy with testosterone restores the marking level of castrates to normal (Price, 1975; Thiessen, Friend & Lindzey, 1968). Figure 4-1 shows the effects of castration and androgen replacement therapy on territorial marking in male gerbils. Note that prolonged treatment of castrated animals with high androgen levels leads to marking levels that are even higher than those of controls.

How do the androgens affect territorial marking? One possibility is that these hormones alter the state of the tissues that produce the critical pheromones. For example, gerbils mark their territories with the ventral gland, which is androgen dependent. However, gerbils still exhibit marking behaviors after the ventral gland has been removed, suggesting that it is not the sole site of androgen action, at least on the behavioral component of marking (Blum & Thiessen, 1970).

It is likely that another site of androgen effects on territorial marking is the neural circuits that control this behavior. Testosterone implants into restricted brain sites are effective in counteracting the effects of castration, which removes the androgens from the total circulation. Therefore, only the neural actions of these hormones are necessary to the display of territorial marking, at least in the gerbil (Thiessen, Yahr & Owen, 1973; Yahr & Thiessen, 1972).

THE FEMALE Although female mammals mark at lower rates than males, they do exhibit territorial marking. The female sex hor-

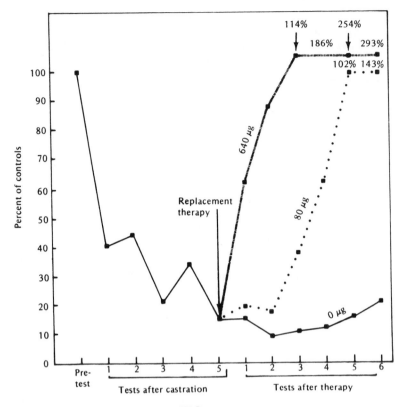

FIG. 4-1

Effects of castration and testosterone propionate therapy on territorial marking (from Thiessen, Friend & Lindzey, *Science*, Vol. 160, p. 432, 26 April 1968, copyright 1968 by the American Association for the Advancement of Science, by permission).

mones appear to be related to territorial marking in some species, such as the gerbil, although the ovarian hormones do not seem to be related to marking in others, such as house mice (Maruniak et al., 1975).

In the female gerbil, there is a rise in territorial marking during late pregnancy and lactation, and this increased rate of marking is counteracted by ovariectomy (Wallace, Owen & Thiessen, 1973). In addition, ovariectomy will reduce the marking rate of nonpregnant females who mark at very high rates, although this operation does not affect marking in those females whose natural marking rate is low (Yahr & Thiessen, 1975). In high-marking female gerbils, estrogen alone or estrogen in combination with progesterone will restore the marking rate of ovariectomized individuals, although these female sex hormones do not affect marking in gerbils who have low natural marking rates, whether or not they have been ovariectomized (Yahr & Thiessen, 1975). On the other hand, testosterone treatment will increase the marking rate of ovariectomized, low-marking gerbils (Owen & Thiessen, 1973). Figure 4-2 presents the effects of estrogen alone, testosterone alone, and estrogen in combination with testosterone on the marking rates of ovariectomized, low-marking female gerbils. Thus, in the female gerbil: (1) ovariectomy reduces the marking rate of animals with high natural marking rates, and (2) treatment with estrogen or estrogen and progesterone will restore their marking rates to normal. (3) On the other hand, ovariectomy does not affect the marking of female gerbils with low marking rates (perhaps this is because they cannot mark at a lower rate), and (4) estrogen or estrogen plus progesterone treatment does not affect the marking rate of these low-marking animals. (5) Testosterone treatment, however, will increase the marking rate of ovariectomized female gerbils whose natural rate is low. Therefore, there may be different hormonal mechanisms controlling marking in female gerbils that have different natural marking rates.

Pheromones in Agonistic Interactions

Many laboratories have shown the importance of olfactory or pheromonal signals in determining patterns of agonistic responding. Some animals are attacked more readily than other animals, and this quality of "attackability" seems to depend on the pheromones that the animals produce. In addition, an intact olfactory appara-

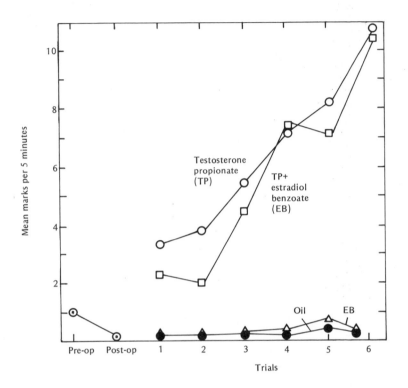

FIG. 4-2

Response of ovariectomized female gerbils to testosterone propionate and estradiol, alone or in combination (from Owen & Thiessen, *Physiology and Behavior*, 1973, 11, 443, by permission of Brain Research Publications).

tus appears to be critical to the display of aggressive reactions to other individuals, emphasizing that a critical quality of an opponent as a stimulus for aggression is its odor (e.g., Devor & Murphy, 1973, for the hamster; Rieder & Lumia, 1973, for the gerbil; Ropartz, 1968, for the mouse).

There appear to be two types of pheromones operating in agonistic situations, and both seem to be dependent on the animal's hormonal state. One type is characteristic of males, and its presence seems to facilitate aggressive attacks by an opponent. It has been termed *aggression-promoting*. The second type is characteristic of females, and it seems to inhibit attack by an opponent. This type of pheromone has been termed *aggression-inhibiting*. Interestingly, the same pheromones that act in agonistic interactions also may serve other, attractant functions in sexual interactions (Bronson, 1971). This possibility will be discussed later in this chapter.

AGGRESSION-PROMOTING PHEROMONES The aggression-promoting pheromone of the male mouse appears to be a substance released into the urine, perhaps by the preputial glands (Mugford & Nowell, 1970; Vandenbergh, 1975), and the presence of this pheromone seems to depend on the animal's androgen status. Castrated mice and hamsters are attacked less than intact rodents, and replacement therapy with testosterone restores the attackability of castrates to the level of intact animals (Evans & Brain, 1974; Mugford & Nowell, 1970). Moreover, smearing castrated mice with the urine from intact males increases the attackability of the castrates, as does smearing castrates with the preputial secretion of intact animals (Mugford & Nowell, 1970; Vandenbergh, 1975). In addition, the developmental stage when a male is castrated does not seem critical to its responsiveness to androgen replacement therapy, because testosterone treatment is equally effective in restoring the attackability of neonatal castrates, juvenile castrates, and adult castrates (Figs. 4-3a, b, and c). This finding suggests that the presence of androgens at the time of testing is all that is critical for an animal to be attacked readily; the duration of castration or the stage of development when castrated may be irrelevant (Mugford, 1974).

How do the androgens affect the aggression-promoting pheromone(s)? There have been no studies designed to answer this question directly, although three lines of indirect evidence suggest

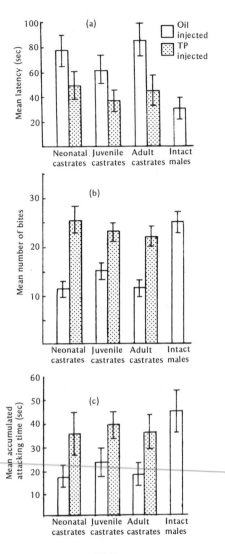

FIG. 4-3

The effects of testosterone propionate on (a) mean ± standard error latency to the first bite of different opponents, (b) mean ± standard error number of bites directed against opponents during a 4-minute observation period, and (c) mean ± standard error accumulated attacking times in a 4-minute period (modified from Mugford, *Hormones and Behavior*, 1974, 5, 98-99, by permission of Academic Press).

that the androgens affect this pheromone peripherally, at the level of its production and release (at the level of the producing gland), rather than through effects on the brain. First, as just discussed, the developmental stage at castration is not critical to the pheromone's responsiveness to androgen. Therefore, early neural organization or sensitization is not necessary for the release of the aggression-promoting pheromone, so long as androgens are present at the time of testing. Even if an animal (and presumably its brain) is "feminized" by early castration, it will exhibit aggression-promoting properties if androgen is provided in adulthood. Second, the aggression-promoting pheromone of normal males is not released in a pulsatile fashion (only at selected times), as is the case in territorial marking. The aggression-promoting pheromone is constantly present, and even anesthetized animals have it. These findings suggest that elaborate neural activity is not necessary for the release of the aggression-promoting pheromone. Third, the glands suggested as sites of pheromone production and release are androgen-dependent tissues (Vandenbergh, 1975). For example, the preputial glands of castrated mice are smaller than those of intact mice, and all that is needed for replacement therapy is androgen treatment at the gland site. These findings argue that typical, male-like, androgen-dependent neural organization and activity are not demanded for the activity and/or release of the pheromone.

There also is a pheromone released into the urine of male mice that seems to have aversive properties (it discourages investigation), and the degree of its aversiveness seems related both to dominance status (aggressiveness?) and to androgen status. The urine of dominant mice is much more aversive than that of subordinate mice (Jones & Nowell, 1973a), and the relationship between dominance and androgen levels discussed in Chapter 3 would argue that the aversive pheromone may be androgen-related. In fact, castrating male mice decreases the aversiveness of their urine for other mice, and testosterone replacement therapy increases the aversiveness of the urine of castrates to the level of controls (Jones & Nowell, 1973b). It is interesting to speculate whether this dominance-related pheromone is the same as the aggression-promoting pheromone, or whether it is another substance released to mark off territories. The latter explanation seems more likely, since the aggression-promoting pheromone elicits approach (attack), whereas the aversive pheromone elicits avoidance. However, it is unknown how many pheromones a mouse releases in its urine, and we do not even know whether an animal can control which pheromone would be released under what circumstances.

AGGRESSION-INHIBITING PHEROMONES The females of many mammalian species seem to produce pheromones that inhibit attack by males, and there appear to be different degrees and forms of hormonal dependence in different species. The aggression-inhibiting properties of the mouse do not seem to vary with the estrous cycle, and even ovariectomy does not appreciably alter the aggression-inhibiting qualities of female mice (Mugford & Nowell, 1971; Dixon & Mackintosh, 1975). On the other hand, in the female hamster, ovariectomy does seem to lead to a slight reduction in aggression-inhibiting qualities (Payne, 1974).

It may be that the aggression-inhibiting pheromone of female rodents does not depend heavily on the presence of female sex hormones, but, rather, results from the absence of high androgen levels. If female rodents are treated with even very little androgen, their aggression-inhibiting qualities are diminished, and they are attacked quite readily (Mugford & Nowell, 1971, 1972; Payne, 1974). This latter finding raises an interesting question as to whether androgen-treated females are attacked because their aggression-inhibiting pheromones have been diminished, or whether they are attacked because the androgen has induced the production of the aggression-promoting pheromone normally found only in males. In either case, one cause for the aggression-inhibiting quality of females may be the absence of high androgen levels.

Sex Recognition and Attraction

Interest in pheromonal communication really originated with the early discovery that some insects use odorous signals as attractants for their mates. In fact, many insect pheromones have been synthesized, and they are used commercially to lure males to traps or to disrupt their mating patterns, thus providing an effective tool for pest control (Vandenbergh, 1975). Many mammalian species, particularly the olfactory-dependent rodents, also seem to use pheromonal signals for sex recognition and attraction, and the production, release, and ability to recognize these signals often seem related to hormonal factors.

THE ATTRACTIVE FEMALE Although many other kinds of signals can be used to denote reproductive states, the females of many species seem to emit an odor during periods of estrus that is attractive to males, and this pheromonal sex attractant is not present during nonestrous states. This quality has been observed during estrus in species as diverse as mice and rats, dogs, sheep, cows, and even some primates (e.g., Beach & Gilmore, 1949; Dixon & Mackintosh, 1975; Hart, Mead & Regan, 1946; Lindsay, 1965; Michael & Keverne, 1968). The fact that the attractiveness of a female and her odors usually varies with her reproductive cycle suggests that the sex-attractant pheromone is related to ovarian hormone states. However, the majority of evidence remains correlational, since there have been very few experimental studies to determine the causality in such relationships, at least in typical laboratory rodent species.

Some recent studies of the rhesus monkey have yielded somewhat conflicting evidence about the importance of pheromonal attractants in the reproductive interactions of this primate species. Michael and co-workers have conducted a series of studies with a group of rhesus monkeys that have suggested that the female rhesus might secrete an odorous substance from the vagina in response to increases in estrogen levels, that is particularly attractive to males (Keverne & Michael, 1971; Michael & Keverne, 1968; Michael et al., 1972). However, Goldfoot et al. (1976) conducted a series of studies using somewhat different measures of sexual behavior, and the results suggest that if there is an attractant quality to the vaginal secretions of female rhesus monkeys, it does not stimulate all males of this species. In their studies, Goldfoot and colleagues found very little effect on male sexual responses when the vaginal secretions of estrogen-treated animals were applied to the vaginal area of spayed females.

Some recent studies also have begun to examine the attractiveness of human vaginal secretions, and their variations across the menstrual cycle. Michael, Keverne, and Bonsall (1971) had suggested that the rhesus' attractant was a particular combination of aliphatic acids that increased naturally during the periovulatory period. Interestingly, they also observed a periovulatory increase in volatile aliphatic acids during the late follicular phase in humans, suggesting the possibility of an attractant in the vaginal secretions of the human female (Michael, Bonsall & Warner, 1974). In addition, Doty et al. (1975) reported that men found periovulatory vaginal secretions less aversive than those of the premenstrual or menstrual periods.

Some of these findings seem somewhat suggestive of a primate sex pheromone. However, the studies have been contradictory, and the data certainly are not clear. In addition, in Doty's study, very few of the men found vaginal secretions to be at all attractive, no matter when they were collected. Therefore, one must conclude that the possibility of a primate sex pheromone is an interesting one that demands additional study. However, any conclusions would be premature at this time.

Not only may hormonal states affect the production and emission of the sex attractant pheromone of the female, but the hormonal state of the male seems to affect his receptivity to that attractant. This issue, of course, is reflected clearly in the general sexual responsiveness of males and its hormonal dependence, and will be discussed in more detail in Chapter 5. However, it might be useful to note in this discussion of pheromonal communication that the hormonal state of the receiver also affects the utility or effectiveness of the sex attractant of the female. As stated above, intact males of many species prefer the odor of estrous females to that of nonestrous females. Castration of the male can reduce that preference for estrous odors, although it does not affect the male's ability to discriminate estrous and nonestrous odors (Carr, Loeb & Wylie, 1966; Carr, Solberg & Pfaffmann, 1962). In addition, replacement therapy with testosterone restores the preference of castrated males for estrous female odors. This androgen dependency of male preference for female pheromonal attractants has been observed in at least two rodent species: rats (Carr, Wylie & Loeb, 1970) and hamsters (Gregory, Engel & Pfaff, 1975).

THE ATTRACTIVE MALE In addition to the female's emitting an attractant pheromone, the males of many rodent species appear to release odorous signals that are attractive to females. At least in mice, this sex pheromone seems to be secreted from the preputial glands, since male preputial secretions are quite attractive to female mice (Bronson & Caroom, 1971).

Two lines of evidence suggest that the male sex attractant pheromone is dependent on circulating androgens. First, urine of dominant male animals is more attractive to females than is that of submissive animals (Jones & Nowell, 1974). As discussed earlier in this chapter and in Chapter 3, there also is evidence that dominance status is correlated with androgen levels. Therefore, the correlation between dominance status and odor attractiveness really may reflect one between androgen levels and attractiveness.

The second line of evidence is a more potent argument for androgen dependency because it includes experimental demonstrations that the attractiveness of the male to the female is reduced by withdrawing androgens. Female rats and mice clearly prefer and are more attracted to the odor of intact animals than to that of castrated animals (Carr, Wylie & Loeb, 1970; Scott & Pfaff, 1970).

Similar to the case of the female's sex attractant pheromone, the hormonal state of the female receiver seems to be related to her preferences for and attraction to male pheromones. Female rodents show greatest attraction to male pheromones during periods of estrus, and lesser attractions during nonestrous states (Carr, Loeb & Dissinger, 1965; Doty, 1973). Because the female's sexual motivation is dependent on her hormonal state (see Chapter 5), it is reasonable to expect that the female's attraction to male sex odors would be related to her hormonal state. This kind of relationship between the female's hormonal state and her attraction to male odors would be predicted, of course, because one would assume that the primary purpose of the male's attracting a female is to facilitate reproduction, and, therefore, it is more adaptive to be attractive to estrous females than to either all females or nonestrous females. As mentioned for the case of the male receiver when discussing the female attractant pheromone, the relationship between female reproductive states and the female's perception of or reaction to males as sexual stimuli is more involved than mere preferences for or gross attraction to olfactory signals. Therefore, this particular issue will be discussed in more detail in Chapter 5, which is concerned with the role of hormonal factors in sexual responding.

The Maternal Pheromone

It recently has been discovered that lactating rats and mice emit a pheromone that is attractive to their young (e.g., Breen, 1976; Leon & Moltz, 1972). This *maternal pheromone* seems to be emitted with the feces, and it probably is produced in the caecum.

The emission and effectiveness of the maternal pheromone appear to be dependent on prolactin levels. Although ovariectomy, adrenalectomy, or a combination of these operations does not affect the release or effectiveness of the maternal pheromone, blocking prolactin secretion with the drug ergocornine does diminish the pheromone. In addition, administering additional prolactin to ergocornine-treated lactating rats restores the maternal pheromone (Leon & Moltz, 1973), and treating virgin rats with prolactin induces the maternal pheromone in these obviously nonlactating females (Leon, 1974).

Leon (1974) has suggested a mechanism through which prolactin may be stimulating the production and release of the maternal pheromone. As mentioned before, this pheromone seems to be produced in the caecum and it seems to be released in or with a substance released with the feces, the caecotrophe. According to Leon's hypothesis, stimulation from the presence of the young induces the secretion of prolactin (see Chapter 6) which, in turn, causes a large increase in food intake. This increased amount of food is processed in the caecum and, therefore, there is an increase in the amount of caecotrophe that is defecated. The odor emitted in this way, then, can serve to attract the young to the mother. This kind of explanation suggests that some of the effects of prolactin on the maternal pheromone are indirect, i.e., due to the effects of this hormone on food intake, not directly on the pheromone-producing gland. As usual, however, additional studies will be needed to clarify further the role of hormonal factors in the production and release of this newly-discovered pheromonal factor that serves to attract young to their mothers.

PRIMER PHEROMONES

The second major class of pheromones includes the *primer pheromones*. These are odorous signals that result in neuroendocrine changes in the receiver. In most cases, the primer pheromones have been studied in regard to reproductive physiology, and the case of the female receiver has received almost all of the experimental attention. However, there is some recent evidence that females can emit primer pheromones that affect the state of the male; for example, exposure to the vaginal discharge of the female hamster will induce increases in testosterone secretion in male hamsters (Macrides et al., 1974).

It should be noted at the outset, however, that almost all studies of primer pheromonal effects have used rodent subjects. Therefore, the generality of these effects across species has not been determined.

The primer pheromones of male rodents appear to have three kinds of effects on female reproductive physiology. The first effect is to accelerate development: exposure to an adult male will lead to an earlier onset of first estrus. The second effect is to induce "estrus synchronization." This phenomenon, often called the "Whitten effect," refers to the induction of estrous cycling in females that normally are not cycling regularly. The third primer effect is pregnancy block, the "Bruce effect," where the odor of a strange male disrupts the pregnancy of recently impregnated females.

Puberty Advancement

If prepubertal female mice (and, interestingly, pigs, Brooks & Cole, 1970), are exposed to adult males, they exhibit their first estrous cycles earlier than if they are not exposed to males (Kennedy & Brown, 1970; Vandenbergh, 1967). This primer effect appears to be a result of a pheromonal signal from the male, since the physical presence of the male is not essential; the female need only be exposed to the odors of the male to exhibit advanced puberty (Vandenbergh, 1969). In addition, the male's estrus-accelerating pheromone appears to be androgen dependent. The odors of either immature or castrated males are ineffective in accelerating puberty (Vandenbergh, 1969; Zarrow et al., 1970).

The mechanism by which male pheromones advance puberty in a female appears to be through changes in neuroendocrine activity.

When prepubertal female mice are exposed to males or their odors, there is an almost immediate increase in LH levels in the female that is followed by a marked rise in estradiol levels. On the third day of exposure, adult-like periovulatory changes in LH, FSH, estradiol, and progesterone occur (Bronson & Desjardins, 1974). Thus, the estrus accelerating effect of male odors seems to be accomplished by inducing cyclic pituitary-ovarian hormone secretion in the receiver.

Estrus Synchronization

When female rodents are housed together, they exhibit relatively few and certainly irregular estrous cycles. If they are housed in the presence of a male, however, they show quite regular cycles (Bronson & Whitten, 1968; Whitten, 1957). This phenomenon of a male's synchronizing female estrous cycles appears to be a result of a pheromonal signal emitted by the male, and this phenomenon has been called the "Whitten effect." It is clear that the effect is a result of a pheromone because, first, the signal can be carried in the air: if females are placed downwind from males, estrus synchrony occurs. If, on the other hand, the females are placed upwind from males, simple proximity of males will not induce synchrony (Whitten, Bronson & Greenstein, 1968). Second, the signal appears to be released through the urine. Merely dropping male urine onto the bedding of females is sufficient to induce synchronous cycling (Bronson & Dezell, 1968; Bronson & Whitten, 1968).

As with other male-emitted pheromones, the estrus synchronizing pheromone appears to be androgen dependent. First, the urine of males is effective in synchronizing cycles, but the urine of females is ineffective (Marsden & Bronson, 1964). Second, castrating males decreases the effectiveness of their urine as a synchronizing substance (Bronson & Whitten, 1968; Bruce, 1965). Finally, treating ovariectomized females with androgens makes their urine effective in synchronizing the cycles of other females (Bronson & Whitten, 1968). Thus, the male emits an androgen-dependent pheromone through the urine that is effective in synchronizing the cycles of females.

Pregnancy Block

The third primer effect of male pheromones on female reproductive physiology has been termed the "Bruce effect." If a pregnant female mouse is exposed to a strange male mouse within 24-48 hours after insemination, implantation is blocked, and, therefore, pregnancy is terminated (Bronson & Eleftheriou, 1963; Bruce, 1959). This pregnancy block by a strange male does not demand the physical presence of the male, and removing the olfactory bulbs from the female provides protection from the Bruce effect. Therefore, it is most likely that pregnancy block is the result of exposure to an odorous signal released by the male (Bruce, 1970; Bruce & Parkes, 1960).

As is true of other male pheromones, the pregnancy blocking pheromone appears to be androgen dependent. Prepubertal males do not block pregnancy, and castrating adult males prevents their odors from exerting the blocking effect (Bruce, 1965). In addition, both intact and ovariectomized females are ineffective in blocking pregnancy, but if females are treated with androgens, they acquire blocking potential (Bruce, 1970; Dominic, 1965). Thus, like the other primer pheromones of the male, the pregnancy blocking pheromone appears to depend on androgen for its potency.

As for the receiver, some evidence has suggested that pregnancy block occurs because the pheromone blocks or diminishes the prolactin rise that normally accompanies early pregnancy. If pregnant female mice are treated with exogenous prolactin, they are protected from the blocking effects of strange males (Parkes & Bruce, 1961).

ULTRASONIC COMMUNICATION

In the past decade, a new and exciting area of research has evolved that is directed toward understanding the bases and functions of another form of social communication used by the members of many species, particularly rodents. Some mammals have been found to emit high-frequency calls or "ultrasounds" that serve social communication functions and may, at times, operate in combination with pheromonal signals. The instances of ultrasonic communication studied to date in rodents include the ultrasonic calls emitted by very young rats, probably to attract the mother (e.g., Noirot, 1964, 1970), the "postejaculatory song" of the male rat, which seems to be a desist-contact signal that the male emits following ejaculation (Barfield & Geyer, 1972), and the series of calls used by both male and female rodents in reproductive interactions (e.g., Floody & Pfaff, 1977a, b). Although the relationship between endocrine function and ultrasonic communication has not been studied extensively, some recent evidence suggests that hormonal factors may be important in the determination of calling rates and patterns.

Both male and female hamsters emit ultrasonic calls, and the form of their ultrasounds are different (Floody & Pfaff, 1977a). In addition, estrous females emit more ultrasounds than nonestrous females, suggesting a correlation between gonadal hormone states and rates of calling (Floody, Pfaff, Lewis, 1977). The emission of calling by estrous females seems to be facilitated by the attractant pheromones emitted by the male, because both anesthetized males and the bedding from cages of males increase the frequency of calling by estrous females (Floody, Pfaff & Lewis, 1977).

Experimental studies have suggested some causality in the observed correlation between estrous states and female hamster calling rates. Floody and Cahill (personal communication) have found that, whether measuring spontaneous calling, calling in response to males, or calling in response to the taped playbacks of male calls, ovariectomized females call less than intact estrous females. In addition, ovariectomized females treated with estrogen call more than nontreated ovariectomized females, and those given a combination of estrogen and progesterone call even more than estrogen-treated ovariectomized females. Thus, the calling rates of female hamsters seem to depend on the ovarian hormones.

Calling by males has been studied less extensively, and the role of hormones in male ultrasonic communication is unclear. In mice, calling by males first appears developmentally at the same time that testosterone levels begin to rise, the time of puberty (Whitney et al., 1973). This suggests at least a correlation between androgen levels and male calling. On the other hand, the postejaculatory calls of the male rat do not seem related to the presence of androgens, since castration does not affect the postejaculatory calls of at least sexually experienced male rats (Parrott & Barfield, 1975).

Of particular relevance to the main topic of this chapter, Floody and Pfaff (1977b) have suggested that ultrasonic communication operates in combination with pheromonal signals to facilitate reproductive interactions in the hamster. They have proposed a descriptive model, reproduced in Figure 4-4, which proposes a particular sequence of events. According to this model, the female patrols, flank-marks and vaginal-marks her territory. The male then enters and explores the female's territory. When he encounters the female's scent marks, the form of the mark determines his next action. If he encounters a vaginal-mark, he will emit ultrasounds. If he encounters flank-marks, he will flank-mark. In this latter case, when the female encounters the male's flank-marks, she decreases her flank-marking and increases vaginal-marking. This increase in vaginal-marking increases the probability that the male will encounter this sex attractant and then emit ultrasounds. When the female senses the male's presence, perhaps through his flank-

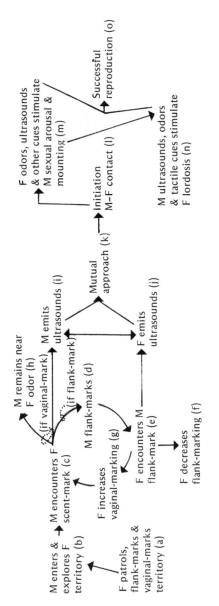

FIG. 4-4

A hypothetical model of social communications leading to reproduction among golden hamsters. Male's behavior (M) above; female's (F) below. Lower-case letters in parentheses code behavior. Many of the "links" in this chain of social behaviors and signals depend on gonadal hormones. In particular, testosterone facilitates male responses at least at points d, h, m, and o. Estrogen and progesterone facilitate female responses at least at points a, g, j, k, n, and o (from Floody & Pfaff. *Journal of Comparative and Physiological Psychology*, 1977b, 91, 826. Copyright 1977 by the American Psychological Association. Reprinted by permission).

marks, she emits ultrasounds, and the combination of both sexes' emitting ultrasounds leads to approach and initiation of male-female direct contact. Reproduction, then, follows because of stimulation received from a combination of odors, ultrasounds, and other (e.g., tactile) cues. Of particular relevance to our discussion, Floody and Pfaff also proposed some sites in this sequence where hormones may be acting in this complex, with testosterone facilitating male responses, and estrogen and progesterone facilitating female responses (see Fig. 4-4 legend). Some of the issues related to the role of these hormones in reproductive responding may become clearer as they are discussed in more detail in Chapter 5.

SUMMARY AND COMMENT

This chapter was concerned primarily with the relationship between endocrine function and pheromonal communication, the use of odorous signals in communication. Two classes of pheromones were reviewed: signaling pheromones and primer pheromones. In the case of the signaling pheromones, we reviewed the use of pheromones in territorial marking, agonistic interactions, sexual interactions, and attracting the mother to her young. In each of these cases, hormonal factors seem to affect pheromonal communication, and they do so at least by exerting local actions on the glands which produce and release the chemical signal. In addition, at least in the case of territorial marking in gerbils, hormones seem to affect the behaviors needed to make the pheromone an effective signal, and they do so by modifying the state of the neural circuits that control marking behavior.

The primer pheromones all seem to affect the neuroendocrine state of the receiver—in the cases reviewed here, the female. We reviewed primer effects of accelerating maturation, synchronizing estrous cycles, and blocking pregnancy. The emission of the primer pheromones seems to be under the same kind of hormonal control as the emission of the signaling pheromones, and hormones probably affect primer pheromones at the level of the pheromone-producing gland.

The final section of this chapter was concerned with another form of social communication that may be used in conjunction with pheromonal signals, the use of ultrasounds. Although there have been only very few studies of hormones and ultrasonic calling, the preliminary data reviewed here suggest that ultrasonic production, and its receipt, may be under hormonal control.

How many different pheromones are there? Many of those discussed here seem to be permanent odorous qualities of the individual. With the exception of the act of territorial marking, the emission of pheromones seems to be primarily a passive phenomenon; the pheromones are always present. The reader may also have noticed that all of the pheromones produced by the male are under androgen control, and most of those of the female appear to be under the control of the ovarian hormones. On the basis of these similarities, Bronson (1971) suggested that there are not many different and discrete pheromones (in the case of our review it would be seven different pheromones). Rather, he suggested that there are three signaling pheromones and one primer pheromone. For signaling pheromones, Bronson suggested that, first, there is one pheromone emitted by the male which serves both to elicit aggression and attract females. Second, there is one pheromone released by the female which serves both to inhibit aggression and to attract males. The reader should recall here, however, that the ovarian hormone dependency of the aggression-inhibiting pheromone has not been established clearly. Third, Bronson suggested there is a third pheromone that is aversive to conspecifics and may serve either to demark territories or warn of danger.

For the case of the primer pheromones, Bronson suggested that a single pheromone emitted by the male can accomplish all three priming functions: advancing puberty, synchronizing estrous cycles, and blocking pregnancy. One might be tempted to suggest that the male's primer pheromone is the same as the sex attraction and aggression-eliciting pheromone. However, recent studies have suggested that the male's primer and signaling pheromones are produced at different sites (Vandenbergh, 1975).

A final note of caution: As research programs have advanced, more and more instances of pheromonal communication have been identified in diverse species. However, almost all of the basic evidence relating hormones and pheromones has been collected from rodent species. Therefore, it might be useful to resist the temptation to generalize too quickly to the case of more advanced species, such as humans, for whom olfaction is not the primary means of communication, a temptation to which the perfume industry (with its "musk" odors) may have fallen prey too soon.

REFERENCES

Barfield, R. J. & Geyer, L. A.   Sexual behavior: ultrasonic postejaculatory song of the male rat. *Science*, 1972, 176, 1349-1350.

Beach, F. A. & Gilmore, R. W.   Response of male dogs to urine from females in heat. *Journal of Mammology*, 1949, 30, 391-392.

Blum, S. L. & Thiessen, D. D.   Effect of ventral gland excision on scent marking in the male Mongolian gerbil. *Journal of Comparative and Physiological Psychology*, 1970, 73, 461-464.

Blum, S. L. & Thiessen, D. D.   The effect of different amounts of androgen on scent marking in the male Mongolian gerbil. *Hormones and Behavior*, 1971, 2, 93-105.

Breen, M. F.   The maternal pheromone in mice. Unpublished Master's Thesis, Bucknell University, 1976.

Bronson, F. H.   Rodent pheromones. *Biology of Reproduction*, 1971, 4, 344-357.

Bronson, F. H. & Caroon, D.   Preputial gland of the male mouse: attractant function. *Journal of Reproduction and Fertility*, 1971, 25, 279-282.

Bronson, F. H. & Desjardins, C.   Circulating concentrations of FSH, LH, estradiol and progesterone associated with acute, male-induced puberty in female mice. *Endocrinology*, 1974, 94, 1658-1668.

Bronson, F. H. & Dezell, H. E.   Studies on the estrus-inducing (pheromonal) action of male deermouse urine. *General and Comparative Endocrinology*, 1968, 10, 339-343.

Bronson, F. H. & Eleftheriou, B. E. Influence of strange males on implantation in the deermouse. *General and Comparative Endocrinology*, 1963, 3, 515-518.

Bronson, F. H. & Whitten, W. K. Oestrus-accelerating pheromone of mice: assay, androgen-dependency and presence in bladder urine. *Journal of Reproduction and Fertility*, 1968, 15, 131-134.

Brooks, P. H. & Cole, D. J. A. The effect of the presence of a boar on the attainment of puberty in gilts. *Journal of Reproduction and Fertility*, 1970, 23, 434-440.

Bruce, H. M. An exteroceptive block to pregnancy in the mouse. *Nature*, 1959, 184, 105.

Bruce, H. M. Effect of castration on the reproductive pheromones of male mice. *Journal of Reproduction and Fertility*, 1965, 10, 141-143.

Bruce, H. M. Pheromones. *British Medical Bulletin*, 1970, 26, 10-13.

Bruce, H. M. & Parkes, A. S. Hormonal factors in exteroceptive block to pregnancy in mice. *Journal of Endocrinology*, 1960, 20, xxix-xxx.

Carr, W. J., Loeb, L. S. & Wylie, N. R. Responses to feminine odors in normal and castrated male rats. *Journal of Comparative and Physiological Psychology*, 1966, 62, 336-338.

Carr, W. J., Loeb, S. L. & Dissinger, M. L. Responses of rats to sex odors. *Journal of Comparative and Physiological Psychology*, 1965, 59, 370-377.

Carr, W. J., Solberg, B. & Pfaffmann, C. The olfactory threshold for estrous female urine in normal and castrated male rats. *Journal of Comparative and Physiological Psychology*, 1962, 55, 415-417.

Carr, W. J., Wylie, N. R. & Loeb, L. S. Responses of adult and immature rats to sex odors. *Journal of Comparative and Physiological Psychology*, 1970, 72, 51-59.

Devor, M. & Murphy, M. R. The effect of peripheral olfactory blockade on the social behavior of the male golden hamster. *Behavioral Biology*, 1973, 9, 31-42.

Dixon, A. K. & Mackintosh, J. H. The relationship between the physiological condition of female mice and the effects of their urine on the social behaviour of adult males. *Animal Behaviour*, 1975, 23, 513-520.

Dominic, C. J. The origin of the pheromones causing pregnancy block in mice. *Journal of Reproduction and Fertility*, 1965, 10, 469-472.

Doty, R. L. Odor preferences of female *Peromyscus maniculatus bairdi* for male mouse odors of *P. m. bairdi* and *P. leucopus noveboracensis* as a function of estrous state. *Journal of Comparative and Physiological Psychology*, 1973, 31, 191-197.

Doty, R. L., Ford, M., Preti, G. & Huggins, G. R.   Changes in the intensity and pleasantness of human vaginal odors during the menstrual cycle. *Science*, 1975, 190, 1316-1318.

Drickamer, L. C., Vandenbergh, J. G. & Colby, D. R.   Predictors of dominance in the male golden hamster (*Mesocricetus auratus*). *Animal Behaviour*, 1973, 21, 557-563.

Evans, C. M. & Brain, P. F.   Some studies on endocrine influences on aggressive behavior in the golden hamster (*Mesocricetus auratus*). *Progress in Brain Research*, 1974, 41, 473-480.

Floody, O. R. & Pfaff, D. W.   Communication among hamsters by high-frequency acoustic signals. I. Physical characteristics of hamster calls. *Journal of Comparative and Physiological Psychology*, 1977, 91, 794-806. (a)

Floody, O. R. & Pfaff, D. W.   Communication among hamsters by high-frequency acoustic signals. III. Responses evoked by playbacks of natural and synthetic "ultrasound." *Journal of Comparative and Physiological Psychology*, 1977, 91, 820-829. (b)

Floody, O. R., Pfaff, D. W. & Lewis, C. D.   Communication among hamsters by high-frequency acoustic signals. II. Determinants of calling by females and males. *Journal of Comparative and Physiological Psychology*, 1977, 91, 807-819.

Gleason, K. K. & Reynierse, J. H.   The behavioral significance of pheromones in vertebrates. *Psychological Bulletin*, 1969, 71, 58-73.

Goldfoot, D. A., Kravitz, M. A., Goy, R. W. & Freeman, S. K.   Lack of effect of vaginal lavages and aliphatic acids on ejaculatory responses in rhesus monkeys: behavioral and chemical analyses. *Hormones and Behavior*, 1976, 7, 1-27.

Gregory, E., Engel, K. & Pfaff, D. W.   Male hamster preference for odors of female hamster vaginal discharges: studies of experiential and hormonal determinants. *Journal of Comparative and Physiological Psychology*, 1975, 89, 442-446.

Hart, B. L.   Gonadal androgen and sociosexual behavior of male mammals: a comparative analysis. *Psychological Bulletin*, 1974, 81, 383-400.

Hart, G. H., Mead, S. W. & Regan, W. M.   Stimulating the sex drive of bovine males in artificial insemination. *Endocrinology*, 1946, 39, 221-223.

Johnson, R. P.   Scent marking in mammals. *Animal Behaviour*, 1973, 21, 521-535.

Jones, R. B. & Nowell, N. W.   Aversive and aggression-promoting properties of urine from dominant and subordinate male mice. *Animal Learning and Behavior*, 1973, 1, 207-210. (a)

Jones, R. B. & Nowell, N. W.   The effect of urine on the investigatory behaviour of male albino mice. *Physiology and Behavior*, 1973, 11, 35-38. (b)

Jones, R. B. & Nowell, N. W.   A comparison of the aversive and female attractant properties of urine from dominant and subordinate mice. *Animal Learning and Behavior*, 1974, 2, 141-144.

Kennedy, J. M. & Brown, K.   Effects of male odor during infancy on the maturation, behavior, and reproduction of female mice. *Developmental Psychobiology*, 1970, 3, 179-189.

Keverne, E. B. & Michael, R. P.   Sex-attractant properties of ether extracts of vaginal secretions from rhesus monkeys. *Journal of Endocrinology*, 1971, 51, 313-322.

Leon, M.   Maternal pheromone. *Physiology and Behavior*, 1974, 13, 441-453.

Leon, M. & Moltz, H.   The development of the pheromonal bond in the albino rat. *Physiology and Behavior*, 1972, 8, 683-686.

Leon, M. & Moltz, H.   Endocrine control of the maternal pheromone in the postpartum female rat. *Physiology and Behavior*, 1973, 10, 65-67.

Lindsay, D. R.   The importance of olfactory stimuli in the mating behaviour of the ram. *Animal Behaviour*, 1965, 13, 75-78.

Macrides, F., Bartke, A., Fernandez, F. & D'Angelo, W.   Effects of exposure to vaginal odor and receptive females on plasma testosterone in the male hamster. *Neuroendocrinology*, 1974, 15, 355-364.

Marsden, H. M. & Bronson, F. H.   Estrus synchrony in mice: alteration by exposure to male urine. *Science*, 1964, 144, 1469.

Maruniak, J. A., Owen, K., Bronson, F. H. & Desjardins, C.   Urinary marking in female house mice: effects of ovarian steroids, sex experience and type of stimulus. *Behavioral Biology*, 1975, 13, 211-217.

Michael, R. P.   Effects of gonadal hormones on displaced and direct aggression in pairs of rhesus monkeys of opposite sex. In S. Garrattini & E. B. Sigg (Eds.), *Aggressive Behaviour*, New York: Wiley, 1969, pp. 172-178.

Michael, R. P., Bonsall, R. W. & Warner, P.   Human vaginal secretions: volatile fatty acid content. *Science*, 1974, 186, 1217-1219.

Michael, R. P., Keverne, E. B. & Bonsall, R. W.   Pheromones: isolation of male sex attractants from a female primate. *Science*, 1971, 172, 964-966.

Michael, R. P., Zumpe, D., Keverne, E. B. & Bonsall, R. W.   Neuroendocrine factors in the control of primate behavior. *Recent Progress in Hormones Research*, 1972, 28, 665-706.

Mugford, R. A.   Androgenic stimulation of aggression eliciting cues in adult opponent mice castrated at birth, weaning and maturity. *Hormones and Behavior*, 1974, 5, 93-102.

Mugford, R. A. & Nowell, N. W.   Pheromones and their effect on aggression in mice. *Nature,* 1970, 226, 967-968.

Mugford, R. A. & Nowell, N. W.   The relationship between endocrine status of female opponents and aggressive behaviour of male mice. *Animal Behaviour,* 1971, 19, 153-155.

Mugford, R. A. & Nowell, N. W.   The dose-response to testosterone propionate of preputial glands, pheromones and aggression in mice. *Hormones and Behavior,* 1972, 3, 39-46.

Noirot, E.   Changes of responsiveness to young in the adult mouse: the effect of external stimuli. *Journal of Comparative and Physiological Psychology,* 1964, 57, 97-99.

Noirot, E.   Selective priming of maternal responses by auditory and olfactory cues from mouse pups. *Developmental Psychobiology,* 1970, 2, 273-276.

Owen, K. & Thiessen, D. D.   Regulation of scent marking in the female Mongolian gerbil *Meriones unguiculatus. Physiology and Behavior,* 1973, 11, 441-445.

Parkes, A. S. and Bruce, H. M.   Olfactory stimuli in mammalian reproduction. *Science,* 1961, 134, 1049-1054.

Payne, A. P.   The aggressive response of the male golden hamster towards males and females of different hormonal states. *Animal Behaviour,* 1974, 22, 829-835.

Parrott, R. F. & Barfield, R. J.   Post-ejaculatory vocalization in castrated rats treated with various steroids. *Physiology and Behavior,* 1975, 15, 159-163.

Price, E. O.   Hormonal control of urine-marking in wild and domestic Norway rats. *Hormones and Behavior,* 1975, 6, 393-397.

Rieder, C. A. & Lumia, A. R.   Effects of olfactory bulb ablation on dominance-related behaviour of male Mongolian gerbils. *Physiology and Behavior,* 1973, 11, 365-369.

Ropartz, P.   The relation between olfactory stimulation and aggressive behaviour in mice. *Animal Behaviour,* 1968, 16, 97-100.

Scott, J. W. & Pfaff, D. W.   Behavioral and electrophysiological responses of female mice to male urine odors. *Physiology and Behavior,* 1970, 5, 407-411.

Thiessen, D. D., Friend, H. C. & Lindzey, G.   Androgen control of territorial marking in the Mongolian gerbil. *Science,* 1968, 160, 432-434.

Thiessen, D. D., Lindzey, G., Blum, S. L. & Wallace, P.   Social interactions and scent-markings in the Mongolian gerbil (*Meriones unguiculatus*). *Animal Behaviour,* 1970, 19, 505-513.

Thiessen, D. D., Yahr, P. I. & Owen, K.   Regulatory mechanisms of territorial marking in the Mongolian gerbil. *Journal of Comparative and Physiological Psychology,* 1973, 82, 382-393.

Turner, J. W.   Influence of neonatal androgen on the display of territorial marking behavior in the gerbil. *Physiology and Behavior*, 1975, 15, 265-270.

Vandenbergh, J. G.   Effect of the presence of a male on the sexual maturation of female mice. *Endocrinology*, 1967, 81, 345-349.

Vandenbergh, J. G.   Male odor accelerates female sexual maturation in mice. *Endocrinology*, 1969, 84, 658-660.

Vandenbergh, J. G.   Hormones, pheromones and behavior. In B. E. Eleftheriou and R. L. Sprott (Eds.), *Hormonal Correlates of Behavior*, Vol. 2. New York: Plenum Press, 1975, pp. 551-584.

Wallace, P., Owen, K. & Thiessen, D. D.   The control and function of maternal scent marking in the Mongolian gerbil. *Physiology and Behavior*, 1973, 10, 463-466.

Whitney, G., Coble, J. R., Stockton, M. D. & Tilson, E. F.   Ultrasonic emissions: Do they facilitate courtship of mice? *Journal of Comparative and Physiological Psychology*, 1973, 84, 445-452.

Whitsett, J. M.   The development of aggressive and marking behavior in intact and castrated male hamsters. *Hormones and Behavior*, 1975, 6, 47-57.

Whitten, W. K.   Effect of exteroceptive factors on the oestrus cycle of mice. *Nature*, 1957, 180, 1436.

Whitten, W. K., Bronson, F. H. & Greenstein, J. A.   Estrus-inducing pheromone of male mice: transport by movement of air. *Science*, 1968, 161, 584-585.

Yahr, P. & Thiessen, D. D.   Steroid regulation of territorial scent-marking in the Mongolian gerbil (*Meriones unguiculatus*). *Hormones and Behavior*, 1972, 3, 359-368.

Yahr, P. & Thiessen, D. D.   Estrogen control of scent-marking in female Mongolian gerbils (*Meriones unguiculatus*). *Behavioral Biology*, 1975, 13, 95-101.

Zarrow, M. X., Estes, S. A., Denenberg, V. H. & Clark, J. H.   Pheromonal facilitation of ovulation in the immature mouse. *Journal of Reproduction and Fertility*, 1970, 23, 357-360.

Chapter 5

SEXUAL BEHAVIOR

The relationship of hormones and sexual behavior has received more attention than any other topic in behavioral endocrinology. Some investigators have come to work in this area apparently because they are interested in sexual behavior per se. Other workers have come to this topic because they are endocrinologists and view sexual behavior as one of many kinds of parameters that hormones can affect. Whatever the reason, most early behavioral endocrinologists and the majority of current workers in this field have been concerned with the role of hormonal factors in sexual responding.

The involvement of hormones in sexual behavior has been studied in almost all vertebrate species, and it has become clear that hormones are related to sexual responding in almost all cases. Interestingly, the degree of dependence of sexual behavior on endocrine factors seems to decrease as one ascends the phylogenetic scale, there being rather minimal hormonal control in many higher-order primates, including humans. That is, the relative contributions of experiential factors and hormonal factors seem to shift in more "advanced" species: whereas in less advanced species, hormonal factors are more important, in the higher-order species, experiential factors become much more important and can overshadow hormonal effects (Beach, 1947; Ford & Beach, 1952; Luttge, 1971; Young, 1941). It was suggested early on that this emancipation from hormonal control has accompanied the evolution of cerebral cortical control of sexual behavior (e.g., Ford & Beach, 1952), a concept which has not really been tested in great detail.

As emphasized in earlier chapters, the relationship between hormones and behavior is multifaceted, and that certainly is true in sexual behavior. For example, not only does the hormonal state in effect at the time of sexual stimulation affect the form and intensity of sexual responses, but it also has marked effects early in development on adult sexual responses. In addition, having certain kinds of sexual experiences can modify endocrine states, which, in turn, might be able to modify future sexual responding. These kinds of relationships have been studied in species ranging from lizards through rodents to nonhuman primates and humans. To review all of that literature would require a separate, multivolumed book, and, therefore, the review that follows will be rather limited in scope. We shall focus here on two rodent species, the rat and the guinea pig, one nonhuman primate, the rhesus monkey, and the human, although examples from other species will be incorporated from time to time. This review also will be restricted, as in earlier chapters, to summarizing the general state of knowledge and theories in the field. A number of excellent, more comprehensive reviews will be suggested as we progress through the topics. However, it might be useful to point out now the excellent and more general reviews to be found in the works by Beach (1965), Bermant and Davidson (1974), Davidson (1972), and Montagna and Sadler (1974), places where the reader interested in more detailed reviews might begin.

The review that follows is organized into sections, and in each section three species, the rat, guinea pig, and rhesus monkey, are considered. The first section is concerned with the effects of hormonal states in effect at the time of stimulation (the baseline hormonal state) on adult sexual behavior. The second section considers the role of hormones in the development and differentiation of gender differences in sexual behavior. The third section is concerned with the effects of sexual experiences on endocrine function. The case of hormones and human sexual behavior is considered in a separate section at the end of the chapter.

ADULT HORMONAL STATES AND SEXUAL BEHAVIOR

This section is labeled "adult hormonal states" to discriminate it from the subsequent discussion, which is concerned with the relationship between the hormonal state early in development and adult sexual behavior patterns. This discussion considers only the role of hormones at the time of the expression of sexual responses; that is, the role of the baseline hormonal state in determining sexual behavior.

The baseline hormonal state affects sexual behavior in both females and males, although in somewhat different ways. We shall first consider the female, and then turn to the male. In each case we shall only be concerned with the behavior patterns primarily characteristic of that gender, so-called *homotypical* behaviors. The issue of hormones and sexual responding similar to that of the opposite sex will be considered in the next general section.

The Female

The earliest studies examined only copulatory probabilities between males and females. Later studies attempted to separate the contributions of male and female behaviors to sexual interactions, and the early emphasis in studying the female was on receptivity. More recent analyses of female sexual behavior, particularly in primates, have shown that there really are many identifiable, somewhat separate elements to female sexual responding, and Beach (1976a) has suggested that the sexual behavioral characteristics of the female can be categorized into three primary classes. The first class is *attractivity*, which refers to the attractiveness of a female for males. In many mammalian species, such as rodents, this quality of attractivity or attractiveness seems to be related to odorous cues that the female emits and, to that extent, already has been discussed somewhat in Chapter 4. The second category, *proceptivity*, refers to the degree of inviting that a female exhibits. Therefore, the category *proceptive behaviors* includes what appear to be appetitive behaviors, such as soliciting approaches from males. The third category, *receptivity*, refers to the responsiveness of females to cues provided by the male. Thus, *receptive behaviors* would include lordosis postures displayed by many mammalian females following contact by a male. This third class, receptivity, or receptive behaviors, has by far received the most experimental attention, although there have been many recent investigations concerned with proceptivity and attractivity, particularly in primate species.

It is common knowledge that many female animals undergo cycles of sexual responsiveness. Some of these cycles are relatively long, such as the passage into and out of breeding seasons that we see in dogs and cats, and some are relatively short, such as the estrous cycles of most laboratory rodents. In both cases such cycles coincide with cycles in gonadal hormonal states, thereby providing correlational evidence that, in the female, the gonadal hormones are somehow related to sexual responding. Sexual behavior cycles tied to gonadal hormone cycles have been observed in species as diverse as lizards, rodents, and primates—and most species in between (see the early reviews by Beach, 1948; Young, 1941, 1961). Of course, the degree of behavioral cyclicity differs greatly among species, and, among the animals to be considered here, the rodents show more pronounced cycles than do most primates. Periods of sexual responsiveness, often called *behavioral estrus* or *heat*, are limited to the periovulatory period in both rats and guinea pigs, and the peak of responsiveness (at least as measured by receptivity) appears to coincide with elevated levels of estradiol followed by a marked elevation in progesterone levels. As an example, the relationship between behavioral estrus and ovarian hormone levels within an estrous cycle is depicted for the female rat in Figure 5-1.

Among the primates, there is some cyclicity in reproductive ac-

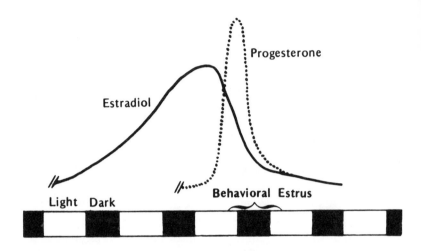

FIG. 5-1

Schematic depiction of estradiol and progesterone patterns during five-day estrous cycles in the rat, with the period of behavioral estrus indicated (from Powers and Moreines, *Physiology and Behavior*, 1976, 17, 494, by permission of Pergamon Press).

tivity, although the degree of cyclicity varies from species to species. In some, such as the gorilla, there is a very close relationship between reproductive (menstrual) cycle status and sexual responsiveness (Nadler, 1975), whereas in others, such as the stumptail macaque, female sexual responsiveness is virtually noncyclic, at least in laboratory settings (Slob et al., unpublished).

As with some other primates, cyclicity is not very strict in the case of the rhesus monkey, although cycles in female sexual responsiveness have been observed in many studies (e.g., Michael & Welegalla, 1968). Also, whether there is a reproductive-cycle rhythm in only one element of sexual responding in the rhesus monkey (that is, attractivity, proceptivity, or receptivity), or rhythms in more than one of those elements is not yet clear. Some investigators (e.g., Eaton, 1973) have found that only attractivity varies with the menstrual cycle, with proceptivity and receptivity remaining relatively constant. On the other hand, other investigators (e.g., Michael, Saayman & Zumpe, 1967; Michael & Welegalla, 1968) have found that both proceptivity (sexual invitations) and receptivity (acceptances of male advances) also vary with the menstrual cycle. These contradictory findings may reflect the fact that different laboratories employ different housing and testing conditions. Social-experiential factors and testing conditions have marked effects on sexual behavior in this species (Goldfoot, 1977). Until the basis of these conflicting findings is discovered, we must be content with the very general statement that some aspect(s) of rhesus monkey sexual behavior does vary with the gonadal hormone (menstrual) cycle.

Having established that there is a correlation between changes in sexual responsiveness and changes in gonadal hormonal states across the reproductive cycle (in most species), we ask the obvious next question concerning the causality in that relationship. A general answer is "Yes, the ovarian hormones exert important effects on female sexual behavior," and that answer is based in part on the often repeated finding that withdrawal of the ovarian hormones by ovariectomy leads to reduced levels of sexual responsiveness, at least in most nonhuman species (e.g., Ball, 1936; Bermant & Davidson, 1974; Goldfoot, 1977). In addition, the reduced sexual responsiveness of ovariectomized females can be expressed in the form of reduced levels of all three elements of sexual responding, attractivity, proceptivity, and receptivity (e.g., Ball, 1936; Michael, 1971; Michael, Herbert & Welegalla, 1967), although the broader effect of ovariectomy on components of sexual responding other than receptivity has been studied extensively only in primates.

That ovariectomy decreases sexual responding shows in a general way that the relationship between the gonadal hormones and sexual responsiveness in the female is causal. But, the more interesting question concerns the particular hormones involved in this relationship. The three groups that have been studied most extensively, the estrogens, progesterone, and the androgens will be considered sequentially.

ESTROGEN EFFECTS The estrogens are the most important gonadal hormones in the control of sexual responsiveness in the females of most species. First, selectively blocking estrogenic actions with chemical anti-estrogens leads to marked reductions in receptivity (Arai & Gorski, 1968; Luttge et al., 1975; Whalen & Gorzalka, 1973). Second, in many species, such as the rat, rabbit, cat, and dog, estrogen treatment alone can restore the level of responsiveness of ovariectomized females to the level of intact estrous controls (Beach & Merari, 1970; Bermant & Davidson, 1974; Davidson et al., 1968; Young, 1941). Thus, selectively blocking estrogenic actions decreases receptivity, and all that is needed to produce receptive females is the presence of estrogen.

It also appears that in some species there is a dose-response relationship between estrogen levels and levels of receptivity. For example, in both rats and guinea pigs, increasing dosages of estradiol can lead to increasing degrees of receptivity (Davidson et al., 1968; Goy & Young, 1957). An example of this kind of dose-response relationship in the rat is presented in Figure 5-2. However, increasing estrogen levels increases the degree of receptivity in ovariectomized females only to a limit, and that limit approximates the level of intact females. Once this level has been reached, further increases in estrogen dosages usually will not lead to further increases in receptivity. Thus, there appears to be a maximum dosage that elicits maximal or optimal levels of receptivity, and, once that level has been reached, further increases in estrogen levels do not lead to further increases in receptivity (Goy & Young, 1957). It should be noted, however, that increasing estrogen levels can prolong the periods during which receptive responses can be elicited.

The role of the estrogens in the sexual responding of female rhesus monkeys is not totally clear. Early studies, considering

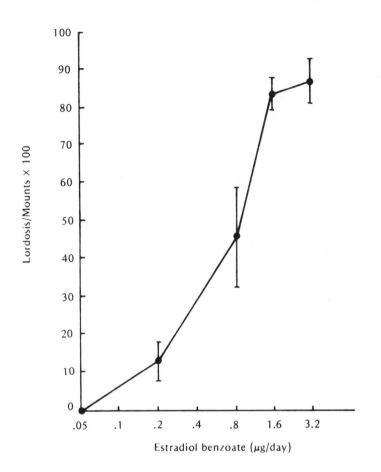

FIG. 5-2

Dose-response relationships between estrogen (estradiol benzoate) administered daily by subcutaneous injection to ovariectomized rats and female receptivity (as measured by lordosis quotient) eight days after onset of treatment. (From Fig. 5-3 in *Biological Bases of Sexual Behavior* by Gordon Bermant and Julian Davidson. Copyright © 1974 by Gordon Bermant and Julian M. Davidson. By permission of Harper & Row, Publishers, Inc. Originally from data of Davidson, J. M., Rodgers, C. H., Smith, E. R., and Bloch, G. J. (1968) Relative thresholds of behavior and somatic responses to estrogen. *Physiology and Behavior* 3: 227-229.

sexual responding in only a general way (e.g., Ball, 1936), found estrogen treatment to be sufficient to restore the sexual behavior of ovariectomized rhesus monkeys to normal levels. However, later studies, attempting to separate the effects of the estrogens on attractivity, proceptivity, and receptivity, have yielded conflicting results. Some (e.g., Johnson & Phoenix, 1976; Michael & Welegalla, 1968) have suggested that the estrogens are involved in the control of receptivity, whereas others (e.g., Dixson et al., 1973) have suggested that other hormones (and not the estrogens) control this aspect of sexual responding. The same kind of conflicting evidence has been found for proceptivity. The one parameter that does seem to be agreed upon as dependent on estrogenic stimulation is attractivity. Ovariectomized rhesus monkeys do not seem very attractive to males, and replacement therapy with estrogens restores their attractivity (Dixson et al., 1973; Goldfoot, 1971).

To summarize, the estrogens are quite important in the control of receptivity in many nonprimate species and of (at least) attractivity in the rhesus monkey. Whether or not the estrogens also are involved in the control of receptivity and proceptivity in the rhesus monkey is not yet resolved.

PROGESTERONE EFFECTS As can be seen from Figure 5-1, the period of maximal sexual responsiveness in some female animals closely follows the marked rise in progesterone levels that precedes ovulation. This kind of correlation suggests that progesterone, like the estrogens, might be involved in the control of sexual behavior in females. However, not all species react to progesterone in the same way. As we shall see, under certain conditions progesterone clearly facilitates sexual responding, whereas under others, it can inhibit female sexual behavior.

Progesterone can facilitate receptivity in many species, including rats, guinea pigs, hamsters, and dogs. Although, as discussed above, estrogen treatment alone can lead to increases in receptivity in ovariectomized animals, treating estrogen-primed ovariectomized females with progesterone decreases both the amount and duration of estrogen treatment needed to induce heat (Beach & Merari, 1970; Boling & Blandau, 1939; Carter & Porges, 1974; Dempsey, Hertz & Young, 1936; Powers, 1970). In addition, preventing the preovulatory rise in progesterone by timed ovariectomy leads to a decrease in receptivity, at least in the rat (Powers, 1970). Thus, progesterone treatment subsequent to estrogen priming can facilitate the effects of estrogen on receptivity. It is significant that these findings are consistent with the correlational studies (compare Fig. 5-1) showing that periods of estrus follow a period of high estrogen levels followed by a sharp rise in progesterone levels.

The relationship between progesterone and receptivity is different from that between the estrogens and receptivity. Whereas estrogen is related to receptivity according to a dose-response relationship (to the limits discussed before), progesterone's effects are "all-or-none." If enough progesterone is administered, it facilitates sexual responding as induced by estrogen. If smaller amounts are given, there is no effect. In addition, further increases in progesterone levels above this threshold amount do not lead to any further increases in receptivity. This finding, coupled with studies of estrogen effects, has led to the conclusion that whereas the estrogens exert some degree of "directive" action on receptivity (that is, the amount of estrogen given contributes to the *degree* of receptivity), progesterone's actions are only "permissive." The presence of some minimal amount of progesterone will facilitate estrogen-induced receptivity, but there is no gradation below this hormone level, and increases in progesterone levels have no greater facilitative effects (Gerall & Kenney, 1970).

The findings just discussed suggest that both the estrogens and progesterone facilitate sexual responding in the female of many species. However, progesterone does not always facilitate receptivity. There are conditions under which progesterone inhibits receptivity in rats, hamsters, guinea pigs, and rabbits, among others (Bermant & Davidson, 1974; Carter et al., 1976). It should be noted at the outset that the evidence concerning an inhibitory action for progesterone is clearer for some of these species than for others.

The guinea pig provides an example where progesterone's inhibitory actions are relatively clear. Interest in the potential inhibitory effects of progesterone on receptivity seems to have emerged from the observation that under conditions where progesterone levels normally are high, such as during the luteal phase of the estrous cycle and during pregnancy, female guinea pigs are relatively unresponsive to the normal heat-inducing effects of sequential estrogen-progesterone treatments (Goy, Phoenix & Young, 1966). This correlation suggested that there might be a biphasic action of progesterone on estrogen-induced receptivity: at some times progesterone would be facilitatory (if it closely follows estrogen treatment), whereas at other times it would be inhibitory.

Wallen, Goy, and Phoenix (1975) have studied in detail the potential inhibitory actions of progesterone on heat in the spayed guinea pig. The results of one of their studies are reproduced in Table 5-1. In this study, they tested a prediction made by the correlations just discussed: that high levels of progesterone at the time of estrogen priming would inhibit the hormonal induction of estrus. In order to test this prediction, they treated guinea pigs with a high dosage of progesterone at varying intervals prior to administering the standard estrogen-progesterone treatments that ordinarily would result in heat. In addition, they measured circulating progesterone levels at varying intervals following progesterone injections. In this way, they could determine the relationship between the presence or absence of progesterone at the time of estrogen priming on the effectiveness of sequential estrogen-progesterone treatments in inducing receptivity. As shown in Table 5-1, if progesterone is administered within 48 hours prior to the estrogen part of the sequence, the normally effective sequential estrogen-progesterone regimen does not induce receptivity. Significantly, it takes nearly this long for progesterone levels to decline

Table 5-1
The Effect on Ovariectomized Female Guinea Pig Lordosis Response
of 1 mg Progesterone Administered from o to 72 Hr Prior to a
Standard Estradiol Benzoate (6 μg) and Progesterone
(0.4 mg) Treatment

Group No.	Hours Prior to EB-P Treatment	N	% Responding	Mean Latency to Heat (hr, ± SEM)[a]	Mean Duration of Heat (hr, ± SEM)[a]
1	0	6	0[b]		
2	2	6	0[b]	—	—
3	4	6	0[b]	—	—
4	8	6	0[b]	—	—
5	16	6	16[c]	6	6
6	24	6	16[c]	7	5
7	48	8	87	5.1 ± .42	7.5 ± .44
8	72	8	87	6.1 ± .37	7.0 ± .37
9	No pretreatment	10	90	4.7 ± .40	7.7 ± .44

[a] Data are for responders only.
[b] Differs significantly from Group 9 ($\chi^2 = 8.96$, $P < 0.005$).
[c] Differs significantly from Group 9 ($\chi^2 = 5.76$, $P < 0.025$).

substantially following the single 1-mg progesterone injection they used. Thus, if progesterone was still present in high amounts, the estrogen-progesterone regimen was not effective, but if progesterone levels had declined, then these treatments were effective in inducing receptivity. These findings, then, support the suggestion that progesterone can exert a biphasic action on receptivity in the guinea pig. If it is present at the time of the estrogen part of the treatment, it inhibits the heat-inducing ability of a sequential estrogen-progesterone regimen. On the other hand, once estrogen's actions have become somewhat effective (following estrogen priming), subsequent progesterone treatment will facilitate estrogen's heat-inducing effects (the often-used regimen of estrogen priming followed by progesterone treatments).

In contrast to the case of the guinea pig, the situation in the rat is not yet clear. As in the guinea pig, estrogen treatments during periods when progesterone levels are high, such as during pregnancy, are ineffective in inducing receptivity in the female rat (Powers & Zucker, 1969). This correlation would suggest that, as in the guinea pig, the presence of high levels of progesterone can inhibit the effectiveness of estrogen in inducing behavioral estrus in the rat. However, experimental studies directed at this issue do not seem to support the suggestion that progesterone usually does reach levels sufficient to inhibit receptivity in the rat, except during those periods when progesterone levels are very high for a very long time, such as in pregnancy (Edwards, Whalen & Nadler, 1968). Progesterone treatments just prior to estrogen treatments do not affect estrogen's ability to induce estrous behavior in the ovariectomized rat, as they do in the guinea pig (Edwards et al., 1968; Zucker, 1967). In addition, ovariectomizing rats when progesterone levels are high, during the late proestrus progesterone peak, does not increase receptivity in response to estrogen treatments, as would be predicted if progesterone normally exerted an inhibitory effect in the rat (Powers & Moreines, 1976). Therefore, the experimental data suggest that although in both the rat and the guinea pig, estrogen is ineffective in inducing heat during the luteal phase of the estrous cycle, when progesterone levels normally are somewhat high, this relationship is not causal in the rat. That is, having high progesterone levels is not the factor responsible for the refractoriness to estrogen's heat-inducing properties during diestrus in the rat, as it seems to be in the guinea pig.

An interesting hypothesis to account for this difference is that since the rat's progesterone levels during nonestrus periods are much higher than those of the guinea pig, the rat is less sensitive to high levels of this hormone. Thus, only very marked and prolonged increases in progesterone levels, such as those that occur during pregnancy, can inhibit estrogen-induced receptivity (Zucker, 1967). Of course, this issue has not been studied completely, and, therefore, these conclusions should be considered tentative.

It should be pointed out that the biphasic action of progesterone on estrogen-induced receptivity, as seen in the guinea pig, is very unusual. It seems strange that a hormone can exert opposite effects depending on when it is administered. The mechanisms by which progesterone might exert these opposite actions is not yet known, but that it does so seems clear. This kind of problem seems to be an interesting starting point for investigators concerned with the mechanisms of hormone action on sexual behavior.

In contrast to the situation in the rat and the guinea pig, progesterone's effects on sexual behavior in the female rhesus monkey appear to be only inhibitory. Treating female rhesus monkeys with progesterone, whether or not these animals have been ovariectomized and/or estrogen-treated, leads to decreases in sexual behavior. More specifically, treating female rhesus monkeys with progesterone leads to decreases in the number of mounting attempts males direct toward these females (a decrease in attractivity) and to increases in the number of refusals that females show when they are approached by males (a decrease in receptivity) (Dixson et al., 1973; Michael, 1968; Michael & Zumpe, 1970).

ANDROGEN EFFECTS There have been some studies directed toward possible roles of the androgens in female sexual behavior in both the rat and the rhesus monkey. There also have been studies implicating the androgens in human female sexual behavior, which will be considered later in this chapter.

In the rat, injections of testosterone propionate are quite effective in inducing receptivity in ovariectomized females (Whalen & Hardy, 1970). In addition, this effect can be blocked by treatment with anti-estrogens (Luttge et al., 1975; Whalen, Battie & Luttge, 1972). The most likely explanation of these androgen effects is that they really are estrogenic effects. Testosterone normally is converted to estrogens quite readily (through a process of aromatization to be discussed in more detail in a later section). And, since its effects can be blocked by anti-estrogens, it seems probable that testosterone affects receptivity in the female rat because it has been converted to estrogens.

The androgens also may facilitate estrogen induction of sexual responding in rhesus monkeys. Both adrenalectomy and dexamethasone treatment, which eliminate the secretion of ACTH-dependent steroid hormones from the adrenal cortex, have been found to decrease both proceptivity and receptivity in ovariectomized, estrogen-treated rhesus monkeys. Further, this effect was shown to be due to some factor other than withdrawal of the adrenal glucocorticoids, since attempts to restore sexual responding with cortisol were ineffective. Rather, it appeared that these effects were the result of decreases in the secretion of the adrenal androgens, because replacement therapy with either testosterone or androstenedione was effective (Dixson et al., 1973; Everitt & Herbert, 1969, 1971; Everitt, Herbert & Hamer, 1972). Thus, there is some evidence that androgens from adrenal origins might be involved in the control of female sexual behavior in the rhesus monkey.

It is important to note that the effects of the androgens on sexual behavior in female rhesus monkeys may not be "pure." Androgens only affect sexual behavior in those animals who have estrogens present. In the studies discussed above, androgen manipulations were made in estrogen-treated ovariectomized animals, and other studies (e.g., Wallen & Goy, unpublished) have shown that only those androgens that can be converted to estrogens, such as testosterone, are effective in facilitating sexual behavior in ovariectomized females not treated with estrogens; dihydrotestosterone has no effect. This might seem to suggest that androgen effects on sexual behavior in the female rhesus monkey really are only a result of conversion to estrogen. However, dexamethasone still decreases some aspects of sexual behavior in monkeys with adequate amount of estrogens, and, therefore, there may be some additional androgen facilitation of estrogen-induced sexual responding in the females of this species that is not dependent on conversion to estrogen (Johnson & Phoenix, 1976). However, the form of the androgen is critical. Even though the androgen's effects go beyond those ascribable to conversion to estrogen, the androgen must be aromatizable.

SUMMARY STATEMENT: THE FEMALE The findings reviewed in this section clearly show that hormones are important to female sexual behavior, and we can make some generalizations about what has been learned so far. First, estrogen facilitates sexual responding, and, in many species, progesterone treatment following a period of estrogen "priming" decreases the amount of estrogen needed to induce receptivity. Thus, progesterone can facilitate the effects of estrogen on receptivity. These findings from experimental studies are consistent with the observation from correlational studies that in these same species the period of maximal receptivity is one following rises in estrogen with a shorter, subsequent rise in progesterone (see Fig. 5-1).

Second, in some species, such as the guinea pig and the rhesus monkey, progesterone also can have inhibitory influences on sexual responding. Although progesterone seems always to be inhibitory in the rhesus monkey, whether it will be facilitatory or inhibitory in the guinea pig (and perhaps the rat) depends on its temporal relationship to increases in estrogen levels: if progesterone levels are high prior to or at the same time that estrogen levels are high, progesterone is inhibitory to sexual responding. However, if estrogen levels are increased first, while progesterone levels are still low, subsequent progesterone increases will result in the facilitation of sexual responding.

Finally, there is some evidence that androgenic substances secreted from the adrenal cortex may affect sexual behavior in both the rat and the rhesus monkey. In the case of the rat, it appears that these androgens affect sexual behavior only because they are readily converted to estrogens. In the case of the rhesus monkey, the situation is not yet clear. A preliminary hypothesis is that certain androgens can facilitate some of estrogen's effects on sexual behavior in the female of this species.

The Male

As in the case of the female, there is some correlational evidence showing that cycles of male reproductive activity covary with cycles in gonadal hormone levels. As would be expected, the critical gonadal hormones in the case of the male appear to be the androgens. These behavioral and hormonal cycles are long in duration compared to those of most females, and the male's cycles are usually expressed in the form of "breeding seasons." But, to our point, breeding-season changes in reproductive behavior are strongly correlated with changes in androgen levels in many species (compare Beach, 1948; Robinson et al., 1975; Young, 1961), suggesting that the androgens are somehow related to sexual behavior in males.

Interestingly, although there is a marked correlation between gross changes in circulating androgen levels and changes in levels of sexual responding, it appears unlikely that individual differences in levels of sexual responding are correlated with individual differences in circulating androgen levels. For example, Harding and Feder (1976a) reported that groups of guinea pigs rated as being either highly active or not very active in terms of sexual responding show no differences in plasma testosterone levels. Moreover, individual differences in sexual responding persist in both guinea pigs and rats even after circulating testosterone levels have been equated, by castrating the animals and administering the same testosterone dosage to all (Beach & Fowler, 1959; Grunt & Young, 1952, 1953). Thus, it seems improbable that differences in testosterone levels, at least in the general circulation, are related to the fine-grain differences between individuals in levels of sexual responding. Some alternative explanations will be considered in a later section.

What of the causality in this relationship? Do the androgens exert determining effects on sexual behavior in the male? Or, does engaging in sexual activity affect androgen levels? Both appear to be the case, although we are concerned in this section only with the first question: the effects of the androgens on male sexual behavior. The effects of engaging in sexual behavior on androgen levels will be discussed in a later section.

THE EFFECTS OF MANIPULATING ANDROGEN LEVELS As mentioned in Chapter 1, it has been known for centuries that decreasing androgenic stimulation by castration leads to a reduction in sexual responding. Interestingly, that reduction in sexual activity is not immediate; sexual responsiveness lasts long after circulating androgen levels have declined to undetectable levels (e.g., Bloch & Davidson, 1968; Stone, 1927). Furthermore, it is clear, at least in rodents, that the maintenance of postcastration sexual responsiveness is not due to the secretion of androgens from the adrenals, since removing this extratesticular source of androgens does not facilitate the decline in sexual responding that accompanies castration (Bloch & Davidson, 1968). Thus, although the androgens clearly are important to sexual responding, this class of behavior is not totally dependent on the presence of these hormones; sexual responding can occur in the absence of the androgens.

Once sexual responding has declined following castration, replacement therapy with androgens results in a reinstatement of sexual responsiveness. However, although, as shown in Figure 5-3, graded dosages of testosterone do lead to consecutive increments in copulatory behavior in castrated males (Beach & Holz-Tucker, 1949), further increasing of androgen dosages above a certain optimal or maximal level usually will not result in further increases in sexual responding; replacement therapy usually will only restore sexual performance to precastration levels (Grunt & Young, 1953; Larsson, 1966). This latter finding suggests that although androgen effects are in one sense "directive," there is a limit. A certain

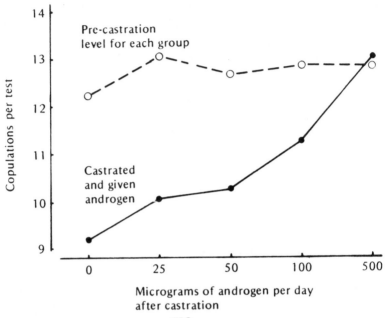

FIG. 5-3

The effects of graded dosages of testosterone propionate on the frequency of copulations per test compared to precastration levels for each group in the rat (modified from Beach & Holz-Tucker, *Journal of Comparative and Physiological Psychology*, 1949, 42, 439).

amount of androgen is necessary to achieve one's "sexual potential," but subsequent increases in androgen levels usually will not lead to increases in sexual performance above this level. This relationship between androgen levels and sexual behavior in the male is similar to that of estrogen levels and sexual behavior in the female.

The situation in the rhesus monkey is basically the same as that in the rodents just discussed. However, there appears to be even less strict androgen dependency in this primate. Castration does lead to some reduction in sexual activity, although there are some monkeys who continue to engage in sexual behavior for years after castration (Michael & Wilson, 1974; Phoenix, Slob & Goy, 1973). As in other animals, sexual responsiveness certainly persists long after testosterone levels have declined (Resko & Phoenix, 1972). In addition, there is some evidence (Michael & Wilson, 1975) that the seasonality in rhesus-monkey sexual behavior persists after castration, suggesting that even the correlation between hormone levels and levels of sexual activity across breeding seasons may not reflect hormonal dependence; seasonality in sexual activity may occur even in the total absence of the androgens.

In those rhesus monkeys who do show decreased sexual activity after castration, replacement therapy with testosterone restores their performance to normal levels (e.g., Michael & Wilson, 1974; Phoenix, Slob & Goy, 1973). Thus, although sexual behavior may not depend totally on androgen stimulation in this species, the level of the androgens can affect sexual activity.

THE NATURE OF ANDROGEN EFFECTS: THE QUESTION OF AROMATIZA-TION TO ESTROGEN In the early 1940s it was discovered that if cas-trated male rats are treated with an estrogen, they exhibit almost all of the normal male sexual responses (Beach, 1942). In addi-tion, it later was found that certain androgens, such as dihydrotes-tosterone, are not effective as replacement therapy for castrated male rates (e.g., Feder, 1971; Whalen & Luttge, 1971). Signifi-cantly, those androgens that are effective in activating sexual be-havior in the male rat also are readily converted to estrogens, through a process called "aromatization" (e.g., Naftolin, Ryan & Petro, 1972), and those androgens that are ineffective are non-aromatizable. These findings led to the hypothesis that androgens normally are converted to estrogens before affecting sexual be-havior in the male rat.

It should be noted at the outset that this discussion of the *aromatization hypothesis* is restricted to the rat. Estrogen treatment is not effective in restoring the sexual responsiveness of either castrated guinea pigs or castrated rhesus monkeys. Furthermore, in both of these species the nonaromatizable androgen dihydrotestosterone is effective, and in much the same way as is testosterone (Alsum & Goy, 1974; Phoenix, 1973, 1974). Therefore, it is unlikely that the androgens affect sexual behavior in the guinea pig and rhesus monkey because they have been converted to estrogens.

Returning to the rat, it seems unlikely that all of testosterone's effects on male sexual behavior are a result of conversion to estrogen. Although estrogen-treated castrated male rats show almost complete sexual behavior, their sexual responses are not complete. These animals often show deficiencies in both intromission and ejaculation performance (e.g., Beach, 1942; Johnson & Tiefer, 1974; Larsson, Södersten & Beyer, 1973). In addition, the deficiencies in these measures can be corrected by treating estrogen-injected castrated male rats with dihydrotestosterone (Baum & Vreeburg, 1973; Feder, Naftolin & Ryan, 1974). Therefore, complete sexual responses in the male rat can only be activated by estrogen treatment if it is combined with androgen treatment, whether or not the androgen is aromatizable. This suggests that some androgen effects may be due to conversion to estrogen, but that some others are "pure"; these effects depend on androgenic activity per se. Furthermore, the "pure" androgen effects appear to be a result of peripheral stimulation of accessory sex organs, since treatment with an androgen that has peripheral physiological effects but no independent behavioral effects, such as fluoxymesterone, is capable of restoring completely the sexual performance of castrated rats that have been treated with estrogens (Johnson & Tiefer, 1974).

Further support for the aromatization hypothesis comes from studies of the effects of chemical anti-estrogens on male sexual responding. Although one anti-estrogen, MER-25, was found to be ineffective in blocking male sexual responding (Baum & Vreeburg, 1976), another anti-estrogen, CI-628, has been shown to effectively block androgen-induced sexual behaviors (Luttge, 1975). Thus, there is some additional evidence that at least some androgen effects on male sexual behavior in the rat may be due to the conversion of these hormones to estrogens.

Comment: Adult Hormonal States and Sexual Behavior

It might be useful to interrupt our discussion to reexamine and compare the effects of different circulating hormones in adulthood on sexual behavior. The effects of those different hormones are in some ways similar but in some ways different. For example, in the case of the female, there is generally a dose-response relationship between estrogen levels and levels of sexual responding, so long as estrogen levels remain below a certain optimal level. Once that optimal estrogen level has been reached, further increases in estrogen levels typically will not lead to further increases in sexual responding. The relationship in the case of the male and circulating testosterone levels is basically the same: increasing androgen levels leads to increases in sexual behavior, but usually to a limit. Increasing androgen levels above that optimal level typically will not lead to further increases in sexual responsiveness.

The case of progesterone effects in those species where this hormone facilitates sexual behavior is somewhat different: they are "all-or-none." If progesterone is present in sufficient amounts, there is facilitation of sexual responding, but at levels below that threshold amount, there is not even partial facilitation. Thus, there is no gradation of progesterone effects at all.

There are some other kinds of differences in the effects of different hormones on sexual behavior. One critical difference concerns the duration of hormone exposure necessary to affect the behavior (Young, Goy & Phoenix, 1964). For example, females need be exposed to estrogens for only relatively short periods of time (often less than one day) before the effects are seen. On the other hand, males often need to be exposed to androgens for weeks before effects become evident. The basis of these differences in critical exposure times for hormone action is unknown, although the existence of such differences may raise important questions about the mechanisms by which hormones affect sexual behavior.

The findings discussed in this section are basically consistent with the proposition raised in Chapter 1 and reiterated in later chapters that the baseline hormonal state affects the form and/or intensity of the behaviors emitted following environmental stimulation. In both males and females, the baseline hormonal state appears critical to at least the intensity of sexual responses displayed when the individual is stimulated (the issue of the form of sexual responses will be considered in a later section). This statement is based on the observations that changes in the baseline hormonal state, whether endogenously produced (such as across reproductive cycles) or experimentally induced, lead to changes in the level of sexual responding.

As an often-repeated caution, however, it should be noted that in both females and males, the level of the gonadal hormones in the circulation does not determine totally the level of sexual responding in any species studied. For example, although circulating gonadal hormones may determine levels of sexual responding in a gross way, there is no clear relationship between fine-grain differences in levels of sexual responding (such as those between different individuals) and levels of the gonadal hormones in the general circulation. Thus, factors other than circulating hormone levels must be contributing to the determination of levels of sexual responding.

Mechanisms of Hormone Actions on Sexual Behavior

Our review so far has shown clearly that hormones do exert important effects on sexual behavior in many species. The next question we might ask concerns the mechanisms by which hormones affect sexual behavior. As discussed in earlier chapters, the ways hormones can affect behavior include: effects on effectors, on sensory or perceptual receptors, and on the state of the critical circuits in the central nervous system (compare Beach, 1948, 1974; Lehrman, 1961). But, what are the important mechanisms in the case of sexual behavior? Evidence has been accumulating implicating at least two kinds of mechanisms: by affecting the state of peripheral structures, such as sensory receptor areas, and by affecting the states of certain areas in the brain and spinal cord.

Some studies have suggested that hormones can exert some of their effects on sexual behavior by modifying the states of peripheral structures. For example, in the female rat, estrogen treatment increases the size of the receptive field around the vagina (Komisaruk, Adler & Hutchinson, 1972; Kow & Pfaff, 1974). Therefore, some of estrogen's facilitatory effects on female sexual responding might be a result of increasing the probability that genital contact will be stimulating to the female. In addition, in the male, changes in sexual behavior after castration and subsequent replacement therapy with testosterone closely follow morphological changes in the male rat's penis (Beach & Levinson, 1950). Furthermore, as discussed before, androgenic compounds that have effects on peripheral accessory sex organs but, purportedly, no effects on the brain can facilitate sexual responding in male rats that have been treated with estrogens (Johnson & Tiefer, 1974). Thus, there is some evidence that in both females and males some of the effects of hormones on sexual behavior are through peripheral structures.

There also is some limited evidence that some effects are a result of hormonal effects on the state of the spinal cord, at least in the male rat. Male rats subjected to spinal transection show only very low level sexual reflexes, such as erection, and the same is true of castrated males. Significantly, the deficiencies in these reflexes in castrated rats can be restored by either systemic testosterone injections or testosterone injections directly into the spinal cord (Hart & Haugen, 1968).

Many hormonal effects on sexual behavior appear to be mediated by changes in the activity of the brain. There have been many studies directed toward this mechanism of hormone action, and the reader interested in pursuing it in more detail might consult the excellent reviews in Bermant and Davidson (1974) and Lisk (1973).

As mentioned in Chapter 1, there is great similarity in the central neural areas of maximal hormonal uptake and the areas shown in lesion and stimulation studies to be important in the control of sexual behavior (Bermant & Davidson, 1974; Pfaff, 1971). This similarity, then, provides a first implication that the brain sites critical to sexual responding also are particularly sensitive to hormones.

As discussed before, one important test of the neural mediation of hormonal effects on behavior is injecting hormones directly into the brain. We shall consider separately each of the major hormones studied. Beginning with the estrogens and female sexual behavior, there have been many studies showing that brain implants of estradiol are virtually as effective as systemic injections in inducing receptivity in ovariectomized female rats. Of course, not all brain sites are equally effective for such results, and most of the sites found to be most effective are in the hypothalamus. Sites in which estrogen implants are particularly effective include the ventromedial arcuate nucleus, the anterior hypothalamus, and the preoptic area, among others. On the other hand, most of the sites in the midbrain seem uninvolved (e.g., Lisk, 1962; Morin & Feder, 1974c).

It also is interesting that lesions in the medial preoptic area of the brain decrease the amount of systemically injected estradiol needed to induce receptivity in ovariectomized female rats (Powers & Valenstein, 1972). This finding suggests that one normal function of estradiol might be to reduce the inhibitory actions exerted by this brain area on sexual behavior. It could be that if the medial preoptic area is present, more estradiol is needed in order to counteract its inhibitory influences (perhaps through working in other brain sites). Or, it could be that in some way, estradiol directly diminishes the inhibitory activity of this brain area. In either case, the medial preoptic area appears to act in a way that is counter to the effects of estradiol.

What of progesterone? Recall that, in some species, progesterone exerts facilitatory effects, whereas in others the effects include inhibition of sexual responding. Both of these kinds of effects appear to be mediated by the actions of progesterone on the brain. For example, in both the rat and the guinea pig, progesterone implants into the basal hypothalamus facilitate the effects of systemically injected estradiol in inducing estrus (Morin & Feder, 1974b; Powers, 1972). On the other hand, if progesterone is implanted into areas of the midbrain, its effects are inhibitory, at least in the guinea pig (Morin & Feder, 1974a). Thus, both kinds of progesterone effects on sexual behavior can be exerted by implanting progesterone only into the brain, and the critical brain sites for each kind of effect are different.

In the case of males, androgen effects also seem to be at least partly mediated by the effects of these hormones on critical brain sites. It has been shown repeatedly that implanting testosterone into the preoptic area of the brain is sufficient to restore the sexual performance of castrated male rats (e.g., Davidson, 1966; Lisk, 1967).

As would be predicted from studies testing the aromatization hypothesis with systemic hormone injections, injections of estradiol into the preoptic area also can restore somewhat the sexual behavior of castrated male rats (Christensen & Clemens, 1974). These neural estrogen implants become totally effective if they are coupled with systemic injections of dihydrotestosterone (Davidson & Trinpin, 1975). Therefore, it may be that in male rats, testosterone is converted to estrogen in the preoptic area in order to affect male sexual responding. One critical question that might be asked concerns whether or not aromatization can or does naturally occur in this brain area, and, importantly, the answer is "yes" (Naftolin, Ryan & Petro, 1972).

It might be useful to note here that the fact that hormone implants directly into the brain can fully restore the sexual behavior of ovariectomized or castrated animals does not mean that hormones cannot also have some peripheral actions. This fact only means that those peripheral actions are not totally necessary. Thus, hormones can affect sexual behavior in many ways, and peripheral hormonal actions should be viewed as complementary.

Earlier in this chapter, we discussed whether fine-grain differences in levels of sexual responding, such as those between intact individuals, might be related to circulating levels of the androgens, and we concluded from the studies reviewed that there was no real relationship. One alternative hypothesis that has been proposed to account for these differences is that they are a result of differential sensitivity to or utilization of androgens in the brain (e.g., Beach & Fowler, 1959). This hypothesis has not been studied extensively, although there has been at least one test in the guinea pig. Harding and Feder (1976b) compared the rate of testosterone uptake into the brain in guinea pigs rated as highly active, moderately active, or not very active sexually. Significantly, they found no differences in the rate of uptake or utilization among these guinea pigs. Of course, although this study does argue against a "neural sensitivity" hypothesis, it is only the first of many studies needed to test this hypothesis adequately.

A final question that might be asked about the neural mediation of hormonal effects on sexual behavior concerns how hormones affect the brain to affect sexual behavior. More simply put: what do hormones do to the brain to alter sexual activity? As discussed in earlier chapters, there are many possibilities, since the effects of hormones are quite pervasive and can be quite varied in different tissues. One interesting hypothesis has been that hormones alter protein synthesis in critical brain areas, thereby modifying the substrates of sexual behavior. Studies supporting this hypothesis for the case of female sexual behavior and estrogen and progesterone facilitatory effects have been conducted in the rat. Injections of protein synthesis inhibitors into critical brain areas decrease the effectiveness of hormones in inducing or facilitating sexual responding (e.g., Quadagno & Ho, 1975; Terkel, Shryne & Gorski, 1973; Whalen et al., 1974).

A related hypothesis suggests that hormones affect sexual responding by modifying the state of neurotransmitter systems in the brain. These hormonal effects may or may not be mediated by the just-discussed changes in protein synthesis, since protein synthesis is, of course, critical to neurotransmitter activity. A discussion of this possible mediational mechanism really is beyond the scope of this book. The interested reader might consult the reviews to be found in Carter (1977), Naftolin, Ryan and Davies (1976) and Sandler and Gessa (1975).

BISEXUALITY AND THE ROLE OF
HORMONES EARLY IN DEVELOPMENT

Our discussion so far has been concerned solely with the behavior patterns most typical of that gender, so-called *homotypical* behavior patterns. We have only considered the effects of hormones present in adulthood on the tendency of males to exhibit "male-like" sexual responses and on the tendency of females to exhibit "female-like" sexual responses. This discussion might give the spurious impression that sexual behavior is in fact dimorphic; that is, that each gender only displays one type of sexual response. However, as mentioned in the introduction to this chapter, this is not the case. Most animals are at least partly *bisexual*. There are many cases of females exhibiting so-called male patterns of behavior, such as mounting, and many cases of males exhibiting female behavior patterns, such as lordosis responses. Responding in the manner most characteristic of the opposite gender often is referred to as *heterotypical* responding, and the role of hormones in determining whether an animal will behave homotypically or heterotypically is the subject of this section.

The frequency of heterotypical responses varies from species to species, and, within a species, between the genders. For example, in rats, females frequently are observed to mount estrous females, whereas males only rarely exhibit lordosis responses (Beach, 1938; Beach & Rasquin, 1942). On the other hand, female hamsters rarely mount other females, but males do show the lordosis posture rather frequently (Beach, 1971; Goy & Goldfoot, 1973).

It should be noted at the outset that hormones certainly do not exert total control over whether an animal will behave homotypically or heterotypically, or how much of each kind of behavior it will show. For example, Goy and Goldfoot (1973) discuss at least five factors that can affect the form of sexual responses, and only two of these involve hormones at all. These two kinds of hormonal factors include the hormonal state in effect at the time the behavior is emitted and the hormonal state early in development. We shall discuss the effects of hormones in adulthood on heterotypical sexual responding first, and then turn to the effects of hormones present early in development on adult patterns of sexual behavior. As in earlier discussions, the literature on these topics is vast and will not be reviewed completely here. The reader interested in pursuing this topic further might consult the excellent reviews by Beach (1971), Goldfoot (1977), Goy and Goldfoot (1973), and Whalen (1968).

The Effects of the Adult Hormonal State on Heterotypical Sexual Behavior

Among the males of the species discussed in this chapter, only the male rat both shows female-like sexual responses and has been studied extensively. The male guinea pig almost never exhibits heterotypical sexual responses, and attempts to induce female-like behavior in the males of this species have been wholly unsuccessful (e.g., Phoenix et al., 1959). In the case of the rhesus monkey, the male often emits female-like responses, but the effects of hormones in adulthood on these responses has received almost no attention.

Therefore, for the case of heterotypical responding in the male, our discussion will be restricted to the male rat.

Although they do not do so very frequently, male rats have been observed to exhibit female-like lordosis postures. In those males that do exhibit lordosis responses, the adult hormonal state seems to be important to those behaviors. Castrating male rats leads to a reduction in the amount of female behavior exhibited, and replacement therapy with testosterone is effective in restoring the level of female-like responding of castrated males to precastration levels (e.g., Beach, 1945; Södersten, 1975; Södersten & Larsson, 1974).

Treating castrated male rats with estrogens also restores their female-like sexual responses, and, in fact, estrogen treatment is even more effective than is testosterone treatment (Beach, 1945; Davidson & Block, 1969; Södersten & Larsson, 1974). Furthermore, treating male rats with the anti-estrogen MER-25 descreases the frequency of female-like responses, at least those in response to manual stimulation of the genital areas (Södersten & Larsson, 1974). These findings would seem to suggest that testosterone might naturally be aromatized to estrogens to stimulate female-like behavior in male rats (see discussion of aromatization above) (Paup, Mennin & Gorski, 1975). However, intact male rats that do and do not show female-like responses do not differ in circulating estradiol levels, suggesting, at least, that if testosterone is converted to estradiol to induce lordosis responses, this conversion is not reflected in increased blood estradiol levels (Södersten et al., 1974). This finding detracts somewhat from the potency of an aromatization hypothesis to account for heterotypical responding in male rats. But, as in the case of homotypical responding, aromatization could be occurring in the brain and, then, would not necessarily be reflected in measures of peripheral (circulating) estrogen levels. Whether or not aromatization is critical to heterotypical responding, we can say that the presence of either androgens or estrogens is necessary for male rats to exhibit female-like sexual responses.

Turning to the female, the influence of the adult hormonal state on the control of heterotypical sexual behavior varies greatly across species. For example, in the guinea pig, some females exhibit mounting behavior toward other females, and the frequency of this mounting increases around the time of estrus. In addition, ovariectomy leads to a decrease in the frequency of mounting, and treating ovariectomized females with estrogen and progesterone increases their mounting rates almost to the level of intact males (Goy, Bridson & Young, 1964). Thus, in the female guinea pig, heterotypical (male-like) sexual responding is dependent on the presence of the ovarian hormones and is affected much in the same way as is homotypical responding.

In contrast to the case of the guinea pig, estrogen and/or progesterone levels appear unrelated to heterotypical sexual responses in the female rat. Female rats exhibit mounting throughout the estrous cycle, and removing the ovarian hormones by ovariectomy does not alter the frequency of this behavior (Beach, 1968; Beach & Rasquin, 1942). Furthermore, selective depletion of estrogen with the anti-estrogen MER-25 has no effect on mounting by female rats (Södersten, 1974). Thus, the presence of the ovarian hormones is not necessary for such mounting.

On the other hand, treating female rats with testosterone does increase their mounting frequencies (Ball, 1940; Pfaff, 1970), and this androgen effect probably is not a result of aromatization of testosterone to estrogen. Estrogen treatment alone has no effect on mounting by female rats (Beach & Rasquin, 1942). Thus, the androgens, but not the ovarian hormones estrogen and progesterone, do affect male-like responding in the female rat. It should be noted, however, that it is unclear whether the androgens naturally control mounting in female rats, because androgen effects only have been studied through exogenous androgen manipulations. No studies have yet examined the effects of withdrawing androgens from female rats, as would be accomplished by combining ovariectomy with adrenalectomy. Thus, although the androgens can affect male-like responding in the female rat, it is unclear whether these hormones ordinarily do control this behavior.

The role of hormones in male-like sexual behavior in female rhesus monkeys has not been studied in any depth, although the female rhesus monkey clearly is quite capable of emitting these behaviors. One study by Michael, Wilson, and Zumpe (1974) suggests that the ovarian hormones may be related to mounting behavior in female rhesus monkeys, since these investigators observed a greater frequency of mounting by females around the time of menstruation. However, this relationship would be different from that for homotypical responses and ovarian hormone levels, because the two classes of sexual behavior peak at different times in the menstrual cycle.

In summary, the findings discussed in this section show that the members of many species are quite capable of behaving either homotypically or heterotypically. However, the reader may have noticed that in some cases, as in the female guinea pig, heterotypical responding depends on the same adult hormonal state as does homotypical responding. What, then, determines which type of behavior will be emitted in these cases? The probability that an animal will react homotypically usually is greater than the probability that it will react heterotypically. Beach (1976b) has labeled this greater tendency to react homotypically as *sex-linked prepotency*. Although many nonhormonal factors can contribute to this sex-linked prepotency, one of the factors that clearly contributes to the tendency to react homotypically does involve hormones. This hormonal factor is the endocrine state during certain critical stages early in development.

Hormonal States Early in Development and Adult Sexual Behavior

Although it had been known for some time that the early hormonal environment is important to the determination of adult morphology and reproductive physiology, the first study focusing on the influences of the early hormonal state on adult sexual behavior was published by Phoenix et al. in 1959. In this study, female guinea pigs were treated throughout most of the prenatal period with testosterone propionate, which was accomplished by injecting the mothers with this hormone. When these female guinea pigs matured, they were found to be "defeminized" and "masculinized." That is, they were less likely to exhibit normal female-like responses in the presence of estrogen and progesterone and more likely to exhibit male-like mounting responses than non-treated females. These findings led to the hypothesis that the hormonal state early in development *organizes* the central neural circuits that will control adult sexual responses. We shall return to the question of how that organization might take place later in this section.

Before discussing this topic further, it is important to mention one issue. The original *organization hypothesis* suggested that hormones present during the critical developmental stages lead to both defeminization and masculinization (compare Phoenix et al., 1959). However, later studies have shown that masculinity and femininity do not always vary in opposite ways; they are not opposite ends of a single continuum, and they can be manipulated separately (compare Whalen, 1974). For example, withdrawing androgens during the critical period by prenatal treatment of male guinea pigs with the anti-androgen cyproterone acetate leads to demasculinization (decreased mounting), as would be predicted, but this treatment does not lead to feminization (increased lordosis behavior) (Goldfoot, Resko & Goy, 1971). Therefore, although masculinity and femininity usually do vary in opposite ways and often are affected oppositely by early hormonal manipulations, as the organization hypothesis would predict, this is not always the case.

Many later studies have replicated the basic finding that the hormonal state early in development is important in the determination of adult sexual responses, and the relationship has by now been studied in a wide variety of species (e.g., Barraclough & Gorski, 1962, Gerall & Ward, 1966, for the rat; Gerall, 1966, for the guinea pig; Goy & Goldfoot, 1975, Goy & Phoenix, 1971, for the rhesus monkey). An initial generalization we might make is that the presence of gonadal hormones during the critical stages in development predisposes an individual to react in a male-like fashion, whereas the absence of gonadal hormones during these critical periods predisposes the individual to react in a more female-like manner (compare Young, 1961, 1965). However, it is important to note that not all gonadal hormones present during these critical developmental stages act in the same ways, and that such parameters as duration of hormone exposure, timing of treatments, and concentrations of hormones administered can be important (see Edwards & Thompson, 1970; Gerall, Dunlap & Wagner, 1976; Goldfoot & van der Werff ten Bosch, 1975; Mullins & Levine, 1968). But, even with this qualification, the generalization is appropriate as a generalization: the presence of gonadal hormones during critical developmental stages does predispose the animal to behave in a more masculine fashion, and the absence of those hormones does lead to an increased propensity to behave in feminine ways.

As a further qualification, it should also be noted that this generalization holds primarily for mammalian species. The statement must be reversed, for example, for birds. Adkins (1975) has shown that the presence of gonadal hormones during critical developmental stages favors female-like rather than male-like behaviors in Japanese quail. But, our discussion is limited only to mammals, and the generalization, as stated, is appropriate.

There are some important differences among mammalian species in the effects of hormones present early in development on adult sexual responding. For example, the critical period for early hormonal influences varies. In both the guinea pig and the rhesus monkey, the critical period is well before birth, during the middle stages of gestation (Goy, Bridson & Young, 1964; Goy & Phoenix, 1971). On the other hand, the critical period in the rat is just around the time of birth; although combined pre- and postnatal androgen treatments are the most effective in masculinizing female rats, postnatal treatment alone is quite effective (Ward, 1969). What determines the timing of the critical period is unknown, although it may be related to the degree of maturity of the young at birth. Both the rhesus monkey and the guinea pig are born relatively well-developed, whereas the rat is born relatively immature.

A second important difference concerns the form of the effects of the early hormonal state. As stated before, in both the rat and the guinea pig, early hormone treatments of females typically lead to both defeminization and masculinization. However, in the rhesus monkey, it appears that early hormonal treatments only produce masculinizing effects; there is no clear evidence of defeminization following early hormonal treatments (Goy & Goldfoot, 1975). Thus, the effects exerted by the hormonal state early in development are not totally uniform, even across mammalian species.

Our discussion so far really has been based only on the effects of treating females with gonadal hormones during early critical periods. For our initial generalization to hold, however, it should also be the case that withdrawing gonadal hormones from males during the early critical period affects their adult sexual responses. Specifically, the generalization would predict that removing androgens during the critical developmental period produces males that are feminized and demasculinized. This issue has been studied in detail in the rat, and the results are consistent with the prediction. Castrating male rats during the neonatal critical period leads both to a decrease in male-like behavior when testosterone is provided in adulthood and to an increase in the emission of female-like behaviors in the presence of estrogen and progesterone (Beach & Holz, 1946; Feder & Whalen, 1965).

A further prediction from our initial generalization would be that if male rats are castrated on the day of birth (thereby demasculinizing them), replacing androgens during the same critical period should "re-masculinize" them. A study by Beach, Noble, and Orndoff (1969) dramatically shows this to be the case. The results of that study are summarized in Figure 5-4. These investigators castrated male rats on the day of birth and then administered exogenous androgens at different times during the next two weeks. As can be seen from Figure 5-4, replacing androgens within two days after birth counteracted the effects of neonatal castration. These males exhibited appropriate male-like responses in the presence of testosterone in adulthood and no female-like responses in the pres-

FIG. 5-4

Adult sexual responses of neonatally castrated male rats given testosterone at different ages. Male-like behavior is represented by ejaculations and female-like behavior by the lordosis quotient (from Beach, Noble & Orndoff, *Journal of Comparative and Physiological Psychology*, 1969, 68, 493. Copyright 1969 by the American Psychological Association. Reprinted by permission).

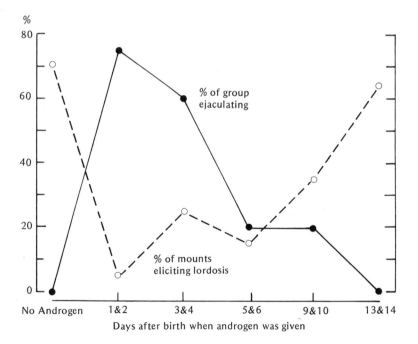

ence of estrogen and progesterone. As the time between withdrawal of the endogenous androgens by castration and replacement with testosterone increased, the effectiveness of early androgen replacement in remasculinizing neonatally castrated males decreased dramatically. This study, then, emphasizes the fixedness of the early critical period for gonadal hormone exposure in determining adult sexual responses.

How does the hormonal state early in development modify adult sexual behavior? By what mechanism(s) does this temporally delayed hormonal effect occur? The original paper published by Phoenix et al. (1959) contained the suggestion that hormones present early in development somehow permanently modify or organize the developing nervous system in a more masculine and less feminine way. This view has come to be called the *organization hypothesis*. Inherent in this hypothesis is the belief that adult male and female brains are different in some fundamental way, and that those differences are dependent on the hormonal state during early developmental stages. The exact form of those neural changes was not specified in the original paper, although there has been much discussion about this issue since.

Before specifying the mechanisms by which early hormonal treatments can modify the brain to alter adult sexual behavior, it is important to show that the hormonal effects on behavior are in fact neurally mediated. As in other cases where neural mediation of hormonal effects on behavior have been shown, the critical test has been to examine whether implanting hormones only into the brain would have the same effects as systemic hormone injections. These tests have been conducted, and it does appear that the effects of hormones present during early developmental stages on adult sexual behavior are mediated by changes in the functioning of the brain. As one example, in an elaborate series of studies, Nadler (1968, 1972, 1973) showed that implanting testosterone propionate pellets into the brains of neonatal female rats does lead to a facilitation of male-like behaviors and an inhibition of female-like behaviors exhibited in adulthood. Therefore, at least one part of the organization hypothesis seems to be accurate: that hormones present early in development can somehow modify the state of the developing brain circuits that control sexual responding.

What, then, do hormones present early in development do to the brain so that adult sexual responses will be modified? The original organization hypothesis implied that there were some kinds of structural changes induced by the presence of hormones during the early critical periods (see Phoenix et al., 1959). An alternative hypothesis has been that hormones present early in development produce only functional changes in neural activity, not structural changes. Specifically, it was suggested (e.g., Beach, 1971) that hormones present early in development alter the sensitivity of the critical brain circuits to the gonadal hormones circulating in adulthood. This "sensitivity" position was based, at least in part, on the findings that the presence of androgens early in development seems to lower the amount of androgen needed to activate male-like responses.

An example of these changes in sensitivity to adult hormones is provided in part by a study by Gerall and Kenney (1970). Some of the results of their study are presented in Figure 5-5. In this study, female rats were treated neonatally with either no hormone or one of several increasing dosages of testosterone propionate. Then, the effects of different dosages of estrogen or testosterone on adult sexual responses were examined, much in the same way as in those studies examining the dose-response relationships between adult gonadal hormone levels and sexual responding discussed in the preceding section. As can be seen from Figure 5-5, as neonatal androgen dosages were increased, the amount of female-like behavior displayed in the presence of varying estrogen dosages decreased. Specifically, the "oil" group shows the usual dose-response relationship between estrogen levels and receptivity, but as neonatal androgen dosages increase, the curves become flatter and flatter; more estrogen is demanded to elicit the same amount of female-

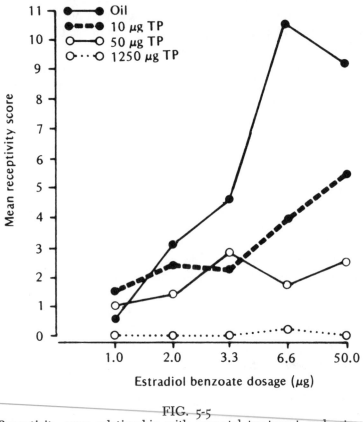

FIG. 5-5

Receptivity score relationship with neonatal treatment and estrogen dosage in adulthood (from Gerall & Kenney, *Endocrinology*, 1970, 87, 562, by permission of J. B. Lippincott Company).

like behavior. Thus, neonatal androgen treatment can be said to be desensitizing the females to estrogen encountered in adulthood.

In turn, proponents of the organization hypothesis have argued that mere sensitivity changes cannot account for all of the behavioral effects of hormones present during early critical periods.

There are some behaviors that are different in the two genders and can be affected by hormones present during the early critical periods, but they are not dependent on hormones circulating in adulthood. Therefore, the effects of early hormones on the adult display of these behaviors cannot be a result of altered sensitivity to circulating gonadal hormones. For example, the characteristic male-like urination posture of dogs is not usually shown by females. In addition, the display of this behavior in males does not depend on the presence of androgens in adulthood. But, female dogs treated with androgen during early developmental stages do display male-like urination postures, whether or not they are again treated with androgens in adulthood (Beach, 1975). Therefore, a sensitivity explanation would not be sufficient to account for the effects of hormones early in development in this case; no adult sensitivity to hormones is demanded—the behavior can occur in the absence of gonadal hormones. Similarly, there are marked gender differences in the display of rough-and-tumble play and chasing play in juvenile rhesus monkeys, and these gender differences do not seem to depend on which hormones (if any) are present at the time the behavior is displayed. But, treating female rhesus monkeys prenatally with androgens leads to these females' displaying male-like play responses, suggesting, again, that the early hormonal state can affect sexually dimorphic behaviors which are not affected by hormonal treatments at the time of their emission (Goy, 1968; Goy & Resko, 1972). On the basis of these kinds of findings, then, the proponents of the organization hypothesis have suggested that there must be some changes in brain function caused by the presence of hormones early in development that go beyond changes in sensitivity to hormones circulating at the time the behavior is displayed.

There is some evidence that the hormonal state early in development can influence the structure of the brain, and, thereby, might be the mechanism for some effects on adult responses. Neonatal androgen treatments seem to modify the structure and concentration of neurons in areas around the hypothalamus (Greenough et al., 1976; Raisman & Field, 1973). However, these findings are only preliminary, and, surely, identification of the precise mechanism(s) by which hormones present early in development can affect later behaviors will have to await further investigations.

Comment

Let us return to the question of the role of hormones in determining the form of adult sexual responses; that is, whether an animal will behave homotypically or heterotypically. There are some cases, such as the female rat, where the adult hormonal state might predispose the animal to react in one way or the other. Increasing testosterone levels in the female rat does increase the tendency to mount estrous females. But, there also are cases where the adult hormonal states controlling homotypical and heterotypical responses are the same, such as in the female guinea pig. What, then, determines the sex-linked prepotency, or the tendency to react homotypically? The data just reviewed argue strongly that the hormonal state early in development is the critical hormonal factor. Males are exposed to androgens during the critical developmental stages, and they react primarily in a male-like way in adulthood. On the other hand, females are not exposed to gonadal hormones during these critical developmental stages, and they react in female-like ways in adulthood. Reversing the hormonal conditions during the early developmental stages decreases the probability that the animal will behave homotypically and increases the probability that it will behave heterotypically. Therefore, the early hormonal state appears to be one factor that is very important in determining the form of adult hormonal responses, and the presence of the homotypical hormonal state during the critical developmental periods appears to contribute to the sex-linked prepotency for sexual responses.

EFFECTS OF SEXUAL STIMULATION
ON ENDOCRINE FUNCTION

We now have reviewed fairly extensively the effects of hormones on sexual responding. However, as mentioned in the beginning of this chapter, the relationship between hormones and sexual behavior is not unidirectional. There also are some marked effects of sexual contact on endocrine function. Some of these kinds of effects were discussed in Chapter 4, where the effects of exposure to certain stimulus properties of other animals on endocrine function were considered. Engaging in sexual activities also can lead to changes in hormonal states, and that is the topic of the discussion in this section.

The Female

It is well known that in some species, such as the cat and rabbit, engaging in coitus can lead to ovulation. In fact, in many of them, ovulation will not occur without copulation. Those animals in whom ovulation is dependent on sexual activity are called *reflex ovulators*. Of significance to our discussion is the likelihood that the behavioral induction of ovulation is hormonally mediated. For example, engaging in coitus leads to a rise in LH levels in female rabbits (e.g., Dufy-Barbe, Franchimont & Faure, 1973; Kanematsu et al., 1974), and this rise is similar in form to the ovulation-inducing LH surge observed in many nonreflex ovulators. Because this LH surge intervenes temporally between coitus and the occurrence of ovulation, it seems likely that sexual activities induce ovulation at least partly via changes in endocrine function.

What of the nonreflex ovulators? Do sexual activities lead to changes in endocrine function in animals that do not depend on coitus for the induction of ovulation? The answer is "yes." For example, in the female rat, mating often is followed within a short time by increases in the levels of LH, prolactin, and progesterone in the general circulation (Adler, Resko & Goy, 1970; Moss, 1974; Rodgers, 1971). Curiously, these hormonal responses to copulation appear to depend on the timing of the sexual activity. If copulation occurs early in proestrus, there is no LH rise in response to this experience. If, on the other hand, mating occurs later in proestrus, the LH increase does occur (Rodgers, 1971). It also is the case that the intensity of mating activities can affect the magnitude of the hormonal responses to copulation. Adler, Resko, and Goy (1970) observed that female rats receiving more intromissions prior to ejaculation by the male responded with greater progesterone responses than females receiving fewer intromissions.

What are the functions of these hormonal responses to sexual activity? Is there a long-chain hormone–behavior interaction occurring in the case of female sexual behavior? It is clear that in some birds, hormonal changes are important to the dynamic behavioral changes that occur across the complete reproductive cycle (see Lehrman, 1965). Some of these interactions are discussed in Chapter 6. However, the conditions in the mammals discussed in this chapter are less clear. At the least, the hormonal responses to sexual contact seem important to the effectiveness of coitus in resulting in pregnancy, perhaps through facilitating sperm transport (Adler, 1974). In an extensive series of studies, Adler and his colleagues (e.g., Adler, 1969, 1974; Adler & Zoloth, 1970) have shown that the greater the number of intromissions received from males, the greater the probability that pregnancy will ensue. This effect appears to be mediated by the progesterone responses to engaging in coitus. As discussed above, copulation leads to an increase in progesterone levels, and further increasing progesterone levels by experimental manipulations reduces the number of intromissions needed to induce pregnancy (Adler, 1969). Thus, the progesterone increase that normally accompanies copulation may be involved in determining whether coitus will be successful in inducing pregnancy.

But what of behavior? Engaging in coitus leads to a period of relative nonreceptivity in the females of many species (Goldfoot & Goy, 1970; Hardy & DeBold, 1972). Since progesterone can have inhibitory effects on receptivity in some of these species (see discussion above), might not the progesterone response to coitus be involved in the induction of this nonreceptive period? The answer seems to be "no." Both preventing progesterone changes by ovariectomy and augmenting the normal progesterone responses to copulation by exogenous hormone treatments have no effect on coitus-induced decreases in receptivity (Carter, 1972; Goldfoot & Goy, 1970). Furthermore, estrus periods are terminated normally whether or not progesterone levels are high (Morin & Feder, 1973), showing that changes in progesterone levels do not naturally lead to decreases in receptivity.

One effect of sexual stimulation on sexual responding in female rats might be hormonally mediated. Mechanically probing the vagina of female rats seems to lead to increased lordosis responsiveness, and this effect may be a result of an increase in the secretion of luteinizing-hormone release factor (LRF). LRF treatment does increase receptivity in hypophysectomized and/or ovariectomized, estrogen-primed female rats (Moss & McCann, 1973; Pfaff, 1973), and decreasing LRF release by dihydrotestosterone treatment does diminish the effects of vaginal probing on receptivity (Crowley, Rodriguez-Sierra & Komisaruk, 1976). Therefore, it may be that the LRF response to vaginal stimulation is involved in the mediation of the effects of this sensory experience on receptivity (Komisaruk, 1974).

In summary, although there certainly is insufficient evidence to make a generalization with confidence, preliminary findings suggest that the normal hormonal responses to engaging in the usual types of sexual activities do not feed back and modify ongoing sexual behavior characteristics. But, hormones might be involved in mediating some effects of more artificial experiences, such as mechanical vaginal probing, on female sexual responsiveness.

The Male

The effects of sexual contact on endocrine function have been studied less extensively in the male than in the female. However, it is known that copulation can lead to fairly rapid (within minutes) changes in some endocrine parameters. Engaging in copulation has been found to increase testosterone, prolactin, and LH levels in many species (Kamel et al., 1975, Purvis & Haynes, 1974, for the rat; Harding & Feder, 1976a, for the guinea pig; Macrides, Bartke & Dalterio, 1975, for the mouse; Saginor & Horton, 1968, for the rabbit). In addition, the greater the amount of sexual activity, the greater the magnitude of the testosterone responses to that experience (Harding & Feder, 1976a).

What of possible long-chain hormone–behavior interactions? As mentioned for the female, there are some male birds in which there do appear to be these kinds of relationships between the hormonal and behavioral responses to experience (see Lehrman, 1965, and discussion in Chapter 6), but this question has not been studied in male mammals.

HORMONES AND HUMAN SEXUALITY

The data on hormones and sexual behavior in nonhuman animals reviewed in this chapter clearly show the importance of these secretions to normal sexual responding and, at times, the importance of hormones to the form of sexual responses. However, as suggested in the beginning of this chapter, it should be clear by now that hormones are less important in the control of sexual behavior in our primate model, the rhesus monkey, than in the less advanced species discussed. In fact, there are many primates, such as the female stumptail macaque, whose sexual responses are at most only minimally related to their hormonal states (Slob et al., unpublished). But, what of the human? Can we generalize any of the findings from studies of nonhuman animals to the case of the human?

Curiously, there have been very few systematic studies of the role of hormones in human sexuality. But, there is a fairly extensive clinical literature reporting selected case studies of hormonal effects on sexual behavior that are tangential to the parameters that are the focus of the studies. Some of that clinical literature will be summarized here. It should be made clear at the outset that hormones seem to contribute relatively little to the determination of human sexuality, although there may be some effects of hormones on sexual responding in humans. To emphasize this point, it seems significant that in their very extensive discussion of human sexual behavior, Masters and Johnson (1966) devote almost no attention to the possible role of hormones in human sexual behavior. Whalen (1966) has suggested that, at most, hormones only affect the ability of humans to become aroused, their *arousability*. Whalen argues that hormones do not contribute to arousal per se; they are not important factors in the stimulation of sexual activities. This kind of distinction can be contrasted with the case of nonhuman female animals, where hormones can affect both receptivity (arousability?) and proceptivity (arousal?).

The Male

We shall begin with the male. It is well known that castrating adult males leads to an eventual decrease in both sexual performance and sexual desire (see reviews by Beach, 1948; Tauber, 1940). In addition, once sexual activity has decreased following withdrawal of the androgens, replacement therapy with these hormones can be quite effective in restoring sexual activity to normal levels (Gordon & Fields, 1943; Jakobovits, 1970). However, the fact that sexual activity does persist long after androgen levels have declined argues that sexual behavior in the human male, like that in many nonhuman males, does not depend totally on androgen secretion.

Interestingly, prepubertal castration in inexperienced male humans does often lead to sexual apathy in adulthood (Money, 1961a; Money & Ehrhardt, 1972). This finding suggests that experiential factors are prepotent over hormonal factors in male sexual behavior. If a male has not had sexual experiences, castration leads to sexual apathy. On the other hand, if the man has had sexual experiences, androgen withdrawal is not immediately effective. Thus, even though androgenic stimulation may be important to sexual behavior, the testicular hormones do not exert very strong control over this behavior.

As an interesting side note, castration or treatment with chemical anti-androgens has been used with habitual sex offenders. Although certainly drastic, these kinds of treatments can be quite effective in reducing this kind of criminal activity. Furthermore, reversing these treatments with testosterone injections results in a return of the criminal sexual activity. It has been argued that the effectiveness of these treatments is a result of decreasing the sex offender's sexual desires and, thereby, his criminal behaviors (Hawke, 1950; Money et al., 1975; Stürup, 1972). Thus, androgen manipulations can affect sex-related behaviors in addition to sexual activity per se.

Given that changes in androgen levels can affect sexual activity in human males, we can ask the same question that we asked in the case of nonhuman animals: how do the androgens affect sexual behavior in the human male? There have been no studies directed toward this question, but it is clear that the androgens have marked effects on peripheral physical characteristics, much in the same way as they affect these characteristics in nonhuman animals. Thus, the androgens could affect human male sexual behavior by altering the state of necessary peripheral structures such as the penis or the seminal vesicles—any androgen-dependent tissues. But, in discussing nonhuman animals we suggested that much of the androgenic effects on sexual behavior were mediated by changes in central neural activity. Could this not also be true for the human male? Of course it could, but, as Beach (1976b) points out, given the progressive independence of human sexual behavior from hormonal influences, it would be dangerous to attempt to generalize in the absence of data.

The Female

What of hormones and sexual behavior in the human female? There have been numerous attempts to show correlations between sexual interests and activity and the stage of the female reproductive cycle. These kinds of studies have yielded contradictory results. One group of studies has found increases in sexual interest and activity around the time of ovulation (e.g., Daniels, 1971; Udry & Morris, 1968). An example of this kind of cyclicity in sexual behavior of human females is presented in Figure 5-6. Notice that there is some small rise in sexual activity around the general time of ovulation, but that there also is an increase in sexual activity just prior to menstruation. Other studies have yielded different correlations, often suggesting that there are two peaks in sexual activity, one just prior to menstruation and one just following menstruation (see reviews by Luttge, 1971; Money & Ehrhardt, 1972).

The existence of any correlation between menstrual-cycle status and sexual activity or interest might seem to suggest that the ovarian hormones are related to sexual behavior in human females. However, the inconsistencies in those correlations from study to study detract severely from the power of that suggestion. More importantly, it is well-known clinically that ovariectomy usually does not affect sexual desire in human females (e.g., Filler & Drezner, 1944; Waxenberg, Drellich & Sutherland, 1959), showing that the ovarian hormones are not very important to sexual behavior in the human female.

It has been suggested (e.g., Money, 1961b) that androgens, probably of adrenal origins, are quite important to the control of sexual behavior in human females. This suggestion is based on observations of the sexual behavior of women whose androgen levels

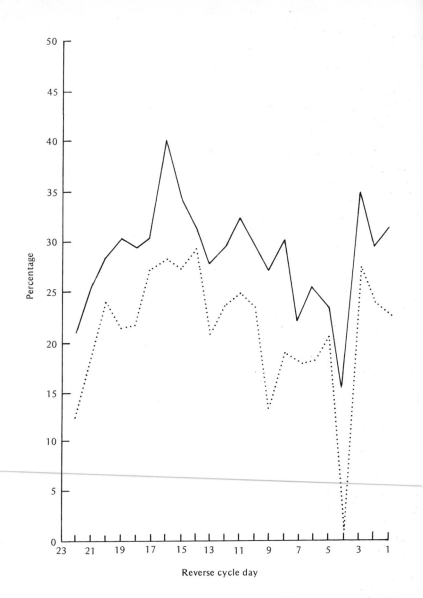

FIG. 5-6
Percentage of 40 women reporting intercourse and orgasm, by reverse day of menstrual cycle. (——) = intercourse, (••••) = orgasm (reprinted from Udry & Morris, *Nature*, Vol. 220, 593, 1968).

were manipulated for a variety of clinical reasons. For example, although ovariectomy does not affect sexual behavior, adrenalectomizing ovariectomized women does lead to a noticeable decline in "libido" (Waxenberg et al., 1960). Furthermore, treating women with androgens has been reported to lead to marked increases in sexual desire (e.g., Salmon & Geist, 1943; Sopchak & Sutherland, 1960). In fact, some studies suggest that androgen treatment is an effective therapeutic tool for cases of frigidity (Burdine, Shipley & Papas, 1957). Thus, there are at least two lines of evidence suggesting that the androgens can affect sexual activity in human females: removing the androgens by adrenalectomy leads to a decrease in sexual desire, and treating women with androgens leads to an increase in libido.

However, these kinds of studies are difficult to interpret clearly. First, adrenalectomy is a very drastic operation, one that has a wide range of metabolic consequences that could account for a decrease in sexual desire. Plainly, the women might feel sick. Second, androgen treatment stimulates clitoral hypertrophy, and this stimulation of the size of the clitoris could be involved in the effects of androgens on sexual interest (see Luttge, 1971). But, by whatever means, manipulating androgen levels does affect sexual behavior while other hormonal manipulations do not. Therefore, the kinds of findings discussed here present an interesting hypothesis that deserves additional experimental investigation.

Comment: Hormones and Human Sexuality

The reader might be somewhat disappointed by the limited amount of information available about the role of hormones in human sexual behavior. However, the study of this question in human subjects is extremely difficult, as is the study of the role of hormones in any human behavior. First, the study of hormones and behavior in animals has taught us that one's experiential history often is such an important factor that its effects can overshadow any influences that hormones might exert. Certainly this would be a problem in studying human sexual interests and activity. Second, we cannot subject humans to the kinds of hormonal manipulations needed to determine precisely the role of hormones in human sexual behavior in the same way that we manipulate the hormonal states of animals. Therefore, we must depend on the findings of studies manipulating hormonal states to correct either endocrinopathies or other disease states. These disorders by themselves could be affecting sexual behavior in any of many ways. But, the kinds of studies reviewed in this section do raise some provocative questions about hormones and human sexual behavior, and we have had some hints of hormonal involvement in these kinds of reactions. It does seem clear that the androgens are necessary both to the initiation (or development) and maintenance of sexual responding in human males. These androgen effects may not be nearly as strong as they are in the rodents we have discussed, but they do seem to be present. We also have learned that the ovarian hormones are not critical to sexual behavior in human females; ovariectomy usually does not alter women's sexual behavior, even after long postoperative time periods. Finally, there are some provocative data suggesting that the androgens, perhaps from adrenal origins, may be important in human female sexual responding.

SUMMARY AND COMMENT

This chapter was concerned with the relationship between hormones and sexual behavior, the most heavily studied topic in behavioral endocrinology. Rather than attempt to summarize what is known about hormones and sexual behavior in all of the species that have been studied, this discussion focused on two rodents (the rat and the guinea pig), one nonhuman primate (the rhesus monkey), and the human. It is hoped that this choice has been sufficient to provide ideas about what has been learned and examples of some of the problems that arise in attempting to study hormones and sexual behavior. One dramatic problem that should by now be quite clear is that there is great variation from species to species. Even the rodents discussed here differ greatly in the way in which hormones are related to their sexual responses.

The first section of this chapter was concerned with the effects of the hormonal state extant at the time the behavior is emitted on homotypical sexual responses. In that discussion, we saw, first, that estrogen levels are important to the activation of female sexual responses in most species. The other major ovarian hormone, progesterone, seems to have different effects on sexual behavior in different species at different times. In some cases, progesterone facilitates sexual responding, whereas in other cases it inhibits such responding. Some interesting preliminary data were discussed suggesting that the androgens, presumably of adrenal origins, might be important to female sexual behavior in the rhesus monkey.

We then turned to the case of the male. The androgens seem important to sexual behavior in all species discussed. It is important to recall, however, that in some cases the androgens may be affecting sexual behavior in part because they are readily converted to estrogens.

Although the three gonadal hormones discussed here, the estrogens, progesterone, and the androgens, all seem to affect sexual behavior, the nature of their effects can vary greatly. In one sense, the estrogens and the androgens appear to affect the appropriate homotypical responses similarly. There is a dose-response relationship between androgen levels and levels of sexual activity, although usually to a limit. Once that limit has been reached, which seems to be the individual's maximum potential for sexual activity, further increases in androgen levels do not lead to even further increases in sexual responding. In contrast, progesterone is related to sexual behavior quite differently. All of the effects of this hormone appear to be "all-or-none." If progesterone is present in sufficient amounts, its effects are evident. On the other hand, if progesterone levels are below the "threshold" level for its effects on sexual behavior, it does not influence sexual responding.

Although androgen and estrogen effects are similar in one sense, they are quite different in another. Specifically, a female needs to be exposed to estrogens for only a very short period of time for her sexual responses to be affected. On the other hand, androgen stimulation must be available for up to weeks in some species for the effects to be seen. Conversely, ovariectomy has a fairly rapid depressive effect on sexual behavior, whereas castration of the male only affects sexual behavior after rather long postoperative time periods.

The final issue raised in discussing hormonal effects on homotypical sexual responses concerned the mechanisms by which hormones affect sexual behavior. It seems that most such effects are mediated by changes in brain function, although some may be mediated by peripheral mechanisms. Areas in the region of the hypothalamus appear involved in the facilitatory effects of the estrogens, the androgens, and progesterone, whereas areas in the midbrain seem important to progesterone's inhibitory effects.

We next considered bisexuality in nonhuman animals, and the roles of two kinds of hormonal factors in determining the form of adult sexual responses. The first factor discussed was the influence of the hormonal state extant at the time the behavior is emitted in determining the probability of an animal's exhibiting heterotypical sexual behaviors. Of the males of the species discussed in this chapter, only the male rat both exhibits heterotypical responses somewhat frequently and has been studied in any detail. In this male, it appears that female-like responses are dependent on the presence of androgens, and these androgen influences may be a result of the conversion of these hormones to estrogens. Interestingly, homotypical sexual responses also depend on androgenic stimulation in the male rat, and, therefore, it is unlikely that the hormonal state in adulthood is responsible for determining whether a male rat will react in a male-like or a female-like fashion.

In the two female rodents discussed, the hormonal basis of heterotypical responding is different. In the female guinea pig, mounting behavior appears dependent on estrogen and progesterone stimulation, much in the same way as is homotypical responding. On the other hand, estrogen and progesterone levels seem irrelevant to heterotypical responding in the female rat. Mounting responses in the female rat appear to depend on androgenic stimulation. It would appear, then, that in the guinea pig, since both homotypical and heterotypical responses depend on ovarian hormones, the determination of the form of sexual responses is not accomplished by the adult hormonal state. Some other factor(s) must be critically involved. However, the adult hormonal state may affect the form of sexual responses in the female rat. If ovarian hormone influences predominate, homotypical behaviors will be displayed; if androgen influences predominate, male-like responses will be exhibited. Of course, as discussed before, hormonal factors existing at the time the behavior is emitted do not exert anywhere near total control over the form of sexual responses; they are only a part of the controlling mechanisms.

Another of these controlling mechanisms also involves hormones. Whether an animal will react homotypically or heterotypically appears to depend heavily on the hormonal state during certain critical developmental periods. If gonadal hormones are present during these critical periods (among the mammals discussed here), it is likely that the animal will behave in more masculine and less feminine ways. If these hormones are absent during those early developmental stages, the reverse behavior patterns are seen. These hormonal states early in development appear to affect adult sexual responses by modifying the state of the brain circuits that are critical for sexual behavior.

The next section discussed the hormonal responses to sexual stimulation. Clearly, engaging in sexual activity leads to some major changes in endocrine states. For example, engaging in sexual activity leads to an increase in LH, prolactin, and androgen levels in male rats and guinea pigs. Whether these hormonal responses to sexual experience feed back and modify either ongoing or subsequent responses in a long-chain hormone–behavior interaction in these animals is not yet known. However, preliminary evidence has not supported the existence of this kind of feedback mechanism, at least in mammalian species.

The final section of this chapter considered the role of hormones in human sexuality. There really have been very few experimental studies bearing on this issue, although there have been some correlational studies and some reports in the clinical literature of side-effects of endocrine treatments for other purposes. First, the human male, like the males of many other species, appears to depend on androgenic stimulation for the initiation and maintenance of sexual responding. However, these androgenic influences appear to be weaker than those in nonhuman species. Sexual activity seems to last much longer following castration in humans than in other species. Thus, there may be less marked hormonal dependence in the human male than in other animals.

The human female's sexual responsiveness appears unaffected by either the presence or absence of ovarian hormones, in contrast to the other species discussed. There is some evidence suggesting that androgens secreted from the adrenal cortex can contribute to the human female's sexual responsiveness, similar to the case of the female rhesus monkey, but the accuracy of this suggestion has not been evaluated adequately.

REFERENCES

Adkins, E. K.   Hormonal basis of sexual differentiation in the Japanese quail. *Journal of Comparative and Physiological Psychology*, 1975, 89, 61-71.
Adler, N. T.   Effects of the male's copulatory behavior on successful pregnancy of the female rat. *Journal of Comparative and Physiological Psychology*, 1969, 69, 613-622.
Adler, N. T.   The behavioral control of reproductive physiology. In W. Montagna & W. A. Sadler (Eds.), *Reproductive Behavior*. New York: Plenum Press, 1974, pp. 259-286.
Adler, N. T., Resko, J. A. & Goy, R. W.   The effect of copulatory

behavior on hormonal change in the female rat prior to implantation. *Physiology and Behavior*, 1970, 5, 1003-1007.

Adler, N. T. & Zoloth, S. R. Copulatory behavior can inhibit pregnancy in female rats. *Science*, 1970, 168, 1480-1482.

Alsum, P. & Goy, R. W. Actions of esters of testosterone, dihydrotestosterone or estradiol on sexual behavior in castrated male guinea pigs. *Hormones and Behavior*, 1974, 5, 207-217.

Arai, Y. & Gorski, R. A. Effect of anti-estrogens on steroid induced sexual receptivity in ovariectomized rats. *Physiology and Behavior*, 1968, 3, 351-353.

Ball, J. Sexual responsiveness in female monkeys after castration and subsequent estrin administration. *Psychological Bulletin*, 1936, 33, 811.

Ball, J. The effect of testosterone on the sex behavior of female rats. *Journal of Comparative Psychology*, 1940, 29, 151-165.

Barraclough, C. A. & Gorski, R. A. Studies on mating behaviour in the androgen-sterilized female rat in relation to the hypothalamic regulation of sexual behaviour. *Journal of Endocrinology*, 1962, 25, 175-182.

Baum, M. J. & Vreeburg, J. T. M. Copulation in castrated male rats following combined treatment with estradiol and dihydrotestosterone. *Science*, 1973, 182, 283-285.

Baum, M. J. & Vreeburg, J. T. M. Differential effects of the anti-estrogen MER-25 and three 5-α-reduced androgens on mounting and lordosis behavior in the rat. *Hormones and Behavior*, 1976, 7, 87-104.

Beach, F. A. Sex reversals in the mating pattern of the rat. *Journal of Genetic Psychology*, 1938, 53, 329-334.

Beach, F. A. Copulatory behavior in prepuberally castrated male rats and its modification by estrogen administration. *Endocrinology*, 1942, 31, 679-683.

Beach, F. A. Bisexual mating behavior in the male rat: effects of castration and hormone administration. *Physiological Zoology*, 1945, 18, 390-402.

Beach, F. A. Evolutionary changes in the physiological control of mating behavior in mammals. *Psychological Review*, 1947, 54, 297-315.

Beach, F. A. *Hormones and Behavior*. New York: Hoeber, 1948.

Beach, F. A. (Ed.), *Sex and Behavior*. New York: Wiley, 1965.

Beach, F. A. Factors involved in the control of mounting behavior by female mammals. In M. Diamond (Ed.), *Perspectives in Reproduction and Sexual Behavior*. Bloomington, Ind.: Indiana University Press, 1968, pp. 83-131.

Beach, F. A. Hormonal factors controlling the differentiation, development and display of copulatory behavior in the ramstergig and related species. In E. Tobach, L. R. Aronson & E. Shaw (Eds.), *The Biopsychology of Development*. New York: Academic Press, 1971, pp. 249-296.

Beach, F. A. Behavioral endocrinology and the study of reproduction. *Biology of Reproduction*, 1974, 10, 2-18.

Beach, F. A. Hormonal modification of sexually dimorphic behavior. *Psychoneuroendocrinology*, 1975, 1, 3-23.

Beach, F. A. Sexual attractivity, proceptivity, and receptivity in female mammals. *Hormones and Behavior*, 1976, 7, 105-138. (a)

Beach, F. A. Cross-species comparisons and the human heritage. *Archives of Sexual Behavior*, 1976, 5, 469-485. (b)

Beach, F. A. & Fowler, H. Individual differences in the response of male rats to androgens. *Journal of Comparative and Physiological Psychology*, 1959, 52, 50-52.

Beach, F. A. & Holz, A. M. Mating behavior in male rats castrated at various ages and injected with androgens. *Journal of Experimental Zoology*, 1946, 101, 91-142.

Beach, F. A. & Holz-Tucker, A. M. Effects of different concentrations of androgen upon sexual behavior in castrated male rats. *Journal of Comparative and Physiological Psychology*, 1949, 42, 433-453.

Beach, F. A. & Levinson, G. Effects of androgen on the glans penis and mating behavior of castrated male rats. *Journal of Experimental Zoology*, 1950, 114, 159-171.

Beach, F. A. & Merari, A. Coital behavior in dogs: V. effects of estrogen and progesterone on mating and other forms of social behavior in the bitch. *Journal of Comparative and Physiological Psychology*, 1970, 70, 1-22.

Beach, F. A., Noble, R. G. & Orndoff, R. K. Effects of perinatal androgen treatment on responses of male rats to gonadal hormones in adulthood. *Journal of Comparative and Physiological Psychology*, 1969, 68, 490-497.

Beach, F. A. & Rasquin, P. Masculine copulatory behavior in intact and castrated female rats. *Endocrinology*, 1942, 31, 393-409.

Bermant, G. & Davidson, J. M. *Biological Basis of Sexual Behavior*. New York: Harper & Row, 1974.

Bloch, G. J. & Davidson, J. M. Effects of adrenalectomy and experience on postcastration sex behavior in the male rat. *Physiology and Behavior*, 1968, 3, 461-465.

Boling, J. L. & Blandau, R. J. The estrogen-progesterone induction of mating responses in the spayed female rat. *Endocrinology*, 1939, 25, 359-364.

Burdine, W. E., Shipley, T. E. & Papas, A. T. Delatestryl, a long-acting androgenic hormone: its use as an adjunct in the treatment of women with sexual frigidity. *Fertility and Sterility*, 1957, 8, 255-259.

Carter, C. S. Unpublished review, 1977.

Carter, C. S. Postcopulatory sexual receptivity in the female hamster: the role of the ovary and the adrenal. *Hormones and Behavior*, 1972, 3, 261-265.

Carter, C. S., Landauer, M. R., Tierney, B. M. & Jones, T. Regulation of female sexual behavior in the golden hamster: behavioral effects of mating and ovarian hormones. *Journal of Comparative and Physiological Psychology*, 1976, 90, 839-850.

Carter, C. S. & Porges, S. W. Ovarian hormones and the duration of sexual receptivity in the female golden hamster. *Hormones and Behavior*, 1974, 5, 303-315.

Christensen, L. W. & Clemens, L. G. Intrahypothalamic implants of testosterone or estradiol and resumption of masculine sexual behavior in long-term castrated male rats. *Endocrinology*, 1974, 95, 984-990.

Crowley, W. R., Rodriguez-Sierra, J. F. & Komisaruk, B. R. Hypophysectomy facilitates sexual behavior in female rats. *Neuroendocrinology*, 1976, 20, 328-338.

Daniels, G. E. Approaches to a biological basis of human behavior. *Diseases of the Nervous System*, 1971, 32, 227-240.

Davidson, J. M. Activation of the male rat's sexual behavior by intracerebral implantation of androgens. *Endocrinology*, 1966, 79, 783-794.

Davidson, J. M. Hormones and reproductive behavior. In S. Levine (Ed.), *Hormones and Behavior*. New York: Academic Press, 1972, pp. 64-104.

Davidson, J. M. & Bloch, G. J. Neuroendocrine aspects of male reproduction. *Biology of Reproduction*, 1969, 1, 67-92.

Davidson, J. M., Rodgers, C. H., Smith, E. R. & Bloch, G. J. Stimulation of female sex behavior in adrenalectomized rats with estrogen alone. *Endocrinology*, 1968, 82, 193-195.

Davidson, J. M., Smith, E. R., Rodgers, C. H. & Bloch, G. J. Relative thresholds of behavioral and somatic responses to estrogen. *Physiology and Behavior*, 1968, 3, 227-229.

Davidson, J. M. & Trinpin, S. Neural mediation of steroid-induced sexual behavior in rats. In M. Sandler & G. L. Gessa (Eds.), *Sexual Behavior: Pharmacology and Biochemistry*. New York: Raven Press, 1975, pp. 13-20.

Dempsey, E. W., Hertz, R. & Young, W. C. The experimental induction of oestrus (sexual receptivity) in the normal and ovariectomized guinea pig. *American Journal of Physiology*, 1936, 116, 201-209.

Dixson, A. F., Everitt, B. J., Herbert, J., Rugman, S. M. & Scruton, D. M. Hormonal and other determinants of sexual attractiveness and receptivity in rhesus and talapoin monkeys. *Symposia of the IVth International Congress of Primatology*, 1973, 2, 36-63.

Dufy-Barbe, L., Franchimont, P. & Faure, J. M. A.   Time-courses of LH and FSH release after mating in the female rabbit. *Endocrinology*, 1973, 92, 1318-1321.
Eaton, G. G.   Social and endocrine determinants of sexual behavior in simian and prosimian females. *Symposia of the IVth International Congress of Primatology*, 1973, 2, 20-35.
Edwards, D. A. & Thompson, M. L.   Neonatal androgenization and estrogenization and the hormonal induction of sexual receptivity in rats. *Physiology and Behavior*, 1970, 5, 1115-1119.
Edwards, D. A., Whalen, R. E. & Nadler, R. D.   Induction of estrus: estrogen-progesterone interactions. *Physiology and Behavior*, 1968, 3, 29-33.
Everitt, B. J. & Herbert, J.   Adrenal glands and sexual receptivity in female rhesus monkeys. *Nature*, 1969, 222, 1065-1066.
Everitt, B. J. & Herbert, J.   The effects of dexamethasone and androgens on sexual receptivity of female rhesus monkeys. *Journal of Endocrinology*, 1971, 51, 575-588.
Everitt, B. J., Herbert, J. & Hamer, J. D.   Sexual receptivity of bilaterally adrenalectomized female rhesus monkeys. *Physiology and Behavior*, 1972, 8, 409-415.
Feder, H. H.   The comparative actions of testosterone propionate and 5-α-androstan-17-β-ol-3-one propionate on the reproductive behaviour, physiology and morphology of male rats. *Journal of Endocrinology*, 1971, 51, 241-252.
Feder, H. H., Naftolin, F. & Ryan, K. J.   Male and female sexual responses in male rats given estradiol benzoate and 5-α-androstan-17-β-ol-3-one propionate. *Endocrinology*, 1974, 94, 136-141.
Feder, H. H. & Whalen, R. E.   Feminine behavior in neonatally castrated and estrogen-treated male rats. *Science*, 1965, 147, 306-307.
Filler, W. & Drezner, N.   The results of surgical castration in women under forty. *American Journal of Obstetrics and Gynecology*, 1944, 47, 122-124.
Ford, C. S. & Beach, F. A.   *Patterns of Sexual Behavior*. New York: Harper & Bros., 1952.
Gerall, A. A.   Hormonal factors influencing masculine behavior of female guinea pigs. *Journal of Comparative and Physiological Psychology*, 1966, 62, 365-369.
Gerall, A. A., Dunlap, J. L. & Wagner, R. A.   Effects of dihydrotestosterone and gonadotropins on the development of female behavior. *Physiology and Behavior*, 1976, 17, 121-126.
Gerall, A. A. & Kenney, A. M.   Neonatally androgenized female's responsiveness to estrogen and progesterone. *Endocrinology*, 1970, 87, 560-566.
Gerall, A. A. & Ward, I. L.   Effects of prenatal exogenous androgen

on the sexual behavior of the female albino rat. *Journal of Comparative and Physiological Psychology*, 1966, 62, 370-375.

Goldfoot, D. A. Sociosexual behavior of nonhuman primates during development and maturity: social and hormonal relationships. In A. Schrier (Ed.), *Behavioral Primatology: Advances in Research and Theory*. Hillsdale, New Jersey: Lawrence Ehrlbaum, 1977, pp. 139-184.

Goldfoot, D. A. & Goy, R. W. Abbreviation of behavioral estrus in guinea pigs by coital and vagino-cervical stimulation. *Journal of Comparative Physiological Psychology*, 1970, 72, 426-434.

Goldfoot, D. A., Resko, J. A. & Goy, R. W. Induction of target organ insensitivity to testosterone in the male guinea pig with cyproterone. *Journal of Endocrinology*, 1971, 50, 423-429.

Goldfoot, D. A. & van der Werff ten Bosch, J. J. Mounting behavior of female guinea pigs after prenatal and adult administration of the propionates of testosterone, dihydrotestosterone, and androstanediol. *Hormones and Behavior*, 1975, 6, 139-148.

Gordon, M. B. & Fields, E. M. Observations on the effect of chorionic gonadotropic hormone and male sex hormone on eunochoidism. *Journal of Clinical Endocrinology*, 1943, 3, 589-595.

Goy, R. W. Organizing effects of androgens on the behaviour of rhesus monkeys. In R. P. Michael (Ed.), *Endocrinology and Human Behaviour*. London: Oxford University Press, 1968, pp. 12-31.

Goy, R. W., Bridson, W. E. & Young, W. C. Period of maximal susceptibility of the prenatal guinea pig to masculinizing actions of testosterone propionate. *Journal of Comparative and Physiological Psychology*, 1964, 57, 166-174.

Goy, R. W. & Goldfoot, D. A. Hormonal influences on sexually dimorphic behavior. In *Handbook of Physiology—Endocrinology II, Part I*. Washington: American Physiological Society, 1973, pp. 169-186.

Goy, R. W. & Goldfoot, D. A. Neuroendocrinology: animal models and problems of human sexuality. *Archives of Sexual Behavior*, 1975, 4, 405-420.

Goy, R. W. & Phoenix, C. H. The effects of testosterone propionate administered before birth on the development and behavior in genetic female rhesus monkeys. In C. Sawyer & R. Gorski (Eds.), *Steroid Hormones and Brain Function*. Berkeley: University of California Press, 1971, pp. 193-201.

Goy, R. W., Phoenix, C. H. & Young, W. C. Inhibitory action of the corpus luteum on the hormonal induction of estrous behavior in the guinea pig. *General and Comparative Endocrinology*, 1966, 6, 267-275.

Goy, R. W. & Resko, J. A. Gonadal hormones and behavior of normal and pseudohermaphroditic nonhuman female primates. *Recent Progress in Hormone Research*, 1972, 28, 707-731.

Goy, R. W. & Young, W. C. Strain differences in the behavioral responses of female guinea pigs to alpha-estradiol benzoate and progesterone. *Behaviour*, 1957, 10, 340-354.

Greenough, W. R., Carter, C. S., Steerman, C. & DeVoogd, T. J. Sex differences in dendrite patterns in hamster preoptic area. *Brain Research*, 1976, in press.

Grunt, J. A. & Young, W. C. Differential reactivity of individuals and the response of the male guinea pig to testosterone propionate. *Endocrinology*, 1952, 51, 237-248.

Grunt, J. A. & Young, W. C. Consistency of sexual behavior patterns in individual male guinea pigs following castration and androgen therapy. *Journal of Comparative and Physiological Psychology*, 1953, 46, 138-144.

Harding, C. F. & Feder, H. H. Relation between individual differences in sexual behavior and plasma testosterone levels in the guinea pig. *Endocrinology*, 1976, 98, 1198-1205. (a)

Harding, C. F. & Feder, H. H. Relation of uptake and metabolism of (1,2,6,7-^{3}H)-testosterone to individual differences in sexual behavior in male guinea pigs. *Brain Research*, 1976, 105, 137-149. (b)

Hardy, D. F. & DeBold, J. F. Effects of coital stimulation upon behavior of the female rat. *Journal of Comparative and Physiological Psychology*, 1972, 78, 400-408.

Hart, B. L. & Haugen, C. M. Activation of sexual reflexes in male rats by spinal implantation of testosterone. *Physiology and Behavior*, 1968, 3, 735-738.

Hawke, C. C. Castration and sex crimes. *American Journal of Mental Deficiency*, 1950, 55, 220-226.

Jakobovits, T. The treatment of impotence with methyltestosterone thyroid. *Fertility and Sterility*, 1970, 21, 32-35.

Johnson, D. F. & Phoenix, C. H. Hormonal control of female sexual attractiveness, proceptivity and receptivity in rhesus monkeys. *Journal of Comparative and Physiological Psychology*, 1976, 90, 473-483.

Johnson, W. A. & Tiefer, L. Mating in castrated male rats during combined treatment with estradiol benzoate and fluoxymesterone. *Endocrinology*, 1974, 95, 912-915.

Kamel, F., Mock, E. J., Wright, W. W. & Frankel, A. I. Alterations in plasma concentrations of testosterone, LH, and prolectin associated with mating in the male rat. *Hormones and Behavior*, 1975, 6, 277-288.

Kanematsu, S., Scaramuzzi, R. J., Hilliard, J. & Sawyer, C. H. Patterns of ovulation-inducing LH release following coitus, electrical stimulation and exogenous LHRH in the rabbit. *Endocrinology*, 1974, 95, 247-252.

Komisaruk, B. R.   Neural and hormonal interactions in the reproductive behavior of female rats. In W. Montagna & W. A. Sadler (Eds.), *Reproductive Behavior*. New York: Plenum Press, 1974, pp. 97-129.

Komisaruk, B. R., Adler, N. T. & Hutchinson, J.   Genital sensory field: enlargement by estrogen treatment in female rats. *Science*, 1972, 178, 1295-1298.

Kow, L-M. & Pfaff, D. W.   Effects of estrogen treatment on the size of receptive field and response threshold of pudendal nerve in the female rat. *Neuroendocrinology*, 1974, 13, 299-313.

Larsson, K.   Individual differences in reactivity to androgen in male rats. *Physiology and Behavior*, 1966, 1, 255-258.

Larsson, K., Södersten, P. & Beyer, C.   Induction of male sexual behaviour by oestradiol benzoate in combination with dihydrotestosterone. *Journal of Endocrinology*, 1973, 57, 563-564.

Lehrman, D. S.   Hormonal regulation of parental behavior in birds and infrahuman mammals. In W. C. Young (Ed.), *Sex and Internal Secretions*. Baltimore: Williams & Wilkins, 1961, pp. 1268-1382.

Lehrman, D. S.   Interaction between internal and external environments in the regulation of the reproductive cycle of the ring dove. In F. A. Beach (Ed.), *Sex and Behavior*. New York: Wiley, 1965, pp. 355-380.

Lisk, R. D.   Diencephalic placement of estradiol and sexual receptivity in the female rat. *American Journal of Physiology*, 1962, 203, 493-496.

Lisk, R. D.   Neural localization for androgen activation of copulatory behavior in the male rat. *Endocrinology*, 1967, 80, 754-761.

Lisk, R. D.   Hormonal regulation of sexual behavior in polyestrous mammals common to the laboratory. In *Handbook of Physiology*, Sec. 7, Vol. 2. Washington: American Physiological Society, 1973, pp. 223-260.

Luttge, W. G.   The role of gonadal hormones in the sexual behavior of the rhesus monkey and human: a literature survey. *Archives of Sexual Behavior*, 1971, 1, 61-88.

Luttge, W. G.   Effects of anti-estrogens on testosterone stimulated male sexual behavior and peripheral target tissues in the castrate male rat. *Physiology and Behavior*, 1975, 14, 839-846.

Luttge, W. G., Hall, N. R., Wallis, C. J. & Campbell, J. C.   Stimulation of male and female sexual behavior in gonadectomized rats with estrogen and androgen therapy and its inhibition with concurrent antihormone therapy. *Physiology and Behavior*, 1975, 14, 65-73.

Macrides, F., Bartke, A. & Dalterio, S.   Strange females increase plasma testosterone levels in male mice. *Science*, 1975, 189, 1104-1106.

Masters, W. H. & Johnson, V. E. *Human Sexual Response*. Boston: Little, Brown, 1966.

Michael, R. P. Gonadal hormones and the control of primate behaviour. In R. P. Michael (Ed.), *Endocrinology and Human Behaviour*. London: Oxford University Press, 1968, pp. 69-93.

Michael, R. P. Hormonal factors and aggressive behaviour in the rhesus monkey. In *Proceedings of the International Society of Psychoneuroendocrinology*, Basel: S. Karger, 1971, pp. 412-423.

Michael, R. P., Herbert, J. & Welegalla, J. Ovarian hormones and the sexual behaviour of the male rhesus monkey (*Macaca mulatta*) under laboratory conditions. *Journal of Endocrinology*, 1967, 39, 81-98.

Michael, R. P., Saayman, G. S. & Zumpe, D. Sexual attractiveness and receptivity in rhesus monkeys. *Nature*, 1967, 215, 554-556.

Michael, R. P. & Welegalla, J. Ovarian hormones and the sexual behaviour of the female rhesus monkey (*Macaca mulatta*) under laboratory conditions. *Journal of Endocrinology*, 1968, 41, 407-420.

Michael, R. P. & Wilson, M. Effect of castration and hormone replacement in fully adult male rhesus monkeys (*Macaca mulatta*). *Endocrinology*, 1974, 95, 150-159.

Michael, R. P. & Wilson, M. I. Mating seasonality in castrated male rhesus monkeys. *Journal of Reproduction and Fertility*, 1975, 43, 325-328.

Michael, R. P., Wilson, M. I. & Zumpe, D. The bisexual behavior of female rhesus monkeys. In R. C. Friedman, R. M. Reichart & R. L. van de Wiele (Eds.), *Sex Differences in Behavior*. New York: Wiley, 1974, pp. 399-412.

Michael, R. P. & Zumpe, D. Aggression and gonadal hormones in captive rhesus monkeys (*Macaca mulatta*). *Animal Behavior*, 1970, 18, 1-10.

Money, J. Sex hormones and other variables in human eroticism. In W. C. Young (Ed.), *Sex and Internal Secretions, Vol. II*. Baltimore: Williams & Wilkins, 1961, pp. 1383-1400. (a)

Money, J. Components of eroticism in man: I. the hormones in relation to sexual morphology and sexual desire. *Journal of Nervous and Mental Diseases*, 1961, 132, 239-248. (b)

Money, J. & Ehrhardt, A. A. *Man and Woman, Boy and Girl*. Baltimore: Johns Hopkins University Press, 1972.

Money, J., Wiedeking, C., Walker, P., Migeon, C., Meyer, W. & Borgaonkar, D. 47,XXY and 46,XY males with antisocial and/or sex-offending behavior: anti-androgen therapy plus counseling. *Psychoneuroendocrinology*, 1975, 1, 165-178.

Montagna, W. & Sadler, W. A. (Eds.), *Reproductive Behavior*. New York: Plenum Press, 1974.

Morin, L. P. & Feder, H. H. Multiple progesterone injections and the duration of estrus in ovariectomized guinea pigs. *Physiology and Behavior*, 1973, 11, 861-865.

Morin, L. P. & Feder, H. H. Inhibition of lordosis behavior in ovariectomized guinea pigs by mesencephalic implants of progesterone. *Brain Research*, 1974, 70, 71-80. (a)

Morin, L. P. & Feder, H. H. Hypothalamic progesterone implants and facilitation of lordosis behavior in estrogen-primed ovariectomized guinea pigs. *Brain Research*, 1974, 70, 81-93. (b)

Morin, L. P. & Feder, H. H. Intracranial estradiol benzoate implants and lordosis behavior of ovariectomized guinea pigs. *Brain Research*, 1974, 70, 95-102. (c)

Moss, R. L. Relationship between the central regulation of gonadotropins and mating behaviour in female rats. In W. Montagna & W. A. Sadler (Eds.), *Reproductive Behavior*. New York: Plenum Press, 1974, pp. 55-76.

Moss, R. L. & McCann, S. M. Induction of mating behavior in rats by luteinizing hormone-release factor. *Science*, 1973, 181, 177-179.

Mullins, R. F. & Levine, S. Hormonal determinants during infancy of adult sexual behavior in the female rat. *Physiology and Behavior*, 1968, 3, 333-338.

Nadler, R. D. Masculinization of female rats by intracranial implantation of androgen in infancy. *Journal of Comparative and Physiological Psychology*, 1968, 66, 157-167.

Nadler, R. D. Intrahypothalamic locus for induction of androgen sterilization in neonatal female rats. *Neuroendocrinology*, 1972, 9, 349-357.

Nadler, R. D. Further evidence on the intrahypothalamic locus for androgenization of female rats. *Neuroendocrinology*, 1973, 12, 110-119.

Nadler, R. D. Sexual cyclicity in captive lowland gorillas. *Science*, 1975, 189, 813-814.

Naftolin, F., Ryan, K. J. & Davies, I. J. (Eds.), *Subcellular Mechanisms in Reproductive Neuroendocrinology*. Amsterdam: Elsevier, 1976.

Naftolin, F., Ryan, K. J. & Petro, Z. Aromatization of androstenedione by the anterior hypothalamus of adult male and female rats. *Endocrinology*, 1972, 90, 295-298.

Paup, D. C., Mennin, S. P. & Gorski, R. A. Androgen- and estrogen-induced copulatory behavior and inhibition of luteinizing hormone (LH) secretion in the male rat. *Hormones and Behavior*, 1975, 6, 35-46.

Pfaff, D.   Nature of sex hormone effects on rat sex behavior: Specificity of effects and individual patterns of response. *Journal of Comparative and Physiological Psychology*, 1970, 73, 349-358.

Pfaff, D. W.   Steroid sex hormones in the rat brain: Specificity of uptake and physiological effects. In C. H. Sawyer & R. A. Gorski (Eds.), *Steroid Hormones and Brain Function*. Berkeley: University of California Press, 1971, pp. 103-112.

Pfaff, D. W.   Luteinizing hormone-release factor potentiates lordosis behavior in hypophysectomized female rats. *Science*, 1973, 182, 1148-1149.

Phoenix, C. H.   The role of testosterone in the sexual behavior of laboratory male rhesus. *Symposia of the IVth International Congress of Primatology*, 1973, 2, 99-122.

Phoenix, C. H.   Effects of dihydrotestosterone on sexual behavior of castrated male rhesus monkeys. *Physiology and Behavior*, 1974, 12, 1045-1055.

Phoenix, C. H., Goy, R. W., Gerall, A. A. & Young, W. C.   Organizing action of prenatally administered testosterone propionate on the tissue mediating mating behavior in the female guinea pig. *Endocrinology*, 1959, 65, 369-382.

Phoenix, C. H., Slob, A. K. & Goy, R. W.   Effects of castration and replacement therapy on sexual behavior of adult male rhesus. *Journal of Comparative and Physiological Psychology*, 1973, 84, 472-481.

Powers, J. B.   Hormonal control of sexual receptivity during the estrous cycle of the rat. *Physiology and Behavior*, 1970, 5, 831-835.

Powers, J. B.   Facilitation of lordosis in ovariectomized rats by intracerebral progesterone implants. *Brain Research*, 1972, 48, 311-325.

Powers, J. B. & Moreines, J.   Progesterone: examination of its postulated inhibitory actions on lordosis during the rat estrous cycle. *Physiology and Behavior*, 1976, 17, 493-498.

Powers, J. B. & Valenstein, E. S.   Sexual receptivity: facilitation by medial preoptic lesions in female rats. *Science*, 1972, 175, 1003-1005.

Powers, J. B. & Zucker, I.   Sexual receptivity in pregnant and pseudo-pregnant rats. *Endocrinology*, 1969, 84, 820-827.

Purvis, K. & Haynes, N. B.   Short-term effects of copulation, human chorionic gonadotrophin injection and non-tactile association with a female on testosterone levels in the male rat. *Journal of Endocrinology*, 1974, 60, 429-439.

Quadagno, D. M. & Ho, G. K. W.   The reversible inhibition of steroid-induced sexual behavior by intracranial cyclohexamide. *Hormones and Behavior*, 1975, 6, 19-26.

Raisman, G. & Field, P. M.   Sexual dimorphism in the neuropil of the preoptic area of the rat and its dependence on neonatal androgen. *Brain Research*, 1973, 54, 1-29.

Robinson, J. A., Scheffler, G., Eisele, S. G. & Goy, R. W. Effects of age and season on sexual behavior and plasma testosterone concentrations of laboratory-housed male rhesus monkeys (*Macaca mulatta*). *Biology of Reproduction,* 1975, 13, 203-210.

Rodgers, C. H. Influence of copulation on ovulation in the cycling rat. *Endocrinology,* 1971, 88, 433-436.

Resko, J. A. & Phoenix, C. H. Sexual behavior and testosterone concentrations in the plasma of the rhesus monkey before and after castration. *Endocrinology,* 1972, 91, 499-503.

Saginor, M. & Horton, R. Reflex release of gonadotropin and increased plasma testosterone concentration in male rabbits during copulation. *Endocrinology,* 1968, 82, 627-630.

Salmon, U. J. & Geist, S. H. Effect of androgens upon libido in women. *Journal of Clinical Endocrinology,* 1943, 3, 235-238.

Sandler, M. & Gessa, G. L. (Eds.), *Sexual Behavior: Pharmacology and Biochemistry.* New York: Raven Press, 1975.

Södersten, P. Effects of an estrogen antagonist, MER-25, on mounting behavior and lordosis behavior in the female rat. *Hormones and Behavior,* 1974, 5, 111-121.

Södersten, P. Mounting behavior and lordosis behavior in castrated male rats treated with testosterone propionate or with estradiol benzoate or dihydrotestosterone in combination with testosterone propionate. *Hormones and Behavior,* 1975, 6, 109-126.

Södersten, P. & Larsson, K. Lordosis behavior in castrated male rats treated with estradiol benzoate or testosterone propionate in combination with an estrogen antagonist, MER-25, and in intact male rats. *Hormones and Behavior,* 1974, 5, 13-18.

Södersten, P., De Jong, F. H., Vreeburg, J. T. M. & Baum, M. J. Lordosis behavior in intact male rats: absence of a correlation with mounting behavior or testicular secretion of estradiol-17 and testosterone. *Physiology and Behavior,* 1974, 13, 803-808.

Sopchak, A. L. & Sutherland, A. M. Psychological impact of cancer and its treatment. VII. Exogenous hormones and their relation to lifelong adaptation in women with metastatic cancer of the breast. *Cancer,* 1960, 13, 528-531.

Stone, C. P. The retention of copulatory ability in male rats following castration. *Journal of Comparative Psychology,* 1927, 7, 369-387.

Stürup, G. K. Castration: the total treatment. In H. L. P. Resnick & M. E. Wolfgang (Eds.), *Sexual Behaviours: Social, Clinical and Legal Aspects.* Boston: Little, Brown, 1972.

Tauber, E. S. Effects of castration upon the sexuality of the adult male. *Psychosomatic Medicine,* 1940, 2, 74-87.

Terkel, A. S., Shryne, J. & Gorski, R. A. Inhibition of estrogen facilitation of sexual behavior by the intracerebral infusion of actinomycin-D. *Hormones and Behavior,* 1973, 4, 377-386.

Udry, J. R. & Morris, N. M.   Distribution of coitus in the menstrual cycle. *Nature,* 1968, 220, 593-596.

Wallen, K., Goy, R. W. & Phoenix, C. H.   Inhibitory actions of progesterone on hormonal induction of estrus in female guinea pigs. *Hormones and Behavior,* 1975, 6, 127-138.

Ward, I. L.   Differential effect of pre- and postnatal androgen on the sexual behavior of intact and spayed female rats. *Hormones and Behavior,* 1969, 1, 25-36.

Waxenberg, S. E., Drellich, M. G. & Sutherland, A. M.   The role of hormones in human behavior: I. Changes in female sexuality after adrenalectomy. *Journal of Clinical Endocrinology,* 1959, 19, 193-202.

Waxenberg, S. E., Finkbeiner, J. A., Drellich, M. G. & Sutherland, A. M.   The role of hormones in human behavior: II. changes in sexual behavior in relation to vaginal smears of breast-cancer patients after oopherectomy and adrenalectomy. *Psychosomatic Medicine,* 1960, 22, 435-422.

Whalen, R. E.   Sexual Motivation. *Psychological Review,* 1966, 73, 161-163.

Whalen, R. E.   Differentiation of the neural mechanisms which control gonadotropin secretion and sexual behavior. In M. Diamond (Ed.), *Perspectives in Reproduction and Sexual Behavior.* Bloomington: Indiana University Press, 1968, pp. 303-340.

Whalen, R. E.   Sexual differentiation: models, methods, and mechanisms. In R. C. Friedman, R. M. Reichart & R. L. van de Wiele (Eds.), *Sex Differences in Behavior.* New York: Wiley, 1974, pp. 467-481.

Whalen, R. E., Battie, C. & Luttge, W. G.   Anti-estrogen inhibition of androgen-induced sexual receptivity in rats. *Behavioral Biology,* 1972, 7, 311-320.

Whalen, R. E. & Gorzalka, B. B.   Effects of an estrogen antagonist on behavior and on estrogen retention in neural and peripheral target tissues. *Physiology and Behavior,* 1973, 10, 35-40.

Whalen, R. E., Gorzalka, B. B., DeBold, J. F., Quadagno, D. M., Ho, G. K-W. & Hough, J. C.   Studies on the effects of intracerebral actinomycin-D implants on estrogen-induced receptivity in rats. *Hormones and Behavior,* 1974, 5, 337-343.

Whalen, R. E. & Hardy, D. F.   Induction of receptivity in female rats and cats with estrogen and testosterone. *Physiology and Behavior,* 1970, 5, 529-533.

Whalen, R. E. & Luttge, W. G.   Testosterone, androstenedione and dihydrotestosterone: effects on mating behavior of male rats. *Hormones and Behavior,* 1971, 2, 117-125.

Young, W. C.   Observations and experiments on mating behavior in female mammals. *Quarterly Review of Biology*, 1941, 16, 135-136 & 311-335.

Young, W. C.   The hormones and mating behavior. In W. C. Young (Ed.), *Sex and Internal Secretions, Vol. II*. Baltimore: Williams & Wilkins, 1961, pp. 1173-1239.

Young, W. C.   The organization of sexual behavior by hormonal action during the prenatal and larval periods in vertebrates. In F. A. Beach (Ed.), *Sex and Behavior*. New York: Wiley, 1965, pp. 89-107.

Young, W. C., Goy, R. W. & Phoenix, C. H.   Hormones and sexual behavior. *Science*, 1964, 143, 212-218.

Zucker, I.   Actions of progesterone in the control of sexual receptivity of the spayed female rat. *Journal of Comparative and Physiological Psychology*, 1967, 63, 313-316.

Chapter 6

PARENTAL BEHAVIOR

Successful reproduction demands more than simply copulation. Fetuses must be brought to term, and, once born, the young must be cared for until they can survive on their own. There are many behaviors associated with the care of the young, called *parental behaviors,* and although there are exceptions, as in some birds, the mother is the primary caretaker in most species. Most studies of the role of hormones in parental behavior have focused on the caretaking activities carried out by the female of the species, *maternal behavior.* The discussion that follows is concerned primarily with the role of hormones in the maternal behaviors of laboratory mammals, because these animals have received the most attention. One section of this discussion, however, is devoted to the case of parental behavior in ring doves, an avian species that has been studied extensively.

MAMMALS

Interest in the relationship between endocrine function and maternal behavior in laboratory animals probably emerged from observations of the coincidence between the rapid onset of maternal behavior and the dramatic hormonal changes that occur around the time of parturition. Probably the first detailed analysis of maternal behavior and its physiological basis was the classic series of studies conducted by Wiesner and Sheard (1933) on the laboratory rat. Later studies have examined maternal behavior in other species, such as the rabbit and the mouse, although the majority has focused on the rat.

Maternal behavior begins to appear even before parturition. For example, although the rat engages in self-licking behavior throughout its lifetime, late in gestation, the female concentrates self-licking in the area of the nipples, presumably in preparation for nursing (Roth & Rosenblatt, 1967). In addition, many animals begin to build maternal nests during late pregnancy, in preparation for the emergence of the young (Slotnick, 1975; Zarrow, Denenberg & Sachs, 1972). Following parturition, the primary maternal responses seem to include nursing behaviors and retrieval of the young when they have strayed (Lamb, 1975; Lehrman, 1961). Each of these behaviors has been studied in relation to endocrine function, and the literature on hormones and maternal behavior is extensive. As has been the case in our earlier discussions, the review that follows is not intended as a comprehensive survey of that literature. Rather, we shall focus here on the major classes of issues and findings. The reader interested in pursuing the relationship between hormones and maternal behavior further is referred to the excellent and more comprehensive reviews by Lamb (1975), Lehrman (1961), Slotnick (1975), and Zarrow, Denenberg, and Sachs (1972).

Before proceeding to our review, it might be useful to summarize briefly the major hormonal events surrounding parturition and lactation. Although there is some variation, the general pattern of hormonal changes is similar across different mammalian species. Figure 6-1 summarizes the changes in the levels of progesterone, the estrogens, and prolactin during pregnancy in rats. Notice that just prior to parturition, there is a marked decline in progesterone levels, followed by sharp increases in the levels of both the estrogens and prolactin. Following parturition, prolactin levels remain high until midway through the lactation period, at which point they slowly decline (Amenomori, Chen & Meites, 1970; Slotnick, 1975).

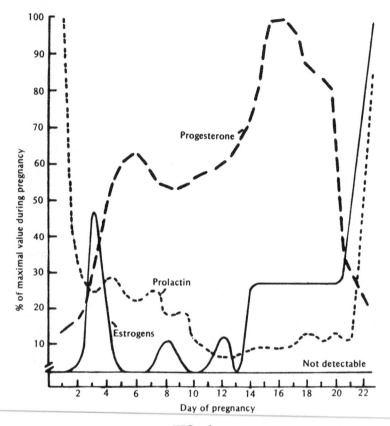

FIG. 6-1

Serum levels of progesterone, estrogen, and prolactin during pregnancy in rats. Serum levels are presented as a percentage of the highest level achieved during pregnancy (modified from Figure 2 of chapter by Slotnick in Eleftheriou and Sprott's *Hormonal Correlates of Behavior.* New York: Plenum Press, 1975, p. 595, by permission).

Hormones have been studied in relation to both the initiation of maternal responsiveness and the maintenance of maternal behavior once initiated. Because the role of hormones appears different in these two aspects of maternal responding, the initiation and maintenance of maternal reactions will be treated separately here. However, in both cases the critical question seems to be the same: Is a particular hormonal state necessary for maternal behavior, and, if so, which hormonal state?

Initiation of Maternal Behavior

The majority of research has used the laboratory rat as the experimental subject. Therefore, this review will begin with the findings derived from those studies of the rat. At the end, we shall discuss the results of studies using other mammals as subjects.

THE RAT The first question one might ask about the role of hormones in the initiation of maternal behavior concerns whether or not the particular hormonal state that coexists with the initiation of maternal responding is essential to that behavior. That is, does the correlation between the hormonal changes around late pregnancy and parturition and the onset of maternal responding represent a truly causal relationship? The answer, simply, is "no." Very early on, Wiesner and Sheard (1933) noted that if virgin rats are kept with newborn pups, the virgins eventually begin to show such maternal behaviors as retrieving and crouching over the young. This phenomenon, wherein nonlactating animals begin to show maternal responding following exposure to young, has been termed *sensitization* or *concaveation*. Concaveation can occur in intact virgin females, ovariectomized virgin females, hypophysectomized virgin females, intact males, and castrated males (Rosenblatt, 1967). Therefore, no combination of pituitary-gonadal hormones can be considered essential to the initiation of maternal responding.

However, parturient females exhibit maternal behavior immediately upon presentation of young, whereas concaveated subjects require between four and seven days of pup exposure before they will behave maternally. Therefore, although the particular hormonal state surrounding late pregnancy and parturition may not be essential to maternal behavior, it may serve some facilitatory function in the initiation of maternal responsiveness.

Whether hormones facilitate the onset of maternal behavior has been asked in both general and specific ways. In the general case, there have been attempts to induce maternal responding in nonlactating animals by treating them with the blood of maternal rats. The earliest attempt by Stone (1925) was unsuccessful. He created a parabiotic preparation by connecting the skins of two female rats. One rat was then impregnated, carried the young to term, and eventually became maternal. Stone reasoned that if the initiation of maternal behavior is affected by the newly parturient female's hormonal state, then the nonparturient, parabiotic partner should become maternal at the same time as the parturient partner. However, the nonparturient female showed no evidence of maternal behavior.

Stone's preparation probably was inadequate, since later studies by Terkel and Rosenblatt succeeded in altering maternal responsiveness in virgin females by transfusing the blood of parturient animals into them. In their first study, Terkel and Rosenblatt (1968) injected plasma taken from females 48 hours after parturition into virgin females. They found that the concaveation latency was significantly shortened in the recipient virgins. Thus, it appeared that some factor in the blood of newly parturient females could facilitate the onset of maternal behavior in virgin females. In a second study, Terkel and Rosenblatt (1972) created a parabiotic preparation wherein blood was continuously cross-transfused between freely moving parturient and virgin females. Again, they found that the blood from newly parturient females shortened the concaveation latency in virgins. Therefore, it appears that there is a blood-borne characteristic of late pregnant and/or newly parturient females that facilitates the initiation of maternal responding.

Having established that a blood-borne factor can facilitate the initiation of maternal behavior, the specific question arises as to the identity of that factor. The first hormone studied was the "primary" hormone of lactation, prolactin. One of the first studies was by Riddle, Lahr, and Bates (1935) who found that injecting an extract of pituitary tissue could induce maternal behavior in virgin females, even without the use of the concaveation procedures. These investigators also reported (Riddle, Lahr & Bates, 1935, 1942) that the same effect of pituitary extracts on maternal behavior could be achieved by injections of prolactin alone. On the other hand, later studies (e.g., Beach & Wilson, 1963; Lott & Fuchs, 1962) found no effect of prolactin treatment alone on maternal behavior. In addition, Obias (1957) reported that hypophysectomizing pregnant rats on the thirteenth day of pregnancy has no effect on their maternal responses following parturition, showing that prolactin is not essential for nor does its absence markedly affect the initiation of maternal responding. As we shall see, however, later studies have shown that prolactin still may have a facilitatory function in the initiation of maternal behavior.

The other major group of hormones studied is the ovarian hormones. In their early studies, Wiesner and Sheard (1933) found no effect of ovariectomy on maternal behavior when the operation was performed either 1-3 days prepartum or 12 hours postpartum. These findings suggested that the ovarian hormones are not important to maternal behavior. However, it may have been that the animals were tested before the ovarian hormones would have been cleared from the bloodstream, and, therefore, those findings could not be considered conclusive. Later studies have examined the effects of the estrogens and progestins separately.

There is conflicting evidence about the effects of manipulating estrogen levels on maternal behavior. Some studies suggest that estrogens can inhibit maternal responding, whereas others suggest that estrogens facilitate the initiation of maternal behavior. In an early study, Riddle, Lahr, and Bates (1942) reported that injecting rats with estrogens blocks maternal retrieving. A later study by Leon, Numan, and Chan (1975) also suggested an inhibitory effect of estrogens on the initiation of maternal responding. These investigators found that ovariectomized-adrenalectomized virgins exhibit shorter concaveation latencies than do virgins that have only been ovariectomized. However, if ovariectomized-adrenalectomized animals are treated with estrogens, they behave much like virgins that have only been ovariectomized. Therefore, it appeared that estrogens can inhibit the initiation of maternal responding in ovariectomized-adrenalectomized virgin rats. Leon and his colleagues interpreted these findings as suggesting that the adrenal can suppress maternal behavior by providing an extra-ovarian source of estrogens.

In contrast to the studies showing an inhibitory effect of the estrogens, Siegel and Rosenblatt have provided data suggesting that the estrogens facilitate the initiation of maternal responding. They found, first, that hysterectomizing pregnant rats prior to parturition leads to an early onset of maternal behavior. If, however, the hysterectomized rats also are ovariectomized, the effect of removing the uterus is blocked (Rosenblatt & Siegel, 1975; Siegel & Rosenblatt, 1975a). Then, if the hysterectomized-ovariectomized female is treated with estrogens, she again becomes maternal very quickly. These findings were interpreted as showing that the rise in estrogen that follows hysterectomy (and the rise in estrogen that precedes parturition) facilitates maternal responding: First, preventing that estrogen rise by ovariectomy retards the initiation of maternal behavior in hysterectomized animals. Second, treating hysterectomized-ovariectomized animals with estrogen restores their maternal responsiveness (Siegel & Rosenblatt, 1975a).

Siegel and Rosenblatt (1975d) also have studied the effects of hysterectomy and ovariectomy in virgin female rats. These studies provided results similar to those of their studies of pregnant rats discussed above. If hysterectomized-ovariectomized virgins are treated with estrogens, these animals exhibit maternal behavior much more quickly following pup exposure than nontreated virgins. In addition, Siegel and Rosenblatt (1975c) found that treating ovariectomized female rats with estrogens stimulates maternal responding.

In summary, there is evidence suggesting that the estrogens can both inhibit and facilitate the initiation of maternal behavior. The differences in the findings of these two groups of studies may be related to methodological differences between them (see Siegel & Rosenblatt, 1975c). However, the fact that there ordinarily is a rise in estrogen levels prior to parturition, when maternal responsiveness is increasing, would lead one to expect a facilitatory effect.

What of the other major ovarian hormone, progesterone? Recall that progesterone levels are fairly high throughout pregnancy, and that those levels drop sharply just prior to parturition. Perhaps this drop facilitates the initiation of maternal responsiveness. Most studies have shown, at least, that the presence of progesterone does inhibit maternal behavior. For example, progesterone treatment increases the concaveation latency in ovariectomized-adrenalectomized virgin females (Leon, Numan & Chan, 1975). In addition, it can block the increase in maternal responding in hysterectomized animals (Siegel & Rosenblatt, 1975b). Therefore, in the rat, the presence of progesterone seems to inhibit the initiation of maternal responsiveness, and, perhaps, its withdrawal just prior to parturition facilitates maternal responding.

The studies reviewed so far all have treated particular hormones singly. However, in the natural state the levels of many hormones change around parturition. Therefore, the question arises as to whether one could induce rapid concaveation in virgin rats by administering the correct hormones in combination and in the proper sequence, in a regimen approximating the natural condition around parturition. Attempts to approximate the natural hormonal changes around parturition have been quite successful in decreasing markedly the concaveation latencies of virgin animals. Two groups of investigators (Lubin et al., 1972; Moltz et al., 1970; Zarrow, Gandelman & Denenberg, 1971) have shown that administering particular sequences of exogenous hormones markedly facilitates the onset of maternal responsiveness in both virgin female and intact male rats. The results of one such study by Moltz et al. (1970) are presented in Figure 6-2. In that study, ovariectomized virgin female rats were treated with estradiol benzoate during Days 1-11, progesterone during Days 6-9, and prolactin during Days 9 and 10. Pups were presented to the test animals on the afternoon of Day 10. As shown in Figure 6-2, the animals treated with this hormone regimen all became maternal within 35-40 hours after pup presentation. Animals treated with either estradiol alone, progesterone alone, or estradiol and progesterone in combination concaveated more slowly. Therefore, this study shows that approximating the natural hormonal events surrounding parturition can facilitate the initiation of maternal responsiveness in virgin rats. It provides the strongest evidence that the sequence of changes in the levels of estrogens, progesterone, and prolactin around the time of parturition are important to the initiation of maternal responsiveness in rats. In addition, in contrast to the studies cited earlier in this section, prolactin does appear to facilitate maternal responding in the rat, but only if it is given in combination with estrogens and progesterone.

THE MOUSE Only a few studies have been conducted considering maternal behavior in mice, and these have focused primarily on the nest-building activities that occur during pregnancy. Those studies have shown, first, that progesterone facilitates nest-building in these rodents. Injecting intact virgin mice with progesterone increases maternal nest-building, as does treating estrogen-primed ovariectomized mice with progesterone (Lisk, 1971). On the other hand, estrogen treatment decreases nest-building in both intact and ovariectomized females (Lisk, Pretlow & Friedman, 1969). Significantly, maternal nest-building ordinarily appears during a period of gestation when the mother's progesterone levels are high and

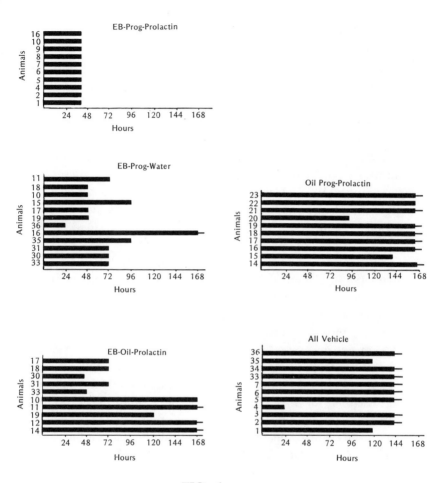

FIG. 6-2

Latency and variability in time of onset for the display of maternal behavior in ovariectomized virgin rats treated with different hormone regimens. Broken bar indicates that the animal failed to act maternally at the conclusion of the observation period. EB = estradiol benzoate; Prog = progesterone (from Moltz, Lubin & Leon, *Physiology and Behavior*, 1970, 5, 1375, by permission of Pergamon Press).

her estrogen levels are low. Therefore, the condition of having high progesterone and low estrogen levels may facilitate the initiation of maternal nest-building in pregnant mice (Lisk, Pretlow & Friedman, 1969).

In contrast to the situation in rats, prolactin treatment alone seems able to facilitate maternal responding in the mouse. Both systemic prolactin administration and prolactin injection directly into the hypothalamus increase retrieving and maternal nest-building in mice (Voci & Carlson, 1973). Therefore, prolactin may be a clear stimulant of maternal behavior in the mouse, and its site of action probably is the hypothalamus.

THE RABBIT Zarrow and his colleagues have conducted an extensive series of studies concerned with the hormonal basis of maternal nest-building in the rabbit. The rabbit builds nests throughout pregnancy, but toward the end, just prior to and during parturition, she pulls out some of her own hair and lines the nest. This type of nest has been termed a "maternal nest," and its construction seems to be affected by the individual's hormonal condition (Zarrow et al., 1961). First, the ovarian hormones do not appear to be essential for maternal nest-building: Although ovariectomy early in gestation will prevent maternal nest-building, during the last few days of pregnancy, it does not affect nest-building in the rabbit (Zarrow, Denenberg & Sachs, 1972; Zarrow et al., 1963). However, as in the rat, there is evidence that although the ovarian hormones may not be necessary for maternal nest-building, the estrogens can facilitate and progesterone can inhibit this behavior. Zarrow et al. (1963) attempted to induce nest-building in nonpregnant rabbits, using nine different hormone regimens. The critical feature of the successful regimen appeared to be producing a shift in the ratio of estrogen and progesterone from progesterone dominance to estrogen dominance. Therefore, Zarrow et al. argued that the reversal in the estrogen/progesterone ratio that occurs prior to parturition is involved in the initiation of maternal nest-building in the rabbit: A condition of high progesterone inhibits, whereas high estrogen facilitates, nest-building.

Zarrow and his colleagues also have implicated a pituitary factor in the control of maternal nest-building. Hypophysectomy during the last third of gestation reduces nest-building in the rabbit, and, although an estrogen and progesterone regimen can induce maternal nest-building in nonpregnant, ovariectomized rabbits, this regimen is ineffective in hypophysectomized rabbits. Therefore, the pituitary gland is necessary for the initiation of maternal nest-building in the rabbit (Anderson et al., 1971).

Which pituitary factor is critical? Preliminary evidence suggests that prolactin is the critical pituitary hormone in the control of maternal nest-building in the rabbit. Treatment with ergocornine, which blocks prolactin secretion, decreases maternal nest-building in pregnant rabbits, and replacement therapy with prolactin is effective in counteracting the effect (Zarrow, Gandelman & Denenberg, 1971). Therefore, prolactin appears essential for maternal nest-building in this species.

SUMMARY: INITIATION OF MATERNAL RESPONDING In this section, we have reviewed what is known about the role of hormones in the initiation of maternal responding in rats, mice, and rabbits. Although there are differences among these species, in each case the hormonal condition that is in effect around the time of the onset of maternal behaviors appears to facilitate the initiation of maternal responding. In the rat, which has been studied most extensively, the hormonal events around parturition appear to facilitate the initiation of maternal responsiveness. For example, the presence of progesterone inhibits maternal responding, and the withdrawal of this hormone just prior to parturition may, therefore, facilitate maternal responding. The situation with the estrogens is somewhat unclear. Some studies suggest that estrogens inhibit maternal responding, whereas others suggest a stimulatory role. That estrogen levels rise just prior to parturition suggests that the

estrogens should facilitate, rather than inhibit, maternal responding. Finally, the pituitary hormone prolactin seems nonessential to
but does facilitate maternal behavior in the rat.

Maternal responding is expressed much earlier in mice than in
rats; maternal nest-building begins quite early in the gestation period. In mice, it appears that the high levels of progesterone present during gestation facilitate maternal nest-building behaviors. In
addition, in contrast to the situation in the rat, increasing the levels
of prolactin alone can facilitate maternal responding.

In the rabbit, maternal nest-building begins just prior to parturition. The experimental data suggest that the decrease in progesterone and increase in estrogen that occur just prior to parturition
facilitate the initiation of this group of responses. In addition, prolactin is essential to the initiation of such responses.

Are there marked species differences in the role of hormones in
maternal responding? The major differences appear to be tied to
the time during gestation or lactation when maternal responses are
first evidenced. For example, in the mouse, maternal nest-building
begins early in gestation and, in this species, high progesterone levels facilitate this behavior. On the other hand, in the rabbit, maternal nest-building begins only just prior to parturition and, therefore, progesterone inhibits the rabbit's tendency to build maternal
nests. One major species difference appears to be related to the
role of prolactin, which seems to have little effect by itself on the
initiation of maternal responding in the rat; but it is clearly important to maternal behavior in both the mouse and the rabbit.

Maintenance of Maternal Responding

As mentioned before, hormones have been studied in relation to
both the initiation of maternal behavior and the maintenance of
maternal responsiveness once it is initiated. We have seen that the
hormonal changes around parturition appear to facilitate the initiation of maternal responding, although these hormonal changes
are not always essential for maternal behavior, since both male and

virgin female rats can be induced to act maternally through concaveation. What of the maintenance of maternal responsiveness?
As has often been the case in our discussions, the issue is unresolved, although preliminary evidence has shown that neither prolactin nor estrogen and progesterone are essential for the maintenance of maternal responding.

The most obvious hormone to study regarding the maintenance
of maternal responding is prolactin. Prolactin levels remain high
during the period of active maternal responding, and as prolactin
levels decline midway through lactation, so do maternal activities
(Amenomori, Chen & Meites, 1970; Rosenblatt & Lehrman, 1963).
This correlation might reflect a direct, causal relationship between
prolactin levels and the maintenance of maternal responsiveness.

Direct experimental tests of this hypothesis, however, have suggested that prolactin is not critical to the maintenance of maternal
responding, at least in the rat. Although blocking prolactin secretion with ergocornine does terminate lactation, it does not affect
ongoing maternal behaviors in the rat (Numan, Leon & Moltz,
1972). Therefore, prolactin is not necessary for the maintenance
of maternal responsiveness. In addition, separating the mother
from her pups reduces both maternal responsiveness and maternal
prolactin levels, but treating the mother with prolactin does not
protect her from the depressive effects of pup separation on maternal responding (Lott & Rosenblatt, 1969). Therefore, prolactin
cannot maintain maternal responsiveness in the absence of continued stimulation by the pups.

Regarding the ovarian hormones, removing estrogen and progesterone from the circulation by ovariectomy does not alter maternal responding once initiated. In addition, progesterone treatment, which inhibits the initiation of maternal behavior in the
rat, has no effect on established maternal responses in this species
(Slotnick, 1975). Thus, neither prolactin nor the ovarian hormones
appear necessary for the maintenance of maternal responding.

Are hormones, therefore, not at all involved in the maintenance of maternal responding? In the same way that hormones are not necessary for but do facilitate the initiation of maternal responding in the rat, it may be that hormones do serve some facilitatory role in the maintenance of maternal behaviors. Concaveated animals exhibit less intense maternal responses, such as retrieving of the young, than do lactating animals (Bridges et al., 1972). This suggests that the hormonal state of lactating animals could be serving to intensify maternal responses. However, the critical experimental tests of this hypothesis have not been conducted, and, therefore, whether hormones can act to facilitate ongoing maternal responses remains speculative.

A variety of nonhormonal factors have been shown to be important to the maintenance of maternal responding. Although a discussion of such factors is outside the realm of this book, it seems worth noting that much of the maintenance of maternal responsiveness does appear to depend on stimulation derived from the young. For example, not dissimilar to the way that presenting pups to nonlactating animals can initiate maternal behavior, separating the pups from maternal animals (whether lactating or sensitized) decreases their maternal responsiveness (Reisbick, Rosenblatt & Mayer, 1975; Rosenblatt & Lehrman, 1963). Significantly, prolactin and the ovarian hormones do not appear to be involved in the maintenance effect of stimuli emanating from the pups (Slotnick, 1975), although it could be that some other hormones are involved in the mediation of such effects.

Maternal Aggression

There is another group of behaviors particular to lactating female rodents that is not a caretaking activity in the same way as are nest-building, nursing, and retrieving. Lactating female rodents (recall from Chapter 3 that most female rodents normally are relatively nonaggressive) will attack and kill a variety of intruders. Specifically, it has been reported that lactating rats, mice, and hamsters will attack both intruding conspecifics and intruding members of other species (see Endröczi, Lissák & Telegdy, 1958, for rats killing frogs; Flandera & Nováková, 1971, for rats killing mice; Gandelman, 1972, for mice attacking other mice; and Wise, 1974, for hamsters attacking other hamsters). The function of this *maternal aggression* is not yet clear, although it may be related to protection of the young from potential predators.

Only the case of mice attacking other mice has been studied extensively. Studies have shown that the hormonal states of both the intruder and the attacker are important to the display of this form of maternal aggression. Beginning with the hormonal state of the intruder, there appears to be a hierarchy of "attackability" among intruders, and the position on that hierarchy depends on the intruder's hormonal state. Although lactating female mice will attack both males and other females, males are attacked much more readily than females (Gandelman, 1972; Rosenson & Asheroff, 1975). Moreover, castrating male mice reduces their attackability, and ovariectomizing female mice reduces the frequency with which they are attacked. Therefore, the gonadal hormones must play a role in determining an intruder's aggression-eliciting qualities. In addition, lactating females are not attacked if they are in the early stages of lactation, although they are attacked if they are in a later lactational stage (Rosenson & Asheroff, 1975). Because of the importance of olfaction to rodent communication, and because of the important role played by hormones in the production and release of the signaling pheromones that allow mice to identify each other (see Chapter 4), it seems reasonable to speculate that the same kinds of pheromones that serve to identify conspecifics in sexual and agonistic interactions also might be operating to identify intruders in the case of maternal aggression.

Maternal aggression does not occur during the entire lactation period of the attacker, but seems to be centered around the earliest part of this period. Maternal aggression first is evident about 48 hours postpartum, peaks during Days 3-8 of lactation, and then declines during Days 9-14 and thereafter (Gandelman, 1972; Svare

& Gandelman, 1973). This particular time course coincides with changes in the levels of both the ovarian hormones and prolactin. Considering the ovarian hormones first, Svare & Gandelman (1975) found that increasing estrogen levels decreases maternal aggression, whereas manipulating progesterone levels has no effect on this behavior. Significantly, maternal aggression first appears at a time when estrogen levels have just fallen, 48 hours postpartum. These findings suggest that estrogens may serve to inhibit maternal aggression, and that their withdrawal after parturition may release maternal aggression from the estrogens' inhibitory influence.

One finding superficially seems to contradict the suggestion that the estrogens inhibit maternal aggression: Hysterectomy, which leads to an increase in estrogen levels, also leads to maternal aggression in pregnant rats. Therefore, it would seem that this is a case where estrogens could stimulate or facilitate rather than inhibit maternal aggression. However, in contrast to the situation with other maternal behaviors, hysterectomy still leads to maternal aggression if the rats also are ovariectomized and cannot respond to hysterectomy with an increase in estrogen levels. Therefore, the effects of hysterectomy on maternal aggression are independent of any concomitant changes in estrogen levels, and the finding that estrogens can inhibit maternal aggression is not necessarily contradicted (Svare, 1975).

Although the evidence is only correlational, some studies have suggested that prolactin may facilitate maternal aggression. First, the time course of changes in maternal aggressiveness over the lactation period is similar to the time course of changes in prolactin levels. Prolactin levels are highest early in lactation and begin to decline midway through the lactation period; maternal aggressiveness follows a similar pattern (Gandelman, 1972). Second, separating mouse mothers from their pups for five hours decreases both prolactin levels and levels of maternal aggressiveness (Svare & Gandelman, 1973). Thus, there are two lines of correlational evidence suggesting that prolactin levels and levels of maternal aggressiveness may be related.

One factor that appears to be essential to maternal aggression is suckling stimulation from the young. If nipple growth is induced in virgin mice by treating them with a specific combination of estrogens and progesterone, foster young will suck at the developed nipples. Significantly, virgins treated in this way exhibit maternal aggression so long as foster young are present. In addition, removing the nipples of lactating mice (thelectomy) abolishes maternal aggression. Therefore, suckling stimulation appears essential to maternal aggression (Svare, 1975; Svare & Gandelman, 1976), but whether the effect is hormonally mediated is not yet known.

Clearly, the role of hormones in maternal aggression has not been fully articulated. However, on the basis of the evidence collected so far, Svare (1975) has proposed that there are three phases to maternal aggression: The first stage is a *substrate preparation phase*, wherein the hormones of late pregnancy prime the animal, through promoting nipple growth and development. The second stage is an *initiation phase* for maternal aggression, instigated by suckling stimulation from the young (and perhaps prolactin). The third stage is the *maintenance phase*, controlled by the frequency of suckling and the presence of other cues emanating from the young.

RING DOVES

In contrast to the case of rodents, where the mother is the primary caretaker of the young, in ring doves, both parents participate in the care of the offspring. Because the parents do remain together throughout the entire reproductive cycle, the division between sexual and parental activities is not always clear. However, we shall use the division suggested by Lehrman (1965) here: that parental behavior begins with the building of nests, followed by egg-sitting or incubation, and then young-sitting and young-feeding.

The earliest reports implicated prolactin in the control of parental behavior in birds. In 1935, Riddle, Bates, and Lahr reported that treating hens with prolactin induces a condition of broodiness (the tendency to incubate eggs). Later, Riddle and Lahr (1944) reported that treating ring doves with either progesterone or testosterone also induces this incubation behavior. Because these investigators observed that progesterone and testosterone both increased the development of the crop sac, a prolactin-dependent tissue, they suggested that these gonadal hormones increase incubation because they stimulate prolactin secretion. Therefore, the earliest observations suggested that prolactin might be responsible for, or at least is involved in, the initiation of parental responding in two avian species, the chicken and the ring dove.

Later studies on the ring dove yielded different results. Lehrman and his colleagues (e.g., Lehrman, 1963; Lehrman & Brody, 1961, 1964) attempted to induce incubation in naive ring doves with prolactin treatment, and they were unsuccessful. In addition, Lehrman and Brody (1961) observed that incubation begins before the crop sac has developed extensively. This finding suggests that incubation normally begins while prolactin levels are still low. Therefore, it is unlikely that prolactin is involved in the initiation of incubation, at least in ring doves (Eisner, 1960; Lehrman, 1965).

Is there no role for prolactin in the parental behavior of the ring dove? Although prolactin seems unable to induce incubation behavior, this hormone does seem to help in its maintenance. If birds have begun to incubate eggs but then are isolated for a 12-day period, they will not incubate eggs immediately upon re-presentation. If, however, the birds have been treated with prolactin during the isolation period, they will incubate the new eggs immediately (Lehrman & Brody, 1964). Therefore, prolactin may be involved in the maintenance of the tendency to incubate, once this behavior has been initiated. In addition, prolactin levels do rise during the period of incubation, and there is some evidence that this hormone may be involved in the control of squab-feeding behaviors (Lehrman, 1965).

In contrast to prolactin, the gonadal hormones clearly seem to be involved in the initiation of parental behaviors, at least in female ring doves. In an early study, Lehrman (1958b) showed that untreated female birds will begin to sit on eggs after 4-10 days of egg exposure. If they have been treated with progesterone, however, those birds will sit on eggs immediately upon egg presentation. In addition, if female ring doves are treated with estrogens, they will incubate eggs after 1-3 days (Lehrman, 1958b). Therefore, it seems that the ovarian hormones might be involved in the initiation of parental responding in the female of this species.

Cheng and Silver (1975) studied in detail the relationship between the effects of estrogens and progesterone on nest-building behavior. They studied the nest-building and incubation behaviors of ovariectomized female and intact male birds when the females were treated with either an estrogen alone, progesterone alone, an estrogen in sequential combination with progesterone, or an oil placebo. The results of their study of the nest-building behavior of these birds following repeated egg presentation are reproduced in Figure 6-3. Notice, first, that ovariectomy markedly reduced nest-building in the female; ovariectomized females show almost no responding when only treated with oil. Second, although estrogen alone or progesterone alone could stimulate some degree of nest-building, sequential treatment with estrogen and progesterone was much more effective than either treatment alone. These findings suggest that the estrogens operate in combination with progesterone to stimulate nest-building in the female. Furthermore, although the male does some nest-building when paired with an ovariectomized female, hormonal treatment of the female facilitates the parental responses of the male.

We might next ask about the factors that can actually cause changes in estrogen and progesterone levels so that the initi-

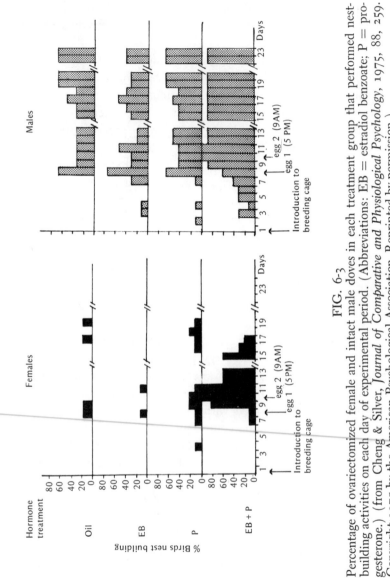

FIG. 6-3

Percentage of ovariectomized female and intact male doves in each treatment group that performed nest-building activities on each day of experimental period. (Abbreviations: EB = estradiol benzoate; P = progesterone.) (from Cheng & Silver, *Journal of Comparative and Physiological Psychology*, 1975, 88, 259. Copyright 1975 by the American Psychological Association. Reprinted by permission.)

ation of nest-building and incubation is facilitated. The evidence suggests that the critical factors include participation in courtship and the presence of a mate, nesting material, and eggs. Presenting the bird with a mate and nesting material will induce nest-building and incubation behaviors, similarly to the effects of the hormonal manipulations discussed above (Lehrman, 1958a; Lehrman, Brody & Wortis, 1961). In addition, the presence of a mate will augment the stimulatory effect of progesterone treatment on incubation (Bruder & Lehrman, 1967). More importantly, participating in courtship and related activities leads to a sequential rise in (first) estrogen and (then) progesterone levels in female ring doves (Korenbrot, Shomberg & Erickson, 1974; Silver et al., 1974), and this kind of hormonal change is the same as the sequence shown by Cheng and Silver to be most effective in stimulating nest-building. Therefore, there appears to be a long-chain hormone–behavior interaction operating in the case of parental behavior in the female ring dove: Engaging in courtship leads to an increase in estrogen and progesterone levels, which feeds back and facilitates nest-building and incubation. The rise in prolactin that accompanies incubation, then, may feed back and help maintain this behavior and stimulate other care-taking activities (see Cheng & Silver, 1975; Lehrman, 1965).

What of the male ring dove? Do the same kind of hormonal factors operate as in the case of the female? Although the same regimen of estrogen and progesterone used by Cheng and Silver for the female might be able to stimulate parental behavior in the male ring dove, there is almost no estrogen present in the male throughout the reproductive cycle (Korenbrot, Shomberg & Erickson, 1974). In addition, progesterone levels do not rise prior to incubation in the male as they do in the female (Silver et al., 1974). Therefore, it is unlikely that these hormones operate naturally in the male; there is almost no estrogen naturally present, and there is no rise in progesterone just prior to parental responding in the male, as there is in the female.

The findings just discussed suggest that the estrogens and progesterone probably do not act naturally in the male, but what of the male sex hormones, the androgens? The answer is unclear. Some investigators (e.g., Silver & Feder, 1973) have found little effect from removing the androgens from the circulation by castration on the initiation of parental responding. In addition, Silver and Feder (1973) found no effect from preventing the courtship-induced rise in androgen levels (by treating castrates with a fixed testosterone dosage). These findings would seem to suggest that the androgens are relatively unimportant to parental responding in the male ring dove. On the other hand, Erickson and Martinez-Vargas (1975) reported that castration dramatically reduces nest-building in male ring doves, suggesting that the androgens are critical to such behavior. Clearly, additional studies are needed to clarify the role of the androgens in male ring dove parental behavior.

SUMMARY AND COMMENT

This chapter was concerned with the role of hormones in parental behavior. We began our discussion with a review of the literature on hormones and maternal behavior in mammals, and then turned to the case of hormones and parental behavior in the ring dove, an avian species that has been studied fairly extensively.

Hormones do not appear to be essential for either the initiation or the maintenance of parental responding in most of the species discussed. Prolonged exposure to critical stimuli, such as rodent pups or nesting material, can induce parental responding in virgin animals. However, it does appear that the hormonal state existing around the time of the onset of parental responding facilitates the initiation of those behaviors. For example, although virgin rats eventually become maternal following repeated exposure to pups, treating them with a sequential regimen of estrogen, progesterone, and prolactin significantly reduces the time needed for concaveation. In addition, although some ovariectomized ring doves respond parentally when exposed to nesting material and eggs, treating them with an estrogen and progesterone regimen accelerates the induction of such responses.

There also is some evidence that hormones might facilitate the maintenance of parental responding. In rats, although removing the pituitary or the ovarian hormones does not disrupt ongoing maternal responses, there still are differences in the intensities of maternal responses between lactating and sensitized animals. In birds, there is some evidence that prolactin may be involved in the maintenance of incubation, perhaps through an interaction with the effects of exposure to critical environmental stimuli. Therefore, it seems that the hormonal state at the time of the expression of parental responses may facilitate both the initiation and the maintenance of those responses.

It may appear, superficially, that different hormones are involved in the parental behaviors of the different species we have discussed. However, in most cases, the behaviors studied in those different species are initiated at different stages of the reproductive cycle. For example, in rats, progesterone appears to inhibit maternal behavior, whereas in mice, it can stimulate maternal responding. However, progesterone inhibits the rat's retrieving and nursing behaviors, whereas progesterone stimulates maternal nest-building in the mouse. Significantly, retrieving only begins around parturition, when progesterone levels are low, whereas maternal nest-building begins during the gestation period, when progesterone levels are high. Therefore, many of the species differences that appear to exist may really be only a result of differences in the time during the reproductive cycle at which the behaviors being studied first appear.

One clear species difference appears to be in the role of prolactin. Although this hormone is essential to maternal behavior in the rabbit, it seems to play only a minor, facilitatory role in the rat. In addition, prolactin does not seem to be involved at all in the initiation of parental responding in the ring dove.

How do hormones exert their effects on parental behavior? Very few studies have examined this question directly, but there seems to be at least two possible mechanisms of action. First, some hormones might alter the state of critical neural circuits. For example, progesterone implants restricted to the preoptic area of the ring dove brain lead to incubation in the same way as do systemic injections of this hormone (Komisaruk, 1967). Therefore, progesterone seems to affect incubation by altering the state of relevant neural circuits.

Second, it is possible that other hormones affect maternal responding because they affect the state of peripheral tissues that are critical to certain parental behaviors. For example, prolactin may affect the initiation of squab-feeding in the ring dove because this hormone stimulates the growth of the crop sac, which will be needed for the feeding of the young (compare Lehrman, 1965). Thus, it is possible that hormones affect parental responding at both the peripheral and the central levels.

The studies reviewed in this chapter all have been conducted using nonprimate subjects. What of the primates? It appears that there have been no systematic studies of hormones and parental behavior in any primate species. Thus, it is difficult to know whether one can generalize from the case of nonprimate animals to the primates, including man. However, the reader may have noticed in previous chapters that the degree of hormonal control of behavior seems to decrease as one ascends the phylogenetic scale. Therefore, it would seem likely that the hormonal state of the individual is less critical or plays a less dramatic role in the parental behavior of primates than it does in nonprimate species.

REFERENCES

Amenomori, Y., Chen, C. L. & Meites, J. Serum prolactin levels in rats during different reproductive states. *Endocrinology*, 1970, 86, 506-510.

Anderson, C. O., Zarrow, M. X., Fuller, G. B. & Denenberg, V. H. Pituitary involvement in maternal nest-building in the rabbit. *Hormones and Behavior*, 1971, 2, 183-189.

Beach, F. A. & Wilson, J. R. Effects of prólactin, progesterone and estrogen on reactions of nonpregnant rats to foster young. *Psychological Reports*, 1963, 13, 231-239.

Bridges, R., Zarrow, M. X., Gandelman, R. & Denenberg, V. H. Differences in maternal responsiveness between lactating and sensitized rats. *Developmental Psychobiology*, 1972, 5, 123-127.

Bruder, R. H. & Lehrman, D. S. Role of the mate in the elicitation of hormone-induced incubation behavior in the ring dove. *Journal of Comparative and Physiological Psychology*, 1967, 63, 382-384.

Cheng, M. F., & Silver, R. Estrogen-progesterone regulation of nest-building and incubation behavior in ovariectomized ring doves (*Streptopelia risoria*). *Journal of Comparative and Physiological Psychology*, 1975, 88, 256-263.

Eisner, E. The relationship of hormones to the reproductive behaviour of birds, referring especially to parental behaviour: a review. *Animal Behaviour*, 1960, 8, 155-179.

Endröczi, E., Lissák, K. & Telegdy, G. Influence of sexual and adrenocortical hormones on the maternal aggressivity. *Acta Physiologica Academiae Scientiarum Hungaricae*, 1958, 14, 353-357.

Erickson, C. & Martinez-Vargas, M. C. The hormonal basis of cooperative nest-building. In P. Wright, P. Caryl & D. Vowles (Eds.), *Neural and Endocrine Aspects of Behaviour in Birds*. New York: Elsevier, 1975, pp. 91-109.

Flandera, V. & Nováková, V. The development of interspecies aggression of rats toward mice during lactation. *Physiology and Behavior*, 1971, 6, 161-164.

Gandelman, R. Mice: postpartum aggression elicited by the presence of an intruder. *Hormones and Behaviour*, 1972, 3, 23-28.

Komisaruk, B. R. Effects of local brain implants of progesterone on reproductive behavior in ring doves. *Journal of Comparative and Physiological Psychology*, 1967, 64, 219-224.

Korenbrot, C. C., Shomberg, D. W. & Erickson, C. J. Radioimmunoassay of plasma estradiol during the breeding cycle of ring doves (*Streptopelia risoria*). *Endocrinology*, 1974, 94, 1126-1132.

Lamb, M. E.   Physiological mechanisms in the control of maternal behavior in rats: a review. *Psychological Bulletin,* 1975, 82, 104-119.
Lehrman, D. S.   Induction of broodiness by participation in court-ship and nest-building in the ring dove (*Streptopelia risoria*). *Journal of Comparative and Physiological Psychology,* 1958, 51, 32-36. (a)
Lehrman, D. S.   Effect of female sex hormones on incubation be-havior in the ring dove (*Streptopelia risoria*). *Journal of Comparative and Physiological Psychology,* 1958, 51, 142-145. (b)
Lehrman, D. S.   Hormonal regulation of parental behavior in birds and infrahuman mammals. In W. C. Young (Ed.), *Sex and Internal Secretions, Vol. 2.* Baltimore: Williams and Wilkins, 1961, pp. 1268-1382.
Lehrman, D. S.   On the initiation of incubation behaviour in doves. *Animal Behaviour,* 1963, 11, 433-438.
Lehrman, D. S.   Interaction between internal and external environ-ments in the regulation of the reproductive cycle of the ring dove. In F. A. Beach (Ed.), *Sex and Behavior,* New York: Wiley, 1965, pp. 355-380.
Lehrman, D. S. & Brody, P.   Does prolactin induce incubation be-haviour in the ring dove? *Journal of Endocrinology,* 1961, 22, 269-275.
Lehrman, D. S. & Brody, P. N.   Effect of prolactin on established incubation behavior in the ring dove. *Journal of Comparative and Physiological Psychology,* 1964, 57, 161-165.
Lehrman, D. S., Brody, P. N. & Wortis, R. P.   The presence of the mate and of nesting material as stimuli for the development of incuba-tion behavior and for gonadotropin secretion in the ring dove (*Strep-topelia risoria*). *Endocrinology,* 1961, 68, 507-516.
Leon, M., Numan, M. & Chan, A.   Adrenal inhibition of maternal behavior in virgin female rats. *Hormones and Behavior,* 1975, 6, 165-171.
Lisk, R. D.   Oestrogen and progesterone synergism and elicitation of maternal nest-building in the mouse (*Mus musculus*). *Animal Be-haviour,* 1971, 19, 606-610.
Lisk, R. D., Pretlow, R. A. & Friedman, S. M.   Hormonal stimulation necessary for elicitation of nest-building in the mouse (*Mus musculus*). *Animal Behavior,* 1969, 17, 730-737.
Lott, D. F. & Fuchs, S. S.   Failure to induce retrieving by sensitiza-tion or the injection of prolactin. *Journal of Comparative and Physio-logical Psychology,* 1962, 55, 1111-1113.
Lott, D. F. & Rosenblatt, J. S.   Development of maternal responsive-ness during pregnancy in the rat. In B. M. Foss (Ed.), *Determinants of Infant Behaviour, IV.* London: Methuen, 1969, pp. 61-67.
Lubin, M., Leon, M., Moltz, H. & Numan, M.   Hormones and ma-

ternal behavior in the male rat. *Hormones and Behavior*, 1972, 3, 369-374.
Moltz, H., Lubin, M., Leon, M. & Numan, M. Hormonal induction of maternal behavior in the ovariectomized nulliparous rat. *Physiology and Behavior*, 1970, 5, 1373-1377.
Numan, M., Leon, M. & Moltz, H. Interference with prolactin release and the maternal behavior of female rats. *Hormones and Behavior*, 1972, 3, 29-38.
Obias, M. D. Maternal behavior of hypophysectomized gravid albino rats and the development and performance of their progeny. *Journal of Comparative and Physiological Psychology*, 1957, 50, 120-124.
Reisbick, S., Rosenblatt, J. S. & Mayer, A. D. Decline of maternal behavior in the virgin and lactating rat. *Journal of Comparative and Physiological Psychology*, 1975, 89, 722-732.
Riddle, O., Bates, R. W. & Lahr, E. L. Prolactin induces broodiness in fowl. *American Journal of Physiology*, 1935, 111, 352-360.
Riddle, O. & Lahr, E. L. On broodiness of ring doves following implants of certain steroid hormones. *Endocrinology*, 1944, 35, 255-260.
Riddle, O., Lahr, E. L. & Bates, R. W. Effectiveness and specificity of prolactin in the induction of maternal instinct in virgin rats. *American Journal of Physiology*, 1935, 113, 109.
Riddle, O., Lahr, E. L. & Bates, R. W. The role of hormones in the induction of maternal behavior in rats. *American Journal of Physiology*, 1942, 137, 299-317.
Rosenblatt, J. S. Nonhormonal basis of maternal behavior in the rat. *Science*, 1967, 156, 1512-1514.
Rosenblatt, J. S. & Lehrman, D. S. Maternal behavior of the laboratory rat. In M. L. Rheingold (Ed.), *Maternal Behavior in Mammals*. New York: Wiley, 1963, pp. 8-57.
Rosenblatt, J. S. & Siegel, H. I. Hysterectomy-induced maternal behavior during pregnancy in the rat. *Journal of Comparative and Physiological Psychology*, 1975, 89, 685-700.
Rosenson, L. M. & Asheroff, A. K. Maternal aggression in CD-1 mice: influence of the hormonal condition of the intruder. *Behavioral Biology*, 1975, 15, 219-224.
Roth, L. L. & Rosenblatt, J. S. Changes in self-licking during pregnancy in the rat. *Journal of Comparative and Physiological Psychology*, 1967, 63, 397-400.
Siegel, H. I. & Rosenblatt, J. S. Hormonal basis of hysterectomy-induced maternal behavior during pregnancy in the rat. *Hormones and Behavior*, 1975, 6, 211-222. (a)
Siegel, H. I. & Rosenblatt, J. S. Progesterone inhibition of estrogen-induced maternal behavior in hysterectomized-ovariectomized virgin rats. *Hormones and Behavior*, 1975, 6, 223-230. (b)

Siegel, H. I. & Rosenblatt, J. S.   Estrogen-induced maternal behavior in hysterectomized-ovariectomized virgin rats. *Physiology and Behavior,* 1975, 14, 465-471. (c)

Siegel, H. I. & Rosenblatt, J. S.   Latency and duration of estrogen induction of maternal behavior in hysterectomized-ovariectomized virgin rats: effects of pup stimulation. *Physiology and Behavior,* 1975, 14, 473-476. (d)

Silver, R. & Feder, H. H.   Role of gonadal hormones in incubation behavior of male ring doves (*Streptopelia risoria*). *Journal of Comparative and Physiological Psychology,* 1973, 84, 464-471.

Silver, R., Reboulleau, C., Lehrman, D. S. & Feder, H. H.   Radioimmunoassay of plasma progesterone during the reproductive cycle of male and female ring doves (*Streptopelia risoria*). *Endocrinology,* 1974, 94, 1547-1554.

Slotnick, B. M.   Neural and hormonal basis of maternal behavior in the rat. In B. E. Eleftheriou and R. L. Sprott (Eds.), *Hormonal Correlates of Behavior,* Vol. 2. New York: Plenum Press, 1975, pp. 585-656.

Stone, C. P.   Preliminary note on the maternal behavior of rats living in parabiosis. *Endocrinology,* 1925, 9, 505-512.

Svare, B. B.   Some factors influencing maternal aggression in mice. Unpublished doctoral dissertation. Rutgers University, 1975.

Svare, B. & Gandelman, R.   Post-partum aggression in mice: experiential and environmental factors. *Hormones and Behavior,* 1973, 4, 323-334.

Svare, B. & Gandelman, R.   Post-partum aggression in mice: inhibitory effect of estrogen. *Physiology and Behavior,* 1975, 14, 31-35.

Svare, B. & Gandelman, R.   Suckling stimulation induces aggression in virgin female mice. *Nature,* 1976, 260, 606-608.

Terkel, J. & Rosenblatt, J. S.   Maternal behavior induced by maternal blood plasma injected into virgin rats. *Journal of Comparative and Physiological Psychology,* 1968, 65, 479-482.

Terkel, J. & Rosenblatt, J. S.   Humoral factors underlying maternal behavior at parturition: cross transfusion between freely moving rats. *Journal of Comparative and Physiological Psychology,* 1972, 80, 365-371.

Voci, V. E. & Carlson, N. R.   Enhancement of maternal behavior and nest-building following systemic and diencephalic administration of prolactin and progesterone in the mouse. *Journal of Comparative and Physiological Psychology,* 1973, 83, 388-393.

Wiesner, B. P. & Sheard, N. M. *Maternal Behavior in the Rat.* Edinburgh: Oliver and Boyd, 1933.

Wise, D. A.   Aggression in the female golden hamster: effects of reproductive state and social isolation. *Hormones and Behavior* 1974, 5, 235-250.

Zarrow, M. X., Denenberg, V. H. & Sachs, B. D.   Hormones and maternal behavior in mammals. In S. Levine (Ed.), *Hormones and Behavior*. New York: Academic Press, 1972, pp. 105-134.

Zarrow, M. X., Farooq, A., Denenberg, V. H., Sawin, P. B. & Ross, S. Maternal behaviour in the rabbit: endocrine control of maternal nest-building. *Journal of Reproduction and Fertility*, 1963, 6, 375-383.

Zarrow, M. X., Gandelman, R. & Denenberg, V. H.   Prolactin: is it essential for maternal behavior in the mammal? *Hormones and Behavior*, 1971, 2, 343-354.

Zarrow, M. X., Sawin, P. B., Ross, S., Denenberg, V. H., Crary, D., Wilson, E. D. & Farooq, A.   Maternal behavior in the rabbit: evidence for an endocrine basis of maternal nest-building and additional data on maternal nest-building in the Dutch-belted race. *Journal of Reproduction and Fertility*, 1961, 2, 152-162.

Chapter 7

AVOIDANCE AND FEAR-MEDIATED BEHAVIORS

Chapters 7 and 8 are concerned with the relationship between endocrine function and emotion. An entire chapter (Chapter 7) is devoted to a special class of emotional responses, the *fear-mediated behaviors*, as studied in nonhuman animals because so much research has been directed to this topic. Chapter 8, on the other hand, is concerned primarily with the relationship between endocrine function and emotion and mood in humans.

The term "fear-mediated behaviors" is used to refer to both *avoidance responses* and *conditioned emotional responses*, or CERs. These behaviors traditionally have been considered to be mediated by fear because they are at least superficially similar to fear-mediated emotional responses as observed in humans; they involve responses made in anticipation of pain. However, we cannot, of course, observe the emotional states of animals directly, and we cannot know whether an animal really is experiencing fear in any way similar to the way a human experiences this emotion. Therefore, the term "fear-mediated behaviors" may not be precise when used to refer to avoidance responses and CERs as studied in animals. The argument about whether these behaviors really are fear-mediated in the emotional sense is outside the realm of this book, and the interested reader is referred to the discussion of this issue by Tarpy (1975). We shall use the term "fear-mediated behaviors" here as operationally defined in the literature and only to provide a general way of referring to avoidance responses and CERs as a single class of responses.

There are two basic classes of avoidance responses: *active avoidance* and *passive avoidance*. In active avoidance, the subject must make a particular response in order to avoid exposure to a noxious or aversive stimulus. An example of an active avoidance task is the shuttlebox situation. The shuttlebox is a two-compartment chamber, and the subject must shuttle from one side to the other in order to avoid being shocked. On the other hand, in passive avoidance, the subject must inhibit, rather than emit, a response in order to avoid an aversive stimulus. For example, a rat placed into a small chamber connected to a larger chamber typically moves quite readily into the larger chamber. But, if it is shocked for entering the larger chamber, the animal will learn to stay in the small chamber. Therefore, the subject learns to inhibit the response of entering the larger chamber in order to (passively) avoid the shock.

Conditioned emotional responses are assumed to be reflected in the effectiveness of a conditioned stimulus (CS) associated with pain in disrupting an ongoing response. That is, when a CS is presented that disrupts or suppresses a behavior, this disruption is thought to be the result of the CS's eliciting an emotional response from the subject. For example, if one first exposes a rat to a series of light–shock pairings, the light becomes a CS, acquiring some of the stress-inducing properties of the shock. One then might present the light while the animal is engaged in another behavior, such as drinking, and determine whether and how much this CS presentation disrupts the ongoing drinking response. The greater the disruption or suppression of drinking, the greater the magnitude of the CER assumed to be elicited by the CS.

Interest in the relationship between hormones and fear-mediated behaviors arose out of the early observations that experiencing stress or fear leads to marked changes in the levels of some hormones. Early in this century, Cannon proposed his Emergency Theory of the adrenal glands, suggesting that the secretion of epinephrine (adrenalin) is increased following exposure to stress, as a means of adapting to that stress (e.g., Cannon, 1915). Later, Selye described the General Adaptation Syndrome (GAS), emphasizing the role of the hormones of the pituitary-adrenocortical axis in the adaptation to stress (e.g., Selye, 1956). Some theorists have argued that the hormonal responses to stressors or fear-provoking stimuli serve as more than simply physiological adaptations to stress. They have suggested that these hormonal responses feed back and modify the behavioral responses of the individual to those stressful stimuli, thereby facilitating behavioral (as well as physiological) adaptations (e.g., Brush & Froehlich, 1975; Levine, 1968). This proposition is another example of a long-chain hormone–behavior interaction, as discussed in Chapter 1 and illustrated in later chapters.

More recent studies of the effects of stressful or emotional experiences on endocrine function have shown that these experiences lead to modifications in the levels of many hormones, not only those of the adrenal medulla and the pituitary-adrenocortical axis. Perhaps the most extensive studies on this subject have been conducted by Mason and his colleagues who used an "endocrine screen" to show the multihormonal response to the experience of being maintained on a Sidman avoidance schedule for 72 hours (e.g., Mason, 1968, 1974). The effects of 72 hours of avoidance on a wide range of hormones in the rhesus monkey is reproduced in Figure 7-1. Notice that the hormones studied follow one of two patterns: Some hormones first increase during the avoidance period, and then decrease in the days following removal from the avoidance situation. Others first decrease during avoidance and then increase following withdrawal from the avoidance situation. Mason (1968, 1974) has suggested that these two patterns reflect two general classes of hormonal actions on metabolic processes.

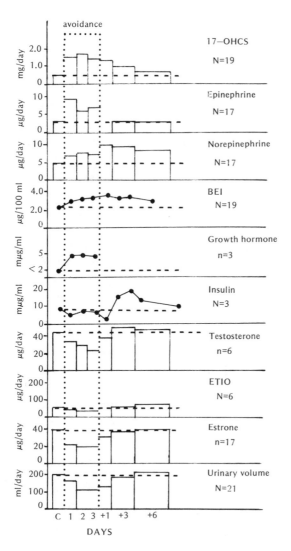

FIG. 7-1

Pattern of multiple hormonal responses to 72-hour avoidance sessions in the monkey. 17-OHCS = 17-hydroxycorticosteroids, a measure of adrenocortical activity; BEI is a measure of thyroid activity; ETIO = etiocholanolone; dotted line refers to pretesting control levels (from Mason, *Psychosomatic Medicine*, 1968, 30, 775, by permission of the American Psychosomatic Society).

Those hormones which first increase are those that are primarily catabolic in action; they lead to the breakdown of tissues, resulting in an increase in available energy. Those that first decrease are anabolic in action, and the decrease in their levels provides an inhibition of tissue synthesis during stress, thereby preserving circulating metabolites for energy production. These anabolic hormones then increase following withdrawal of the stress, providing for an increase in tissue synthesis as a means of recovery.

The studies by Mason and others suggest that many hormones might be related to fear-mediated responding, and the review that follows considers the relationship between a number of hormones and fear-mediated responding. Included in this review are the adrenal medullary hormones, the pituitary-adrenocortical hormones, the posterior pituitary hormones, and the gonadal hormones. These groups of hormones have received the most experimental attention. As we progress through this review, the reader may notice that, as has been the case in earlier chapters, three aspects of the relationship between hormones and fear-mediated behaviors have been studied: the form of the hormonal responses to fear-provoking stimuli, the relationship between baseline hormonal states and levels of fear responding, and a feedback relationship between the hormonal responses to stressful or fear-provoking stimuli and levels of fear responding.

It should be noted before proceeding that we do not know yet whether the findings to be discussed here really can serve as the bases for general statements about the role of hormones in fear responding. Most of the studies have used laboratory rats as subjects, and we have not had sufficient opportunities to assess whether these findings would be consistent across different species or whether they would even hold for rats living under more natural conditions. In addition, most of these studies have used electric shock as the motivating stimulus, and we do not know whether the observed relationships would hold across different fear-provoking stimuli. Thus, although there is a vast literature relating endocrine function and fear responding in the laboratory rat, we should be cautious about attempting to generalize too quickly to other species or to other kinds of situations.

ADRENAL MEDULLARY HORMONES

Interest in the role of the adrenal medullary hormones, the cate-cholamines, in fear-mediated behaviors originated with Cannon's early proposition that there is a marked increase in epinephrine output following exposure to stressors. This suggestion was later translated into a question about the possible roles of the catechol-amines in the elicitation of fear. However, although it is true that engaging in fear-mediated behaviors leads to increases in periph-eral catecholamine levels (Mason et al., 1961; Mason et al., 1968), it is not necessarily true that just because a hormone is released in response to a fearful situation, that hormone also will be involved in the elicitation of fear. In one case we are studying a *response* to fear, and in the other we are studying a *cause* of fear. In any event, this kind of translation of Cannon's view seems to have been the original basis for the many later studies examining the role of the adrenal medullary hormones in fear responding.

Before turning to a review of the experimental literature, it might be useful to announce the limits of that review. First, as the reader may know, the catecholamines really have two kinds of actions; they may function either as hormones (usually periph-erally) or as neurotransmitters. We are concerned here only with the hormonal actions of these substances. The interested reader is referred to the excellent review of the role of central catechol-amines in avoidance learning by Gorelick, Bozewicz & Bridger (1975). Second, the functioning of the adrenal medulla is intri-cately related to the functioning of the sympathetic nervous sys-tem. Some studies have been conducted examining the effects of interrupting sympathetic activity on avoidance behavior, and yielded conflicting results. Because this topic is not directly related to hormones, the interested reader is referred to the review articles by Pappas (1974) and Van-Toller and Tarpy (1974).

Assuming that exposure to stressors or fear-provoking stimuli can lead to increases in the release of catecholamines from the adrenal medulla, we shall consider here only experimental studies intended to demonstrate the role of the catecholamines in the determination of avoidance responding or CERs. Two basic techniques have been used. The first includes removing catecholamines from the general circulation by adrenal demedullation, and the second involves injecting epinephrine systemically. It should be noted at the outset that any effects of manipulating systemic catecholamine levels probably are a result of nonneural actions of these hormones, since exogenous catecholamines (and probably endogenous catecholamines as well) do not pass the blood-brain barrier (Vernikos-Danellis, 1972); therefore, systemic manipulations probably only affect peripheral hormone levels.

The Effects of Adrenal Demedullation

Typically, the first step in determining whether a particular hormone or class of hormones is involved in the determination of a particular pattern or class of responses is to withdraw that hormone from the circulation. In the case of the adrenal medullary hormones, this is not an easy task. In addition to being produced in the adrenal medulla, the catecholamines are produced in noradrenergic nerve endings, and may be produced in accessory chromaffin tissue located around the sympathetic chain glanglia. However, most of an individual's epinephrine is produced in the adrenal medulla, and, therefore, a deficiency in epinephrine can be produced by removing this gland.

The effects of adrenal demedullation are not consistent from study to study and from laboratory to laboratory. It appears to have no effect on one-way active avoidance responses (Moyer & Bunnell, 1959; Silva, 1974) or on one-trial passive avoidance conditioning (Silva, 1973). On the other hand, it does seem to inhibit acquisition of two-way shuttlebox avoidance responses, although only under conditions that produce very efficient learning of that response (Conner & Levine, 1969; Levine & Soliday, 1962). Finally, adrenal demedullation appears to have no effect on the acquisition of conditioned fear responses when those responses are tested using a CER paradigm (Leshner, Brookshire & Stewart, 1971).

An alternative means of decreasing peripheral catecholamine levels is to inject substances that block its synthesis. For example, DiGiusto (1972) injected rats with 6-hydroxydopamine, which blocks norepinephrine and epinephrine synthesis, and found that this manipulation decreased performance of a passive avoidance task. Furthermore, in the same study, adrenal demedullation was without effect. Because adrenal demedullation leads to a reduction primarily in epinephrine levels, whereas treatment with 6-hydroxydopamine would lead to a depletion of both norepinephrine and epinephrine, one might suggest that the effects of drug treatment were due to the depletion of norepinephrine but not epinephrine.

The Effects of Exogenous Catecholamines

The notion introduced in the beginning of this chapter that the hormonal responses to fear-provoking stimuli might feed back and facilitate appropriate fear responses seems particularly attractive for the case of the adrenal medullary hormones, since they are released almost immediately following exposure to stress. Although one might decide to test this suggestion by preventing the critical hormonal responses by removing their source (as in the case of adernal demedullation), one might also test that hypothesis by studying the effects of producing elevated catecholamine levels even before stress exposure. This manipulation should lead to even greater levels of responding because the hormone levels are high at an earlier point in time. Therefore, some studies have been directed to the effects of exogenous catecholamines on fear-mediated behaviors. As in the case of adrenal demedullation, such studies have yielded conflicting results.

A few studies have found that low or moderate dosages of epinephrine increase fear-mediated responding. Latané and Schachter (1962) found that low dosages, but not high dosages, facilitate acquisition of a shuttlebox avoidance response. Kamano (1868) found that if rats are trained in a shuttlebox at 23 days of age and then tested for retention 21 days later, the injection of epinephrine just prior to retention testing will enhance the performance of that fear response. Finally, injecting rats with epinephrine alters their preference for novel over familiar environments. Rats ordinarily prefer novel to familiar chambers, but if they are injected with epinephrine, they prefer familiar chambers. This finding has been interpreted as reflecting a stimulation or facilitation of fear (avoidance of novel places) in epinephrine-injected animals (Leventhal & Killackey, 1968).

Alternatively, some studies have found that injected epinephrine does not affect fear-mediated responding. It has been observed to be without effect in runway avoidance situations (Moyer & Bunnell, 1958), shuttlebox avoidance situations (Stewart & Brookshire, 1967), and CER situations (Stewart & Brookshire, 1968). In addition, injected epinephrine does not appear to affect the extinction of a previously learned runway avoidance response (Leshner & Stewart, 1966).

It does appear that in those situations where adrenal demedullation retards avoidance acquisition, such as the shuttlebox, replacement therapy with a low dosage of epinephrine restores the performance of adrenal demedullated rats. Curiously, the same low dosage that seems to restore the acquisition performance of demedullated rats also decreases the performance of intact rats (Conner & Levine, 1969). This decreased performance of intact animals injected with adrenalin may be a result of the motor impairment that high epinephrine dosages can produce.

There is some evidence that more directly supports the hypothesis that the catecholamine responses to stress might feed back and facilitate subsequent behavioral fear responses. Gold and van Buskirk (1975) conducted a study where they treated rats with varying dosages of epinephrine immediately after training in a one-trial passive avoidance situation, thereby potentiating the normal hormonal response to shock stress. In this situation the animal was shocked for licking at a drinking tube and, therefore, would avoid the tube in subsequent tests. Those animals treated with an inter-mediate dosage of epinephrine exhibited longer latencies to drink during retention tests conducted 24 hours later than either con-trol animals, animals treated with a very low dosage of epineph-rine, or animals treated with a very high dosage of this hormone (Fig. 7-2). In addition, the training–injection interval was critical: the greater the time interval between training experience and epi-nephrine treatment, the less retention was facilitated (Fig. 7-3). These studies, then, show that if the normal catecholamine re-sponses to shock stress are exaggerated by injecting extra epineph-rine, retention of the fear response is facilitated. In addition, the exaggeration of epinephrine responses must occur in close tem-poral proximity to the normal, endogenous hormonal response to the training stressor in order for retention to be increased. Thus, increasing the magnitude of epinephrine responses to stress facili-tates later performance of the fear response.

Summary Statement: The Adrenal Medullary Hormones

The preceding review of the role of the adrenal medullary hor-mones in the control of fear-mediated behaviors certainly must leave the reader with a lack of closure on this topic. Some studies have shown definite effects from manipulating peripheral cate-cholamine levels, whereas others have found no effects. As has been the case before, we must consider the evidence presented here as only preliminary and hope that additional studies will yield more definitive answers.

The reader should keep in mind that this review has been de-

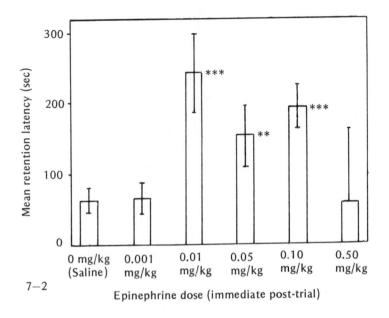

7–2

FIG. 7-2
Mean ± standard error latencies to lick during the retention test for animals which received saline or epinephrine immediately after training. *** = $p < 0.001$; ** = $p < 0.01$ (from Gold and van Buskirk, *Behavioral Biology*, 1975, 13, 148, by permission of Academic Press).

voted solely to the case of fear-mediated responding in nonhuman animals. The adrenal medullary hormones also have been implicated in other kinds of emotional situations, particularly in human subjects. These issues will be considered in Chapter 8.

PITUITARY-ADRENOCORTICAL HORMONES

In the middle 1950s Hans Selye described the General Adaptation Syndrome (GAS), implicating the hormones of the pituitary-adrenocortical axis, ACTH and the glucocorticoids, in the response to stress. According to Selye's GAS, exposure to a stressor

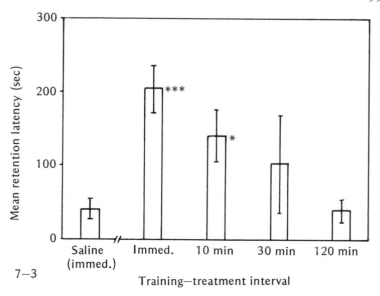

FIG. 7-3

Mean ± standard error latencies during the retention test for animals which received saline after training or epinephrine after various delays after training. *** = $p < 0.001$; * = $p < 0.05$ (from Gold and van Buskirk, *Behavioral Biology*, 1975, 13, 149, by permission of Academic Press).

leads, first, to an immediate (within 30 seconds) rise in ACTH levels, the *Alarm Reaction*. This rise in ACTH is followed (within 3-5 minutes) by a rise in glucocorticoid secretion that ordinarily lasts as long as the stressor is present, the *Phase of Resistance*. If the stress lasts too long, however, the adrenals lose their ability to sustain the high level of glucocorticoid output, and the individual suffers severe physical debilitation, even death. This third stage is called the *Phase of Exhaustion* (Selye, 1956). Later studies provided general support for Selye's basic proposition by showing that a great variety of stressors can elicit increases in pituitary-adreno-cortical activity (e.g., Manogue, Leshner & Candland, 1975).

Included among such stressors are direct shock treatments and having to maintain avoidance responding (even if the animal no longer receives any shocks) (Friedman et al., 1967; Mason, Brady & Tolliver, 1968). The identification of this pituitary-adrenocortical response to shock stress or having to engage in avoidance behaviors led some investigators (e.g., Levine, 1968) to postulate that the hormonal responses to these kinds of stressors might feed back and facilitate fear-mediated responding, as a behavioral adaptation to stress. In order to test this proposition, many studies have been directed toward determining the role of the pituitary-adrenocortical hormones in fear responding. As is usually the case, these studies have been of the two basic types: correlational and experimental.

Correlational Studies

Studies concerned with the pituitary-adrenocortical hormones and fear responding have examined two types of correlations: (1) correlations between resting or baseline hormone levels, determined either before exposure to the behavioral situation or long after withdrawal from the situation; and (2) correlations between the magnitude of pituitary-adrenal responses to stress and levels of fear-mediated responding. The rationale for examining the first type of correlation would be to reveal a relationship between baseline hormonal states and levels of responding. This goal is quite similar to that of most experimental studies that employ hormonal manipulations made prior to exposure to a behavioral situation. The rationale for the second type study is the original proposition that the pituitary-adrenal response to stress would feed back and facilitate fear responding. That is, if the pituitary-adrenal responses to stress have this kind of feedback effect on fear-mediated responding, one should examine the correlation between stress-induced pituitary adrenal hormone levels and fear responding, not only that between resting hormone levels and levels of responding.

Studies of the relationship between resting pituitary-adrenal hormone levels (usually assessed by measuring circulating glucocorticoid levels) and levels of fear-mediated responding have yielded conflicting findings. Some studies (e.g., Bohus, Endröczi & Lissák, 1964) have found a positive correlation between resting glucocorticoid levels and levels of avoidance performance, whereas others (e.g., van Delft, 1970) found a negative correlation between these variables. A third group of studies has provided support for there being a positive correlation between the two variables, although these studies have used a somewhat different approach. Rather than examine the relationship between individual differences in hormone levels and individual differences in levels of fear responding, the investigators used an "intra-individual approach," asking whether there is a correlation between circadian rhythms in pituitary-adrenal hormone levels and rhythms in avoidance responding. These studies (e.g., Gold & van Buskirk, 1976; Pagano & Lovely, 1972; Schneider, Weinberg & Weissberg, 1974) have found that rats exhibit greater fear-mediated responses late in the day, when pituitary-adrenal hormone levels are high, than they do early in the morning, when the levels of these hormones are low. Thus, there is a positive correlation between variations in endogenous pituitary-adrenal hormone levels (variations induced by a circadian rhythm) and levels of fear responding.

Correlational studies have also examined the relationship between pituitary-adrenal hormone levels following stress and avoidance performance, and these studies have found a positive correlation between these measures. First, the glucocorticoid response to training in an avoidance situation dissipates with time. Significantly, retention performance also declines as the interval between training and testing increases (to a point, after which retention performance appears to increase again), and the time course of the behavioral dissipation seems to correspond with the time course of the decline in hormone levels. Thus, there is a temporal correlation between pituitary-adrenal hormone levels following the stress of avoidance training and retention of that avoidance response: as pituitary-adrenal hormone levels decline, so does retention of the behavioral response (Levine & Brush, 1967). Second, rats that exhibit larger glucocorticoid responses to ether stress also show more efficient Sidman avoidance performance than rats that exhibit lower adrenal stress responses (Wertheim, Conner & Levine, 1969). Thus, there is a positive correlation between pituitary-adrenal responsiveness to stress and behavioral avoidance responding. This correlation lends support to the feedback notion discussed before. If the pituitary-adrenocortical responses to stress do feed back and facilitate fear responding, then the greater the magnitude of the pituitary-adrenal stress response, the greater should be the facilitation of avoidance performance.

Experimental Studies

There have been a great many experimental studies directed toward clarifying the roles and mechanisms of action of the pituitary-adrenocortical hormones in fear-mediated and avoidance behaviors. As usual, the review that follows is not intended to be a complete survey of those many studies. Rather, it is intended as a summary of the major classes of findings and their implications. The reader interested in pursuing this area further is referred to the excellent reviews by Brush and Froelich (1975), DiGiusto, Cairncross, and King (1971), and Levine (1968).

The first step in determining the role of the pituitary-adrenocortical hormones in fear-mediated responding might be to remove them from the circulation. This can be accomplished by removing the pituitary (hypophysectomy), because this operation reduces the levels of both groups of hormones at the same time. ACTH levels are reduced because the source of their production is removed, and glucocorticoid levels are reduced because the level of the tropic hormone on which they depend, ACTH, is reduced. The reader should keep in mind that the levels of many other hormones also are reduced following hypophysectomy, and, therefore, any observed effects might be the result of removing any of many combinations of hormones.

Hypophysectomy retards acquisition and facilitates extinction of both active and passive avoidance responses (Applezweig & Baudry, 1955; Weiss et al., 1969, 1970). In addition, replacement therapy with ACTH (which restores the levels of both ACTH and the glucocorticoids) can restore the avoidance performance of hypophysectomized rats to normal levels (Applezweig & Baudry, 1955; Weiss et al., 1970). Therefore, withdrawal of the pituitary-adrenal hormones decreases avoidance performance, and restoring their levels restores avoidance performance. These findings seem to suggest that the pituitary-adrenal hormones are necessary for normal avoidance responding. However, it also is the case that partial restoration can be accomplished by treating hypophysectomized rats with a combination of cortisone, testosterone, and thyroxine, suggesting that some of the effects of this drastic operation might be due to the profound metabolic effects produced by the withdrawal of many different hormones (DeWied, 1964, 1969).

The next step might be to increase the levels of the pituitary-adrenocortical hormones. If it is true that the pituitary-adrenal responses to stress feed back and facilitate fear-mediated responding, then increasing pituitary-adrenal hormone levels even before the individual is exposed to the stress should lead to even faster or more effective behavioral facilitation.

This prediction appears to hold true. Injecting intact animals with ACTH, which increases the levels of both ACTH and the glucocorticoids, retards extinction of both active and passive avoidance responses, and it does so in a dose-dependent manner: as shown in Figure 7-4, the greater the ACTH dosage, the greater the resistance to extinction of the avoidance response (DeWied, 1969; Levine & Jones, 1965; Miller & Ogawa, 1962; Murphy & Miller, 1955). On the other hand, the effects of ACTH treatment on acquisition of fear-mediated responses remains unclear. In some studies, ACTH treatment has been found to increase the acquisi-

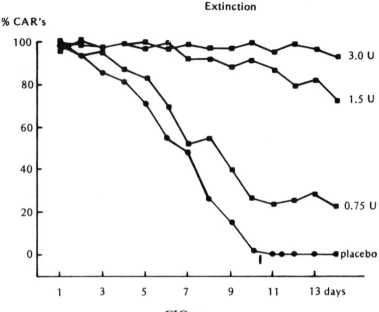

FIG. 7-4

The effects of different dosages of ACTH on the rate of extinction of a shuttlebox avoidance response in intact rats (from chapter by De-Wied in Ganong & Martini's *Frontiers in Neuroendocrinology.* New York: Oxford University Press, 1969, p. 119, by permission).

tion of avoidance responses, whereas in other studies, such treatment appears to have no effect on avoidance acquisition (e.g., Beatty et al., 1970; Levine & Jones, 1965; Murphy & Miller, 1955).

SEPARATION OF ACTH AND GLUCOCORTICOID EFFECTS The findings discussed so far imply that there is a linear relationship between the level of the pituitary-adrenocortical hormones and fear-mediated responding, at least in situations where the aversive stimulus is electric shock. A question that remains concerns whether both ACTH and the glucocorticoids or only one of the pituitary-adrenal hormones is responsible for the observed effects. Because both hypophysectomy and ACTH treatment result in the same kinds of changes in the levels of both ACTH and the glucocorticoids, it was necessary to turn to manipulations that affect these pituitary-adrenal hormones differently in order to separate their effects.

One such technique is adrenalectomy, which results in a decrease in glucocorticoid levels but an increase in ACTH levels. This operation leads to increases in both the acquisition and the retention of active and passive avoidance responses (Beatty et al., 1970; Silva, 1974; Weiss et al., 1969). Therefore, the effects of adrenalectomy are basically the same as those of ACTH treatment; both lead to increases in fear-mediated responding. Because both increasing (via ACTH treatment) and decreasing (via adrenalectomy) glucocorticoid levels lead to the same facilitation of avoidance responding so long as ACTH levels are high, it seems most likely that the hormone responsible for the effects of raising both ACTH and glucocorticoid levels simultaneously is ACTH. That is, so long as ACTH levels are high, it does not seem to matter whether glucocorticoid levels are high or low, which suggests that increases in ACTH levels, rather than glucocorticoid levels, are responsible for the effects of treatments that increase the levels of both hormones.

What of the condition when both ACTH and glucocorticoid levels are low? Does the level of the glucocorticoids matter for fear responding in this condition? Recall that when both ACTH and glucocorticoid levels are reduced simultaneously (e.g., when the animal is hypophysectomized), fear-mediated responding is reduced. One technique used to examine this question involves treating intact animals with high dosages of the glucocorticoids, which leads to high levels of these steroid hormones but reduces ACTH levels.

Treatment of intact rats with either natural or synthetic glucocorticoids generally leads to a decrease in the acquisition and retention of fear-mediated responses (e.g., Endröczi & Fekete, 1973; Levine & Levin, 1970; Wimersma Greidanus, 1970). These effects of corticoid treatment are similar to those of hypophysectomy; both treatments lead to decreased fear-mediated responding. Therefore, so long as ACTH levels are low, it does not matter whether glucocorticoid levels are low (as induced by hypophysectomy) or high (as induced by corticoid treatment). These findings suggest that the effects of treatments that lower the levels of both hormones simultaneously are a result of decreases in ACTH levels alone; it does not matter whether or not glucocorticoid levels also are low.

These two sets of findings, those from studies of adrenalectomy and of glucocorticoid treatment of intact animals, suggest that there might be an extra-adrenal effect of ACTH on fear-mediated responding. That is, that ACTH can affect fear responses independently of its tropic actions on glucocorticoid secretion. Yet another line of evidence supports this view. There are fractions of the ACTH peptide (ACTH analogues) available that appear to have some of the same effects as the whole ACTH molecule on fear-mediated responding without having any physiological effects on glucocorticoid secretion. DeWied and his colleagues have conducted an extensive series of studies using these ACTH fractions, and all studies have shown that many ACTH analogues can facilitate avoidance performance, even though they do not affect glucocorticoid secretion (e.g., DeWied, 1966, 1969). Thus, all that is needed for ACTH to exert its effects on fear-mediated responding is a fraction of the molecule, and it does not matter whether glucocorticoid levels also are affected or not.

What of the glucocorticoids? Have they no role in fear-mediated responding? Some evidence has been provided that suggests that the increase in glucocorticoid levels that follows an increase in ACTH secretion may serve to restore a normal level of responding following excitation by ACTH. That is, the glucocorticoids may be able to inhibit fear responding independently of their effects on ACTH levels. Corticosterone treatment will further reduce the fear responding of hypophysectomized rats, who do not have any

ACTH. Therefore, the glucocorticoids could inhibit fear responding independently of their effects on ACTH levels (DeWied, Bohus & Greven, 1968; Weiss et al., 1970).

GENERALITY OF PITUITARY-ADRENOCORTICAL EFFECTS The studies discussed in this section all have used shock as the aversive stimulus, and one might question whether the observed relationships are also true of situations where the aversive stimulus is different. Some evidence has been accumulated suggesting that the relationship between the pituitary-adrenocortical hormones and avoidance responding might be different when different aversive stimuli are used. Leshner, Moyer, and Walker (1975) studied the effects of a series of pituitary-adrenal manipulations on avoidance responding by mice in a passive avoidance situation where the aversive stimulus was attack by a trained fighter, an avoidance-of-attack situation. They found that some manipulations affect avoidance-of-attack differently from the way they affect avoidance-of-shock. For example, although adrenalectomy and ACTH treatment increased avoidance-of-attack in the same way as they increase avoidance-of-shock, hypophysectomy and corticosterone treatment also increased avoidance-of-attack, whereas they decrease avoidance-of-shock. Therefore, there appears to be a different relationship between pituitary-adrenal hormone levels and avoidance-of-attack and avoidance-of-shock. In the case of avoidance of attack, there is a bimodal relationship between the levels of these hormones and avoidance responding (both decreases and increases in pituitary-adrenal hormone levels lead to increased avoidance). However, in the case of avoidance of shock, there appears to be a linear relationship between the levels of these hormones and avoidance responding (as pituitary-adrenal hormone levels rise, so do levels of avoidance responding).

It also appears that different pituitary-adrenocortical hormones are critical in the avoidance-of-attack and avoidance-of-shock situations. Moyer and Leshner (1976) reported that corticosterone treatment alone is sufficient to return the avoidance performance of hypophysectomized mice to normal levels; restoring ACTH levels is not necessary. In addition, they reported that although ACTH treatment increases avoidance-of-attack in intact mice (which can respond to this treatment with increases in glucocorticoid levels), this treatment does not affect avoidance-of-attack in mice with controlled levels of corticosterone (that cannot respond to ACTH with increased glucocorticoid levels). Thus, in the first case, it is not necessary to increase ACTH levels to return the avoidance performance of hypophysectomized mice to normal levels, so long as there is sufficient corticosterone present. In the second case, ACTH treatment only affects mice that can respond with increased glucocorticoid levels; this hormone does not affect avoidance-of-attack in mice whose glucocorticoid response is controlled. These findings suggest that in the avoidance-of-attack situation, the glucocorticoid corticosterone rather than ACTH is responsible for the effects of those manipulations that cause similar changes in the levels of both pituitary-adrenocortical hormones. In addition, these findings begin to question the generality of the relationships between pituitary-adrenal hormone levels and avoidance responding observed in shock-mediated situations, where the most important pituitary-adrenocortical hormone appears to be ACTH; in the avoidance-of-attack situation, the critical pituitary-adrenocortical hormone appears to be corticosterone.

Mechanisms of Action

How do the pituitary-adrenocortical hormones affect fear-mediating responding? One possibility is that varying at least ACTH levels affects avoidance responding because it affects the state of the musculature; ACTH treatment can increase the amplitude of muscle contraction (Strand, Stoboy & Cayer, 1974). However, although in the case of active avoidance responses increased muscle contractility might facilitate the necessary motor behaviors, in passive avoidance responses the individual must inhibit responding. Since ACTH has the same behavioral effect (increases avoidance responding) under conditions where both active and passive responses must be made, it seems unlikely that changes in muscle activity are responsible for the effects of this hormone.

It also could be that the pituitary-adrenal hormones affect fear-mediated responding because they affect the sensitivity of the organism to the aversive stimulus, in most cases shock. One can test sensitivity to shock by determining what is called the "jump-flinch threshold," which is the minimal amount of shock needed to elicit flinching or jumping responses. The results of studies of the effects of pituitary-adrenal manipulations on shock sensitivity have been inconsistent, suggesting that altering pituitary-adrenal hormone levels has no dramatic effect on shock sensitivity. For example, in one study (Paré & Cullen, 1971), adrenalectomy was found to decrease the threshold to shock (increase sensitivity), whereas in another study (Gibbs et al., 1973) adrenalectomy was found to increase the jump-flinch threshold (decrease sensitivity to shock). In addition, in one study (Gibbs et al., 1973), hypophysectomy was found to have no effect on the jump-flinch threshold, whereas in another study (Gispen, Wimersma Greidanus & DeWied, 1970), it was found to lower this threshold. Thus, although it is possible that pituitary-adrenal manipulations could be affecting avoidance behaviors because they alter sensitivity to aversive stimuli (whether at the level of the receptor or at the level of perception of the stimuli), those sensory effects are not very dramatic, and, therefore, they probably cannot account for the consistent and dramatic effects of these manipulations on fear-mediated responding.

It is most likely that the pituitary-adrenal hormones affect fear-mediated responding because they modify the states of critical central neural circuits. First, the pituitary-adrenal hormones are both controlled by and have dramatic effects on the state of the limbic circuits that are critical to fear-mediated behaviors (e.g.,

Endröczi, 1972; Appendix). Therefore, it easily could be that these hormones affect avoidance responding because they alter the state of the neural circuits that control this class of behavior.

Second, some studies employing brain lesions support the suggestion that the pituitary-adrenal hormones affect avoidance responding because they affect brain function. For example, corticosterone affects passive avoidance learning in intact rats, but it has only a marginal effect in septal-lesioned animals. This finding suggests that the septum may be involved in the mediation of glucocorticoid effects on avoidance learning (Endröczi & Nyákás, 1971). In addition, ACTH treatment is ineffective in modifying avoidance retention in rats with lesions in the parafascicular nuclei of the thalamus, suggesting that this brain area may be a site involved in the mediation of ACTH effects (Wimersma Greidanus, Bohus & DeWied, 1974b). Thus, certain brain sites are necessary for the pituitary-adrenal hormones to exert their effects.

Finally, many experimental studies have shown that direct implants of pituitary-adrenal hormones into neural sites can have the same effects as do systemic hormone treatments. Wimersma Greidanus and DeWied (1971) conducted an extensive study mapping the areas where ACTH and ACTH analogues (the fractions discussed before) can act to retard extinction. They found many sites in the caudal diencephalic and rostral mesencephalic regions of the brain in which ACTH implants were effective in modifying avoidance extinction. In addition, glucocorticoid implants can facilitate extinction of avoidance responses when placed in a variety of neural sites. Included in these active sites are the median eminence, the preoptic area, the thalamic parafascicular area, and the mesencephalic reticular formation (Bohus, 1970; DeWied et al., 1972; Endröczi, 1971; Wimersma Greidanus & DeWied, 1969). Thus, direct pituitary-adrenal hormone implants into specific and restricted brain sites exert the same behavioral effects as do systemic hormone treatments.

Comment: *The Pituitary-Adrenocortical Hormones*

The studies reviewed in this section clearly show that the pituitary-adrenocortical hormones can affect fear-mediated and avoidance responding, and they suggest that these hormonal effects are mediated by the effects of the pituitary-adrenal hormones on the state of the brain. At least in shock-mediated situations, it appears that ACTH exerts an extra-adrenal facilitative effect on fear responding, whereas corticosterone can inhibit fear responses. These findings, in combination with those of correlational studies showing a relationship between the magnitude of the pituitary-adrenal response to stress and levels of avoidance responding, lend general support to the hypothesis that the pituitary-adrenal responses to stress can feed back and facilitate fear responding.

One of the questions that remains concerns the specificity of pituitary-adrenal effects on fear-mediated behaviors. That is, do these hormones exert specific actions on fear motivation per se, or do they exert some kind of general effect that could be reflected in other classes of behavior as well? Many different explanations of pituitary-adrenal effects on avoidance responding have been suggested. Included among these are arguments that these hormones affect fear motivation directly (e.g., DiGiusto et al., 1971), that they affect internal inhibition generally (e.g., Levine, 1968), that they affect central nervous system excitability (e.g., Weiss et al., 1970), and that they affect memory processes (Klein, 1972). Many of these interpretations of pituitary-adrenal effects really are not very different from each other (see Brush & Froelich, 1975), and, of course, it is not necessary that the effects of ACTH and/or the glucocorticoids be restricted to any single mode of action. It is clear, however, that these hormones can affect other, non-fear-mediated behaviors as well (e.g., Gray, 1971; Guth, Seward & Levine, 1971; and discussions in Chapters 2 and 3), and, therefore, it is unlikely that their effects are specific to fear.

SOME OTHER PITUITARY PEPTIDES

Not only does the stress of avoidance responding alter ACTH levels, but this stress leads to increases in the levels of at least two other pituitary peptides, melanocyte-stimulating hormone (MSH) and vasopressin (Sandman et al., 1973; Thompson & DeWied, 1973). In addition, removal of the posterior pituitary (and probably the intermediate lobe along with it) leads to a deficit in the retention of avoidance responses, suggesting a role for these other pituitary peptides in the control of fear-mediated responding (DeWied, 1969; DeWied & Bohus, 1966).

Melanocyte-Stimulating Hormone (MSH)

The effects of removing the posterior lobe of the pituitary on avoidance responding can be counteracted by treating rats with either ACTH, MSH, or an extract of posterior pituitary secretions called pitressin. In addition, treating intact rats with MSH will retard extinction of both active and passive avoidance responses (DeWied, 1966; Dempsey, Kastin & Schally, 1972). These findings implicate MSH in fear-mediated responding.

How or why does MSH affect fear-mediated behaviors? The effects of MSH are quite similar to those of ACTH and the ACTH fractions discussed before. Significantly, in rats, MSH and ACTH also are quite similar structurally. In fact, the first 13 amino acids in the peptide sequence are the same for these two hormones, and only the first 10 amino acids in the ACTH sequence are necessary for an ACTH fraction to exert its behavioral effects (DeWied, 1966). Therefore, it seems reasonable to suggest that MSH, which shares the first 13 amino acids with ACTH, might affect fear-responding because of its similarities to ACTH (DeWied, 1966).

Further support for this suggested mode of MSH action is provided by lesion studies showing that the parafascicular nuclei of the thalamus are necessary for MSH to exert its effects on avoidance responding, similar to the case with ACTH. Both MSH and ACTH retard extinction of avoidance responses in intact rats, but neither of these hormones affects avoidance performance in rats with lesions in the parafascicular nuclei of the thalamus (Bohus & DeWied, 1967; Wimersma Greidanus, Bohus & DeWied, 1974a).

Vasopressin

As mentioned in the discussion of MSH, a crude extract of posterior pituitary secretions, pitressin, also is effective in restoring the avoidance performance of neurohypophysectomized rats. In an attempt to specify more clearly the mechanisms of pitressin's action on avoidance responding, DeWied (1965) injected neurohypophysectomized rats with synthetic lysine vasopressin. He found that vasopressin could restore the avoidance performance of these neurohypophysectomized animals; thus yet another pituitary peptide was implicated in fear-mediated responding.

Specific manipulations of vasopressin levels also have shown that this peptide is important in fear-mediated responding. Exogenous vasopressin and vasopressin analogues retard extinction of both active and passive avoidance responses (Ader & DeWied, 1972; DeWied, Bohus & Wimersma Greidanus, 1974). In addition, selectively depleting vasopressin with an anti-vasopressin serum decreases retention of passive avoidance responses. Furthermore, oxytocin antiserum is ineffective in modifying avoidance responding, lending support to the notion that pitressin's actions are due to its vasopressin activities (Wimersma Greidanus, Dogterom & DeWied, 1975).

Yet another way to study vasopressin's action in fear-mediated responding is to capitalize on the fact that some animals suffer hereditary deficiencies in vasopressin. The Brattleboro rat is such an animal. This rat, having hereditary diabetes insipidus, exhibits deficiencies in the acquisition and maintenance of a variety of avoidance responses, providing further support for the proposition that vasopressin is involved in fear responding (Celestian, Carey & Miller, 1975; Wimersma Greidanus, Bohus & DeWied, 1975).

How does vasopressin exert its effects on avoidance responding? One early suggestion was that it might affect fear-mediated behaviors because it facilitates ACTH responses to stress. Slight increases in vasopressin levels increase the magnitude of the pituitary-adrenal stress response (DeWied, 1973; Yates et al., 1971), and the Brattleboro rats who are deficient in vasopressin exhibit reduced pituitary-adrenal responses when stressed (McCann et al., 1966; Wiley, Pearlmutter & Miller, 1974). Therefore, it seemed reasonable to suggest that vasopressin might affect fear-mediated responses through its effects on ACTH secretion.

However, three lines of evidence suggest that vasopressin affects fear-mediated responding independently of this hormone's effects on pituitary-adrenal activity. First, vasopressin still affects avoidance responding in adenohypophysectomized rats, who have no ACTH. Therefore, ACTH is not necessary for vasopressin to affect avoidance responding (DeWied, 1965, 1973).

Second, the time courses of the effects of vasopressin and ACTH are different. ACTH injections will affect extinction of avoidance responses if the animals are tested at two or four hours after injection, but not at 24 hours after injection. On the other hand, lysine vasopressin still exerts its effects at 24 and 72 hours post-injection (DeWied, 1971). In addition, vasopressin exerts a long-lasting effect, well after treatment with this hormone is terminated, and ACTH does not. Figure 7-5 shows the effects of daily treatment with an ACTH analogue, $ACTH_{4-10}$, and lysine vasopressin on the avoidance acquisition of hypophysectomized rats. Note that performance levels decline following the withdrawal of treatment with $ACTH_{4-10}$ but not following termination of vasopressin treatment (Bohus, Gispen & DeWied, 1973). These findings have been interpreted as suggesting that whereas ACTH acts either on fear motivation, short-term memory, or some similar short-term proc-

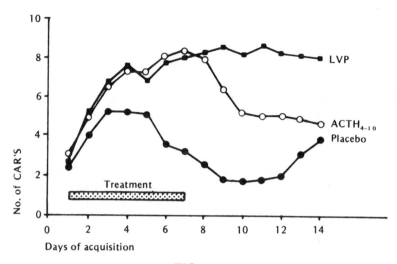

FIG. 7-5
Effect of daily treatment with ACTH$_{4-10}$ (20 μg/day) and lysine vaso-
pressin (LVP) (1 μg/day) for 7 days on avoidance acquisition of
hypophysectomized rats in a shuttlebox (from Bohus, Gispen & De-
Wied, *Neuroendocrinology*, 1973, 11, 139, by permission of S. Karger
AG, Basel).

ess, vasopressin exerts its effects on long-term memory or memory
consolidation (e.g., Wimersma Greidanus, Dogterom & DeWied,
1975).

Third, although it is likely that both vasopressin and ACTH act
by modifying the state of critical brain circuits (Wimersma Greidanus, Dogterom & DeWied, 1975), they seem to be acting at
different neural sites. Recall that ACTH does not retard extinction
in rats with lesions of the parafascicular nuclei, suggesting that this
brain site is critical to ACTH's effects on fear-mediated behaviors.
On the other hand, rats with these lesions still are responsive to
vasopressin treatment. Therefore, at least one brain site that is
critical for ACTH effects is not critical for vasopressin effects.
(Wimersma Greidanus, Bohus & DeWied, 1974a, 1974b).

Summary Statement: Other Pituitary Peptides

The data reviewed in this section suggest that at least two pituitary peptides other than ACTH, namely MSH and vasopressin, can affect fear-mediated responding. Both of these hormones are released following stress, and, therefore, they might be part of the feedback mechanism through which stress exposure facilitates fear-mediated responding. MSH appears to affect fear-mediated responding because of its similarities to ACTH. On the other hand, vasopressin appears to affect such behaviors independently of its effects on ACTH secretion. Because of the differences in the durations of their effects, it is interesting to speculate that ACTH (and perhaps MSH) may be the critical hormone in the short-term retention of fear responses, whereas vasopressin is the critical hormone in the long-term retention of these responses (compare Bohus, Gispen & DeWied, 1973).

GENDER DIFFERENCES

There is a marked gender difference in avoidance responding, at least in rats. Surprisingly, this gender difference is opposite in the cases of active and passive avoidance responses. Females seem to learn active avoidance responses more quickly than males (Beatty, Beatty & Bowman, 1971; Denti & Epstein, 1972), whereas males seem to learn passive avoidance responses more quickly than females (Denti & Epstein, 1972; Klemm, 1969a). In addition, females exhibit greater CER's than males (Leshner, Brookshire & Stewart, 1971).

What factors can account for such differences? The first and most obvious factor to consider might be circulating hormone levels. Males and females certainly differ dramatically in the levels of the gonadal hormones, and these differences might account for the gender differences in avoidance performance. Although Klemm (1969b) did observe that females acquire passive avoidance responses faster during estrous states than during nonestrous states, withdrawal of the gonadal hormones by gonadectomy appears to have no effect on either active or passive avoidance responding (e.g., Archer, 1975; Beatty & Beatty, 1970a; Scouten, Grotelueschen & Beatty, 1975). Therefore, differences in adult gonadal hormone levels do not seem to be responsible for the gender differences in avoidance responding.

A second possibility concerns the role of gender differences in pituitary-adrenocortical activity levels. Female rats have higher levels of pituitary-adrenal activity than males. Because increases in pituitary-adrenal activity levels facilitate avoidance performance (see discussion above), it was reasoned that the gender differences in active avoidance responding might be a result of females having higher pituitary-adrenal hormone levels (e.g., Beatty, Beatty & Bowman, 1971). However, gonadectomy of the female reduces the gender difference in pituitary-adrenal activity levels (e.g., Coyne & Kitay, 1969), but, as just discussed, this operation does not reduce the gender differences in avoidance performance. In addition, animals with increased levels of the pituitary-adrenal hormones exhibit greater passive avoidance responding, whereas females (who have higher levels of these hormones than males) exhibit poorer passive avoidance responding than males. Therefore, it is unlikely that the gender differences in fear-mediated responding are a result of gender differences in the levels of the pituitary-adrenocortical hormones.

A third possible explanation is related to gender differences in general activity levels. Recall from the discussion in Chapter 2 that females generally exhibit higher activity levels than males. The greater activity of females could account for their increased active avoidance performance relative to males (active avoidance demands activity), whereas their greater activity would interfere with the performance of passive avoidance tasks (which demands inhibiting activity) (Denti & Epstein, 1972). This explanation seems plausible but, of course, demands experimental verification.

The final and most probable factor in accounting for gender differences in avoidance performance is the early hormonal environment. Modifications of the early hormonal environment have been successful in reducing and even reversing gender differences, at least in active avoidance responding. Neonatally androgenizing female rats leads to adult avoidance responding similar to that of males (Beatty & Beatty, 1970a, 1970b), and treating males with the anti-androgen cyproterone acetate prenatally and castrating them postnatally makes them respond like females in adulthood (Scouten, Grotelueschen & Beatty, 1975). Thus, although adult hormone levels may not be critical to the gender differences in avoidance responding, the hormonal environment early in development does seem to be important in the determination of those gender differences.

SUMMARY AND COMMENT

This chapter was concerned with the relationship between hormones and fear-mediated responding in nonhuman mammals. The effects of stress or having to maintain avoidance responses on endocrine function were reviewed only briefly, and the main focus was on the role of hormones in the determination or control of fear-mediated responding.

Many studies have attempted to articulate the role of the adrenal medullary hormones in fear-mediated responses. However, they have yielded conflicting results. Some have shown that reducing catecholamine levels reduces fear and increasing catecholamine levels increases fear responding, although many other studies have found no effects of manipulating these hormone levels. Clearly, additional studies, perhaps using different approaches, will have to be conducted in order to clarify the role of the adrenal medullary hormones in fear-mediated behaviors.

The role of the pituitary-adrenocortical hormones in fear-mediated behaviors has received a great amount of attention.

These studies generally show that increasing ACTH levels leads to increases in fear-mediated responding, whereas increasing gluco-corticoid levels decreases fear. Studies of the mode of action of these hormones generally support the view that the pituitary-adrenal hormones affect fear-mediated responding by altering the state of critical circuits in the brain.

Some recent studies also have implicated some of the peptides of the intermediate and posterior lobes of the pituitary in fear-mediated responding. MSH appears to exert effects quite similar to those of ACTH, and this intermediate-lobe hormone may be acting in this way because of its structural similarities to ACTH. The posterior pituitary peptide, vasopressin, however, seems to ex-ert its facilitatory effects on fear-mediated responding independ-ently of its effects on ACTH secretion. Although vasopressin can potentiate pituitary-adrenal responses to stress, it appears to act in different neural sites than does ACTH. In addition, ACTH's and vasopressin's effects on fear-mediated responding appear to follow different time courses. Whereas ACTH exerts fairly short-term ef-fects on avoidance responding, vasopressin exerts rather long-term effects.

Finally, there is a marked gender difference in avoidance re-sponding in rats, although this difference is in opposite directions for active and passive avoidance responses. The gonadal hormones circulating in adulthood do not appear to be important, although the levels of these hormones during early developmental peri-ods appear critical to adult gender differences in fear-mediated responses.

At the beginning of each of the major sections of this chapter, we mentioned that interest in the role of each of the endocrine subsystems studied (except for the gonadal hormones) emerged following the observation that stress leads to a change in the level of the relevant hormones. That observation led to the suggestion that those hormones might feed back following stress and facili-tate fear-mediated responding. This kind of feedback effect is what we previously called a long-chain hormone–behavior interaction. How has this feedback notion fared? The experimental manipulations that increase hormone levels prior to exposure to the stressor or, in most cases, the avoidance situation, all might be viewed as potentiating the normal hormonal responses to experience. That is, although hormonal manipulations made prior to exposure to stress really are preventing natural responses, they also, in many cases, are producing hormonal changes even greater than those that would occur naturally. Therefore, although in most of the studies reviewed here, the hormonal manipulations were made prior to exposing the animal to the fear-provoking stimuli, one could interpret those studies as showing the effects of altering or exaggerating the natural hormonal responses to experience. In that case, the studies reviewed here argue well for there being a long-chain hormone–behavior interaction in the case of the fear-mediated behaviors. Manipulating the levels of many hormones affects fear-mediated responding, and the effects of those manipulations consistently are in the same direction as that predictable from a feedback hypothesis. For example, the feedback hypothesis would argue that the increase in ACTH following stress feeds back and facilitates fear-mediated performance. Significantly, exaggerating the pituitary-adrenal responses to stress by treating the animal with ACTH prior to behavioral testing does facilitate avoidance performance. Therefore, it seems likely that there is some kind of long-chain hormone–behavior interaction in the case of the fear-mediated behaviors.

It might be worthwhile to reiterate the caution raised at the beginning of this chapter: The studies reviewed have been conducted using laboratory animals, primarily rats, as subjects, and most studies have used shock as the fear-provoking stimulus. The few studies conducted using other kinds of aversive stimuli, such as attack by a trained fighter, raise questions about the generality of some of the findings from studies using shock. In addition, it may be that other species, and even rodents living in more natural environments, react differently from these laboratory animals. Therefore, as is often the case, one should remain cautious about generalizing from these studies to all fear-provoking stimuli or to other kinds of animals.

REFERENCES

Ader, R. & DeWied, D. Effects of lysine vasopressin on passive avoidance learning. *Psychonomic Science*, 1972, 29, 46-48.
Archer, J. Rodent sex differences in emotional and related behavior. *Behavioral Biology*, 1975, 14, 451-479.
Applezweig, M. H. & Baudry, F. D. The pituitary-adrenocortical system in avoidance learning. *Psychological Reports*, 1955, 1, 417-420.
Beatty, P. A., Beatty, W. W., Bowman, R. E. & Gilchrist, J. C. The effects of ACTH, adrenalectomy, and dexamethasone on the acquisition of an avoidance response in rats. *Physiology and Behavior*, 1970, 5, 939-944.
Beatty, W. W. & Beatty, P. A. Hormonal determinants of sex differences in avoidance behavior and reactivity to electric shock in the rat. *Journal of Comparative and Physiological Psychology*, 1970a, 3, 446-455.
Beatty, W. W. & Beatty, P. A. Effects of neonatal testosterone on the acquisition of an active avoidance response in genotypically male rats. *Psychonomic Science*, 1970b, 19, 315-316.
Beatty, W. W., Beatty, P. A. & Bowman, R. E. A sex difference in the extinction of avoidance behavior in rats. *Psychonomic Science*, 1971, 23, 213-214.
Bohus, B. Central nervous structures and the effect of ACTH and corticosteroids on avoidance behaviour: A study with intracerebral implantation of corticosteroids in the rat. *Progress in Brain Research*, 1970, 32, 171-183.
Bohus, B. & DeWied, D. Failure of α-MSH to delay extinction of conditioned avoidance behaviour in rats with lesions in the parafascicular nuclei of the thalamus. *Physiology and Behavior*, 1967, 2, 221-223.
Bohus, B., Endröczi, E. & Lissák, K. Correlations between avoiding conditioned reflex activity and pituitary-adrenocortical function in the rat. *Acta Physiologica Academiae Scientiarum Hungaricae*, 1964, 24, 79-83.
Bohus, B., Gispen, W. H. & DeWied, D. Effect of lysine vasopressin and $ACTH_{4-10}$ on conditioned avoidance behavior of hypophysectomized rats. *Neuroendocrinology*, 1973, 11, 137-143.
Brush, F. R. & Froelich, J. C. Motivational effects of the pituitary

and adrenal hormones. In B. E. Elftheriou & R. L. Sprott (Eds.), *Hormonal Correlates of Behavior*, Vol. 2. New York: Plenum Press, 1975, pp. 777-806.

Cannon, W. B. *Bodily Changes in Pain, Hunger, Fear and Rage.* New York: Appleton, 1915.

Celestian, J. F., Carey, R. J. & Miller, M.   Unimpaired maintenance of a conditioned avoidance response in the rat with diabetes insipidus. *Physiology and Behavior*, 1975, 15, 707-711.

Conner, R. L. & Levine, S.   The effects of adrenal hormones on the acquisition of signaled avoidance behavior. *Hormones and Behavior*, 1969, 1, 73-83.

Coyne, M. D. & Kitay, J. I.   Effect of ovariectomy on pituitary secretion of ACTH. *Endocrinology*, 1969, 85, 1097-1102.

Delft, A. M. L. van.   The relation between pretraining plasma corticosterone levels and the acquisition of an avoidance response in the rat. *Progress in Brain Research*, 1970, 32, 192-199.

Dempsey, G. L., Kastin, A. J. & Schally, A. V.   The effects of MSH on a restricted passive avoidance response. *Hormones and Behavior*, 1972, 3, 333-337.

Denti, A. & Epstein, A.   Sex differences in the acquisition of two kinds of avoidance behavior in rats. *Physiology and Behavior*, 1972, 8, 611-615.

DeWied, D.   Influence of anterior pituitary on avoidance learning and escape behavior. *American Journal of Physiology*, 1964, 207, 255-259.

DeWied, D.   The influence of the posterior and intermediate lobes of the pituitary and pituitary peptides on the maintenance of a conditioned avoidance response in rats. *International Journal of Neuropharmacology*, 1965, 4, 157-167.

DeWied, D.   Inhibitory effect of ACTH and related peptides on extinction of conditioned avoidance behavior in rats. *Proceedings of the Society for Experimental Biology and Medicine*, 1966, 122, 28-32.

DeWied, D.   Effects of peptide hormones on behavior. In W. F. Ganong & L. Martini (Eds.), *Frontiers in Neuroendocrinology*. New York: Oxford, 1969, pp. 97-140.

DeWied, D.   Long-term effect of vasopressin on the maintenance of a conditioned avoidance response in rats. *Nature*, 1971, 232, 58-60.

DeWied, D.   The role of the posterior pituitary and its peptides on the maintenance of conditioned avoidance behaviour. In K. Lissák (Ed.), *Hormones and Brain Function*. New York: Plenum Press, 1973, pp. 391-397.

DeWied, D. & Bohus, B.   Long-term and short-term effects on retention of a conditioned avoidance response in rats by treatment with long-acting pitressin and α-MSH. *Nature*, 1966, 212, 1484-1486.

DeWied, D., Bohus, B. & Greven, H. M. Influence of pituitary and adrenocortical hormones on conditioned avoidance behaviour in rats. In R. P. Michael (Ed.), *Endocrinology and Human Behaviour*. New York: Oxford, 1968, 188-199.
DeWied, D., Bohus, B. & Wimersma Greidanus, Tj. B. van. The hypothalamoneurohypophyseal system and the preservation of conditioned avoidance behavior in rats. *Progress in Brain Research*, 1974, 41, 417-428.
DeWied, D., Delft, A. M. L. van, Gispen, W. H., Weijnen, J. A. W. M. & Wimersma Greidanus, Tj. B. van. The role of pituitary-adrenal system hormones in active avoidance conditioning. In S. Levine (Ed.), *Hormones and Behavior*. New York: Academic Press, 1972, pp. 135-171.
DiGiusto, E. L. Adrenaline or peripheral noradrenaline depletion and passive avoidance in the rat. *Physiology and Behavior*, 1972, 8, 1059-1062.
DiGiusto, E. L., Cairncross, K. & King, M. G. Hormonal influences on fear-motivated responses. *Psychological Bulletin*, 1971, 75, 432-444.
Endröczi, E. Pituitary-adrenocortical activity, exploration and avoidance behavior in the rat. In C. H. Sawyer & R. A. Gorski (Eds.), *Steroid Hormones and Brain Function*. Berkeley: University of California Press, 1971, pp. 59-65.
Endröczi, E. *Limbic System, Learning and Pituitary-Adrenal Function*. Budapest: Akademiai Kiado, 1972.
Endröczi, E. & Fekete, T. Correlations between the pituitary-adrenal function and the exploratory activity, learning behaviour and limbic functions. In K. Lissák (Ed.), *Hormones and Brain Function*. New York: Plenum Press, 1973, pp. 399-408.
Endröczi, E. & Nyákás, C. Effect of septal lesion on exploratory activity, passive avoidance learning and pituitary-adrenal function in the rat. *Acta Physiologica Academiae Scientiarum Hungaricae*, 1971, 39, 351-360.
Friedman, S. B., Ader, R., Grota, L. J. & Larson, T. Plasma corticosterone response to parameters of electric shock stimulation in the rat. *Psychosomatic Medicine*, 1967, 29, 323-328.
Gibbs, J., Sechzer, J. A., Smith, G. P., Conners, R. & Weiss, J. M. Behavioral responsiveness of adrenalectomized, hypophysectomized and intact rats to electric shock. *Journal of Comparative and Physiological Psychology*, 1973, 82, 165-169.
Gispen, W. H., Wimersma Greidanus, Tj. B. van & DeWied, D. Effects of hypophysectomy and ACTH$_{4-10}$ on responsiveness to electric shock in rats. *Physiology and Behavior*, 1970, 5, 143-146.
Gold, P. E. & Buskirk, R. B. van. Facilitation of time-dependent

memory processes with post-trial epinephrine injections. *Behavioral Biology*, 1975, 13, 145-153.

Gold, P. E. & Buskirk, R. B. van. Enhancement and impairment of memory processes with post-trial injections of adrenocorticotrophic hormones. *Behavioral Biology*, 1976, 16, 387-400.

Gorelick, D. A., Bozewicz, T. R. & Bridger, W. H. The role of catecholamines in animal learning and memory. In A. J. Friedhoff (Ed.), *Catecholamines and Behavior*, 2. New York: Plenum Press, 1975, pp. 1-30.

Gray, J. A. Effect of ACTH on extinction of rewarded behavior is blocked by previous administration of ACTH. *Nature*, 1971, 229, 52-54.

Guth, S., Levine, S. & Seward, J. P. Appetitive acquisition and extinction effects with exogenous ACTH. *Physiology and Behavior*, 1971, 7, 195-200.

Kamano, D. K. Enhancement of learned fear with epinephrine. *Psychonomic Science*, 1968, 12, 331.

Klein, S. B. Adrenal-pituitary influence in reactivation of avoidance behavior of rats. *Communications in Behavioral Biology*, 1972, 79, 341-359.

Klemm, W. R. ECS effects on one-trial avoidance behavior in intact and gonadectomized male rats. *Communications in Behavioral Biology*, 1969, 4, 455-458. (a)

Klemm, W. R. ECS and estrous cycle interactions in one-trial avoidance behavior of rats. *Communications in Behavioral Biology*, 1969, 4, 459-465. (b)

Latané, B. & Schachter, S. Adrenalin and avoidance learning. *Journal of Comparative and Physiological Psychology*, 1962, 55, 369-372.

Leshner, A. I., Brookshire, K. H. & Stewart, C. N. The effects of adrenal demedullation on conditioned fear. *Hormones and Behavior*, 1971, 2, 43-48.

Leshner, A. I., Moyer, J. A. & Walker, W. A. Pituitary-adrenocortical activity and avoidance-of-attack in mice. *Physiology and Behavior*, 1975, 15, 689-693.

Leshner, A. I. & Stewart, C. N. Effect of epinephrine on extinction of an avoidance response. *Psychonomic Science*, 1966, 5, 89-90.

Leventhal, G. S. & Killackey, H. Adrenalin stimulation and preference for familiar stimuli. *Journal of Comparative and Physiological Psychology*, 1968, 65, 152-155.

Levine, S. Hormones and conditioning. In W. J. Arnold (Ed.), *Nebraska Symposium on Motivation*. Lincoln: University of Nebraska Press, 1968, pp. 85-101.

Levine, S. & Brush, F. R. Adrenocortical activity and avoidance learn-

ing as a function of time after avoidance training. *Physiology and Behavior,* 1967, 2, 385-388.
Levine, S. & Jones, L. E.   Adrenocorticotrophic hormone (ACTH) and passive avoidance learning. *Journal of Comparative and Physiological Psychology,* 1965, 59, 357-360.
Levine, S. & Levin, R.   Pituitary adrenal influences on passive avoidance in two inbred strains of mice. *Hormones and Behavior,* 1970, 1, 105-110.
Levine, S. & Soliday, S.   An effect of adrenal demedullation on the acquisition of a conditioned avoidance response. *Journal of Comparative and Physiological Psychology,* 1962, 55, 214-216.
McCann, S. M., Antunes-Rodrigues, J., Nallar, R. & Valtin, H.   Pituitary-adrenal function in the absence of vasopressin. *Endocrinology,* 1966, 79, 1058-1064.
Manogue, K. R., Leshner, A. I. & Candland, D. K.   Dominance status and adrenocortical reactivity to stress in squirrel monkeys (*Saimiri sciureus*). *Primates,* 1975, 16, 457-463.
Mason, J. W.   Organization of the multiple endocrine responses to avoidance in the monkey. *Psychosomatic Medicine,* 1968, 30, 774-790.
Mason, J. W.   The integrative approach in medicine—implications of neuroendocrine mechanisms. *Perspectives in Biology and Medicine,* 1974, 17, 333-347.
Mason, J. W., Brady, J. V. & Tolliver, G. A.   Plasma and urinary 17-hydroxycorticosteroid responses to 72-hr. avoidance sessions in the monkey. *Psychosomatic Medicine,* 1968, 30, 608-630.
Mason, J. W., Mangan, G., Brady, J. V., Conrad, D. & Rioch, D. McK.   Concurrent plasma epinephrine, norepinephrine and 17-hydroxycorticosteroid levels during conditioned emotional disturbances in monkeys. *Psychosomatic Medicine,* 1961, 223, 344-353.
Mason, J. W., Tolson, W. W., Brady, J. V., Tolliver, G. A. & Gilmore, L. I.   Urinary epinephrine responses to 72-hr. avoidance sessions in the monkey. *Psychosomatic Medicine,* 1968, 30, 654-664.
Miller, R. E. & Ogawa, N.   The effect of adrenocorticotrophic hormone (ACTH) on avoidance conditioning in the adrenalectomized rat. *Journal of Comparative and Physiological Psychology,* 1962, 55, 211-213.
Moyer, J. A. & Leshner, A. I.   Pituitary-adrenal effects on avoidance-of-attack in mice: separation of the effects of ACTH and corticosterone. *Physiology and Behavior,* 1976, 17, 297-301.
Moyer, K. E. & Bunnell, B. N.   Effects of injected adrenalin on an avoidance response in the rat. *Journal of Genetic Psychology,* 1958, 92, 247-251.

Moyer, K. E. & Bunnell, B. N.   Effect of adrenal demedullation on an avoidance response in the rat. *Journal of Comparative and Physiological Psychology*, 1959, 62, 215-216.

Murphy, J. V. & Miller, R. E.   The effect of adrenocorticotrophic hormone (ACTH) on avoidance conditioning in the rat. *Journal of Comparative and Physiological Psychology*, 1955, 48, 47-49.

Pagano, R. R. & Lovely, R. H.   Diurnal cycle and ACTH facilitation of shuttlebox avoidance. *Physiology and Behavior*, 1972, 8, 721, 723.

Pappas, B. A.   Immunological and chemical sympathectomy in the neonatal rodent: effects on emotional behavior. In L. V. DiCara (Ed.), *Limbic and Autonomic Nervous System Research*. New York: Plenum Press, 1974, pp. 165-194.

Paré, W. P. & Cullen, J. W.   Adrenal influences on the aversive threshold and CER acquisition. *Hormones and Behavior*, 1971, 2, 139-147.

Sandman, C. A., Kastin, A. J., Schally, A. V., Kendall, J. W. & Miller, L. H.   Neuroendocrine responses to physical and psychological stress. *Journal of Comparative and Physiological Psychology*, 1973, 84, 386-390.

Scouten, C. W., Grotelueschen, L. K. & Beatty, W. W.   Androgens and the organization of sex differences in active avoidance behavior in the rat. *Journal of Comparative and Physiological Psychology*, 1975, 88, 264-270.

Selye, H.   *The Stress of Life*. New York: McGraw-Hill, 1956.

Schneider, A. M., Weinberg, J. & Weissberg, R.   Effects of ACTH on conditional suppression: a time and strength of conditioning analysis. *Physiology and Behavior*, 1974, 13, 633-636.

Silva, M. T. A.   Extinction of a passive avoidance response in adrenalectomized and demedullated rats. *Behavioral Biology*, 1973, 9, 553-562.

Silva, M. T. A.   Effects of adrenal demedullation and adrenalectomy on an active avoidance response of rats. *Physiological Psychology*, 1974, 2, 171-174.

Stewart, C. N. & Brookshire, K. H.   Shuttle box avoidance learning and epinephrine. *Psychonomic Science*, 1967, 9, 419-420.

Stewart, C. N. & Brookshire, K. H.   Effect of epinephrine on acquisition of conditioned fear. *Physiology and Behavior*, 1968, 3, 601-604.

Strand, F. L., Stoboy, H. & Cayer, A.   A possible direct action of ACTH on nerve and muscle. *Neuroendocrinology*, 1974, 13, 1-20.

Tarpy, R. M.   *Basic Principles of Learning*. Glenview, Illinois: Scott, Foresman, 1975.

Thompson, E. A. & DeWied, D.   The relationship between antidiuretic activity of rat eye plexus blood and passive avoidance behaviour. *Physiology and Behavior*, 1973, 11, 377-380.

Van-Toller, C. & Tarpy, R. M. Immunosympathectomy and avoidance behavior. *Psychological Bulletin*, 1974, 81, 132-137.

Vernikos-Danellis, J. Effects of hormones on the central nervous system. In S. Levine (Ed.), *Hormones and Behavior*. New York: Academic Press, 1972, pp. 11-62.

Weiss, J. M., McEwen, B. S., Silva, M. T. A. & Kalkut, M. F. Pituitary-adrenal influences on fear responding. *Science*, 1969, 163, 197-199.

Weiss, J. M., McEwen, B. S., Silva, M. T. A. & Kalkut, M. Pituitary-adrenal alterations and fear responding. *American Journal of Physiology*, 1970, 218, 864-868.

Wertheim, G. A., Conner, R. L. & Levine, S. Avoidance conditioning and adrenocortical function in the rat. *Physiology and Behavior*, 1969, 4, 41-44.

Wiley, M. K., Pearlmutter, A. F. & Miller, R. E. Decreased adrenal sensitivity to ACTH in the vasopressin-deficient (Brattleboro) rat. *Neuroendocrinology*, 1974, 14, 257-270.

Wimersma Greidanus, Tj. B. van. Effects of steroids on extinction of an avoidance response in rats. A structure-activity relationship study. *Progress in Brain Research*, 1970, 32, 185-191.

Wimersma Greidanus, Tj. B. van, Bohus, B. & DeWied, D. The parafascicular area as the site of action of ACTH analogues on avoidance behavior. *Progress in Brain Research*, 1974, 41, 429-432. (a)

Wimersma Greidanus, Tj. B. van, Bohus, B. & DeWied, D. Differential localization of lysine vasopressin and of $ACTH_{4-10}$ on avoidance behavior: a study in rats bearing lesions in the parafascicular nuclei. *Neuroendocrinology*, 1974, 14, 280-288. (b)

Wimersma Greidanus, Tj. B. van, Bohus, B. & DeWied, D. The role of vasopressin in memory processes. *Progress in Brain Research*, 1975, 42, 135-141.

Wimersma Greidanus, Tj. B. van & DeWied, D. Effects of intracerebral implantation of corticosteroids on extinction of an avoidance response in rats. *Physiology and Behavior*, 1969, 4, 365-370.

Wimersma Greidanus, Tj. B. van & DeWied, D. Effects of systemic and intracerebral administration of two opposite acting ACTH-related peptides on extinction of conditioned avoidance behavior. *Neuroendocrinology*, 1971, 7, 291-301.

Wimersma Greidanus, Tj. B. van, Dogterom, J. & DeWied, D. Intraventricular administration of anti-vasopressin serum inhibits memory consolidation in rats. *Life Sciences*, 1975, 16, 637-644.

Yates, F. E., Russell, S. M., Dallman, M. F., Hedge, G. A., McCann, S. M. & Dhariwal, A. P. S. Potentiation by vasopressin of corticotropin release induced by corticotropin-releasing factor. *Endocrinology*, 1971, 88, 3-15.

Chapter 8

EMOTION AND MOOD

Interest in the role of hormones in emotion and mood stems from a more general interest in the role of physiology in emotion, and there have been numerous theories proposed to account for the role of physiological functioning in emotional experience. One of the first formal statements of the role of physiology in emotion was the strong position advocated by William James in 1884. James suggested that bodily changes directly follow the perception of an exciting "fact," and that "our feeling of the same changes as they occur *is* the emotion" (James, 1892, p. 375). In 1885, Lange suggested, independently, that emotions are vasomotor disturbances following environmental events, and that the cognitive aspects of emotion are secondary to the physiological qualities (Wenger, 1950). In spite of there being some differences in these two theories of emotion, they both advocate a particular sequence of events: the physiological aspect of emotion precedes the cognitive aspect. Because of this similarity, James' and Lange's positions have been considered together historically in what has often been called the "James-Lange theory of emotion."

James' theory of emotion met with a great amount of criticism. Perhaps the most vocal and ardent of his critics was W. B. Cannon, who argued that the real sequence of events in emotion is the opposite of that proposed by James: emotions are cognitive, not visceral, in origin, and cognitive events precede physiological changes (Cannon, 1915, 1927). The disagreement about the sequence of events in emotion often has been called the "James-Cannon controversy." However, both positions could be correct. It is possible that physiological changes both precede and follow cognitive events, or even that some physiological changes occur concomitantly with cognitive reactions (Candland, 1977; Leshner, 1977).

Subsequent theories of emotion all seem to have been derived from either James' or Cannon's basic position. Some of these theories have emphasized the role of physiological antecedents to emotion, whereas others have focused on the physiological reactions to emotional experiences. Perhaps the most well-known theories following in the Jamesian tradition are the *activation theories*, classified as Jamesian because they emphasize the importance of physiological arousal in the intensity of emotional reactions. However, the activation theorists do not seem to believe that the form or source of that arousal affects emotion, as did James. For example, Duffy (1934) argued that emotions differ from other behaviors in degree rather than in kind of physiological reaction, and, therefore, that we should shift our emphasis from studying the role of physiology in specific behaviors to studying the role of physiological arousal in determining the degrees or intensities of behavior. Later activation theorists include Arnold (1950), Bindra (1969), Lindsley (1951), and Malmo (1959).

A second major class of theories of physiology and emotion, derived from Cannon's basic position, have focused on the form of the physiological correlates of or responses to emotional experiences. Some investigators (e.g., Ax, 1953; Funkenstein, 1955) have sought to determine the particular physiological responses that are idiosyncratic to particular types of emotional experiences. Others (e.g., Persky et al., 1958) have argued that the physiological responses to different emotions are all basically similar. In either case, many studies have sought to determine the form of physiological responses to emotional experiences.

The sequence question has been left relatively undecided, perhaps because of the technological difficulties inherent in measuring the time courses of cognitive and physiological events in a reacting system that moves so quickly. One theorist, however, has attempted to specify experimentally the form of the relationship between the cognitive and physiological components of emotion. Stanley Schachter and his colleagues (e.g., Schachter & Singer, 1962; Schachter & Wheeler, 1962) have suggested that emotion, or the recognition of emotion, is a process whereby cognitive labels are attached to physiological states of arousal. The specific label attached depends on the particular environmental conditions. This position can be viewed as an extension of James' view, because it argues that visceral arousal precedes the labeling process (cognition). Schachter's theory also may be viewed as an extension of activation theories because it emphasizes the ambiguity of the information derived from physiological arousal alone; emotional experience demands labeling of that arousal, and the label attached depends on environmental cues. The primary difference from activation theories is that Schachter attempts to articulate why an individual labels a particular arousal state in a specific way, rather than merely focusing on the role of arousal in the intensity of emotional reactions.

What of hormones? Our discussion so far has considered physiology in a very general sense, yet the subject matter of this chapter is hormones, and their relationship to emotion and mood. Hormones have been studied both as a part of the physiological system either affecting or stimulating emotional reactions and as a part of the physiological response system that is activated following (or during) emotional experiences. Studies of hormones and emotion have been of the same basic types as those of hormones and other classes of behavior: Some studies have focused on the effects of hormones on emotion, whereas others have focused on the hormonal correlates of or responses to emotional experiences. Because these groups of studies have remained relatively distinct, they will be considered separately here. In addition, the literature on hormones and emotion is vast, and, therefore, it will only be summarized here. The interested reader is referred to the more comprehensive reviews by Arnold (1960), Black (1970), Frankenhaeuser (1975), and Leshner (1977).

This chapter is concerned solely with the relationship of hormones to emotion and mood as studied in human subjects. There have been some attempts to develop nonhuman animal models of emotion, and some of these have been studied in relation to endocrine function. Many of these animal models have been considered in earlier chapters (e.g., Chapters 3 and 7), and the reader interested in pursuing the issue of animal models of emotion and emotionality further is referred to the reviews by Ader (1975), Archer (1973), and Candland and Nagy (1969).

The review that follows is divided into three major sections. The first section considers the relationship between hormones and relatively short-lived and situation-specific emotional experiences, such as fear, rage, and anger. The second section considers some longer-lasting, more diffuse emotional experiences, mood states. The third section considers long-lasting and debilitating extremes of emotion or mood in the form of the affective disorders.

HORMONES AND EMOTION

The studies to be described in this section all are concerned with relatively short-lived emotional experiences. This review is divided into two subsections. The first is concerned with the effects of hormones on emotional experiences, and the second is concerned with the effects of emotional experiences on endocrine function. Although, as in the case of the behaviors discussed in earlier chapters, it seems reasonable to suggest that there might be long-chain hormone–behavior interactions in the case of emotion (compare, Leshner, 1977), there have been no studies testing this proposition directly. Therefore, the two bodies of literature will be considered separately, and we can only speculate about the possibility of there being a continuous loop between the effects of emotional experiences on endocrine function and the effects of hormones on emotion.

Hormonal Effects on Emotion

The first studies of the effects of hormones on emotion were attempts to test James' hypothesis about the role of physiology in emotion directly. Recall that James' position argued that physiological events precede and determine the cognitive or experiential aspects of emotion. Therefore, these early studies were attempts to produce emotional experiences through physiological manipulations alone. The first attempt was by Marañon (1924). He injected individuals with epinephrine (adrenalin) and asked them to report their feelings. Although most subjects reported feeling aroused, few experienced discrete, identifiable emotional states. Those that did reported only "cold" emotions; no one experienced genuine emotions. That is, the subjects reported feeling *as if* they were afraid, rather than that they *were* afraid. Other investigators (e.g., Cantril & Hunt, 1932; Landis & Hunt, 1932; Lindemann & Finesinger, 1940) conducted similar studies and found, again, that injections of epinephrine could at most induce these cold emotions; their subjects almost never reported feeling genuine emotional states. Therefore, although epinephrine injections could produce physiological arousal, increasing the level of this hormone was not sufficient by itself to produce genuine emotional states.

In another early study, Cantril (1934) compared the effects of epinephrine injections alone with the effects of epinephrine treatment in the presence of environmental emotion-provoking stimuli. He found that some subjects did report feeling somewhat afraid when epinephrine was injected without any additional cues. However, Cantril suggested that these subjects felt fearful because they were concerned about the unidentified state of arousal that they were experiencing. Significantly, when a fear-provoking stimulus, a loud noise, was applied, the subjects reported feeling more intense and genuine fear-like states than when epinephrine was injected alone. On the basis of these findings, Cantril concluded that emotional stimuli from the environment are necessary to the production of genuine emotional states; all that epinephrine does is to affect the intensity of those reactions.

In the early 1960s Schachter and his colleagues began an extensive research program which expanded Cantril's earlier work on the importance of situational conditions in determining emotional reactions. As in the earlier studies, Schachter's group used manipulations of epinephrine levels to alter physiological states. In a typical experiment (Schachter & Singer, 1962), subjects were injected either with epinephrine or with a placebo; and then they were exposed to stooges who were acting either angry or euphoric while "waiting to be tested." The emotional behavior exhibited by the subjects in the presence of the stooges was used as the index of emotional reaction. The experimenters found that if subjects had been forewarned that they would experience some strange physical symptoms, they exhibited no particular emotional behaviors in reaction to the stooges. However, if the subjects had no explanation for their feelings of physical arousal, they acted much like or mimicked the stooges' behavior. When subjects experienced unexplained arousal in the presence of an angry stooge, the subjects acted angry. When they experienced unexplained arousal in the presence of a euphoric stooge, the subjects acted euphoric. Therefore, the same arousal state can lead to different emotional behaviors, depending on the particular environmental situation. Schachter and his colleagues have interpreted these types of studies as showing that one labels unexplained physiological arousal states on the basis of available environmental stimuli that might account for the elicitation of those states. In this way, emotional reactions can be viewed as a function of both a physiological arousal state and a cognition appropriate to the environmental situation.

Gerdes (in press) tested Schachter's hypothesis in a more natural environment, a dental clinic. In her experiment, some subjects had been given the local anesthetic lidocaine with epinephrine in it, whereas other subjects received lidocaine without epinephrine. The presence of epinephrine in the anesthetic was sufficient to cause an increase in physiological arousal. Those subjects given epinephrine reported experiencing greater fear while in the clinic than those not given this hormone, so long as the epinephrine-treated subjects did not know that they had been given this treatment. If they did know that they would feel aroused, however, the subjects reported only the same amount of fear as subjects not treated with epinephrine. Thus, subjects who experience arousal with no explanation for that arousal seem to attribute it to environmental conditions that could produce or evoke arousal. In this case, dental clinics are frightening places and, therefore, if one is unexplainedly aroused, one must be frightened. If, however, there is a rational explanation for that arousal (i.e., in this case if one is told that there is a substance in the anesthetic that will produce arousal), it will not be labeled according to the environmental situation but will be attributed to the real cause.

These studies appear to argue against James' position that the physiological state causes the emotional reaction. James' theory demands that different arousal states cause different emotions, but, in these studies, the same arousal state led to different emotional reactions depending on the environmental circumstances (see Schachter, 1967, 1970). However, these studies have only examined the effects of manipulating epinephrine levels, and this hormone may have been a poor choice. Epinephrine is a sympathomimetic substance, and its effects are very diffuse, producing a generalized state of arousal (Rogoff, 1945; Stein, 1967). Perhaps emotions *can* be differentiated on the basis of specific arousal states, but only if those arousal states are clearly discriminable. Sadly, the critical studies using manipulations that have more specific physiological effects have not been conducted with human subjects. Therefore, final evaluation of James' theory should await more extensive tests involving more specific manipulations of physiological states.

Hormonal Correlates of and Responses to Emotional Experience

This section is concerned with studies examining hormonal states either during or following emotional experiences. These studies differ from those considered in the last section in terms of which variables are manipulated and which are measured. In the studies described in the last section, the physiological state was manipulated, and then the effects of such manipulations on emotional experience were studied. In the studies to be discussed now, however, emotional states were manipulated, and then the effects of these behavioral manipulations on endocrine function were studied. In the same way that the studies reviewed in the last section can be viewed as derived from or based on James' theoretical position, the studies in this section can be viewed as derived from Cannon's position. Recall that Cannon argued that physiological changes follow emotional experiences, and these changes are the topic of these studies.

The primary question examined in these studies is not whether or not there are hormonal changes during and following emotional experiences. Of that there is no question. Rather, the question addressed is whether emotional experiences can be discriminated on the basis of the hormonal changes they produce. That is, are there specific physiological reactions associated with specific emotional experiences?

Studies of the effects of emotional experience on endocrine function have focused on two endocrine subsystems, the sympathoadrenal medullary system and the pituitary-adrenocortical axis. Studies examining the effects of emotion on catecholamine secretion probably are derived from Cannon's early (1929) statement that all emotional reactions are accompanied by increases in the release of these hormones. On the other hand, studies considering the pituitary-adrenocortical responses to emotional experience probably are derived from Selye's (1956) statement about the role of the hormones of this axis in stress-responding (See the more complete discussion of Selye's General Adaptation Syndrome in Chapter 7.)

Arnold (1945) first suggested that emotions could be differentiated on the basis of the physiological reactions they produce. She argued that fear is characterized by sympathetic activation, whereas anger is characterized by parasympathetic activation. Later theorists have argued different ways of characterizing emotional reactions, the most influential being the distinction proposed by Ax (1953) and Funkenstein (1955). They argued that whereas fear is accompanied by a marked increase in epinephrine levels, anger is characterized by increases in both norepinephrine and epinephrine levels (in this later case, norepinephrine influences are assumed to predominate, Stanley-Jones, 1970).

The data concerning the specificity of hormonal responses to emotional experiences are conflicting. Early studies generally supported the position that emotions could be discriminated on the basis of the hormonal reactions they produce. For example, Ax (1953) studied the physiological responses of subjects to either electric shock (fear provoking) or an incompetent technician (anger provoking). On the basis of the form of the subjects' physiological responses to these stimuli, Ax argued that physiological fear reactions are similar to those caused by increases in epinephrine levels, whereas anger reactions are similar to those caused by increases in both epinephrine and norepinephrine levels. Funkenstein (1955) studied the physiological reactions accompanying responses of anger and fear in threatening situations. He used blood pressure changes as an index of whether physiological reactions were epinephrine-like or norepinephrine-like. Those subjects responding to threat with fear exhibited physiological responses similar to the effects of injected epinephrine, whereas those responding with anger exhibited responses similar to the effects of norepinephrine. On the basis of these findings, Funkenstein (1956) argued that different emotions activate different areas of the hypothalamus, which then cause differences in the physiological response pattern.

Some investigators have attempted to discriminate other emotional reactions on the basis of the hormonal responses that characterize them. For example, Elmadjian, Hope, and Lamson (1957, 1958) found that individuals showing aggressive, active emotional displays to an intensive interview situation had increased norepinephrine excretion levels, whereas those showing anxious, passive type responses had increased epinephrine excretion levels.

The studies just reviewed appear to support the position that there are at least different catecholamine responses to different emotional situations. However, a number of more recent studies have found no differences in the hormonal responses to different emotional experiences. At least, the physiological responses idiosyncratic to particular emotional experiences are not easily discriminable. For example, Levi (1965) exposed women to different types of films and found that they responded to both pleasant (amusing) and aggression-provoking films with similar increases in epinephrine secretion. In addition, studying adrenocortical responses to emotional experiences, Brown and Heninger (1975) exposed subjects to either erotic or suspense films and found that all responded with similar increases in plasma cortisol levels. Furthermore, Mason, Rose, and their colleagues (e.g., Mason, 1959; Rose et al., 1969) have reported that a wide variety of stressors and emotion-provoking stimuli all lead to similar increases in pituitary-adrenocortical activity levels. Therefore, although earlier studies did support the position that there are specific physiological (hormonal) responses associated with particular emotional reactions, later studies have not supported this view (see Frankenhaeuser, 1975). It appears that different emotions cannot be discriminated on the basis of, at least, either adrenal medullary or adrenocortical responses.

Finally, some investigators have attempted to describe personality characteristics that might contribute to the form of an individual's hormonal responses to emotional experiences. Roessler, Burch, and Mefferd (1967) found that medical students scoring high in "ego strength" on the MMPI (Minnesota Multiphasic Personality Inventory) show increased catecholamine excretion levels during stressful situations, whereas those scoring low in ego strength show decreased catecholamine excretion levels. Fine and Sweeney (1968) reported that individuals rated as highly aggressive according to a battery of personality tests secrete greater quantities of norepinephrine in response to a cold stress than individuals rated as nonaggressive. Wolff et al. (1964) showed that if parents of fatally ill children exhibit strong defenses against the impending trauma of their children's deaths, these parents also exhibit lower adrenocortical activity than parents with weaker psychological defenses. Thus, it may be that individuals with different personality characteristics exhibit different hormonal responses to emotional experiences.

Comment: Hormones and Emotion

The data reviewed in this section suggest that the relationship between hormones and emotion is not specific. That is, it appears that specific hormones do not affect only specific emotions, and, conversely, having particular emotional experiences does not appear to lead to specific hormonal changes. Rather, it appears that hormones (at least the adrenal medullary hormones) affect emotion more generally, through affecting the arousal state of the individual; and most emotional experiences lead to the same kinds of hormonal responses: increases in the secretion of the catecholamines and the glucocorticoids. This conclusion should remain tentative, however, since only a few hormones have been studied in relation to emotional reactions. It may be that some other hormones do have more specific effects on emotion, and that different emotional experiences would affect other endocrine secretions differentially.

In spite of the generality of the relationship between hormones and emotion, it may still be that there is a long-chain hormone–behavior interaction in operation. For example, increases in epinephrine levels can potentiate emotional reactions, and emotional reactions lead to increases in epinephrine levels. It may be that the increases in epinephrine secretion that follow emotional experiences feed back and facilitate either ongoing responses or responses in subsequent situations (Breggin, 1964; Leshner, 1977). However, this proposition is not based on direct demonstrations of a feedback relationship, and, therefore, it must be considered speculative until the appropriate experimental tests have been conducted.

HORMONES AND MOODS:
THE PREMENSTRUAL SYNDROME

Moods and mood changes are a special class of emotions. Although most emotions are reactions precipitated by and directed toward specific environmental events or stimuli, moods tend to be more diffuse, and there often are no identifiable stimuli associated with mood states. Mood states have dramatic effects on behavior, and they can affect the intensity of our reactions to emotion-provoking stimuli. For example, if one is depressed, relatively mild setbacks can be perceived as drastic. On the other hand, if one is relatively calm, those setbacks may seem minimal.

Most people experience changes in moods or affective states quite regularly. However, some people experience extremes of mood that last for long periods of time. These usually are considered pathological, and the role of hormones in these "affective disorders" will be considered in the next section of this chapter. The discussion in this section is concerned with the role of hormones in the one class of mood changes that has been studied extensively with respect to endocrine function, the mood changes that occur across the menstrual cycle.

Many women report feeling somewhat depressed, anxious, and irritable just before menstruation begins, during the premenstrual period. This pattern of mood changes is so pervasive that it has been termed the *premenstrual syndrome* (Moos, 1968; Parlee, 1973), and many studies have been conducted to determine both the generality and the form of these mood changes. For example, Moos et al. (1969) studied the mood states of 15 women over the course of two menstrual cycles. They found that the women experienced quite consistent mood changes over both cycles: increases in depression during the premenstrual phase and an increase in anxiety during the time of menstruation. Ivey and Bardwick (1968) reported that women are more anxious, hostile, and depressed during the premenstrual period than during other menstrual cycle stages; and Marinari, Leshner, and Doyle (1976) found that women exhibit greater reactivity to stress, as measured by adrenocortical responses, during the menstrual phase of the cycle than during the midcycle phase. The reader interested in pursuing the form and generality of menstrual-cycle mood changes further is referred to the excellent reviews by Parlee (1973) and Smith (1975).

These changes in mood states are coincident with changes in the levels of the gonadal hormones across the menstrual cycle. Therefore, there is a correlation between mood states and gonadal hormone levels. Although there are many nonphysiological factors that might account for the cyclicity of these mood states (Parlee, 1973; Rakoff, 1968), some experimental studies have suggested that there may be causality in the correlation between changes in gonadal hormone levels and changes in mood states across the menstrual cycle. Most of these studies have used the birth control pill as a device for preventing dramatic hormonal changes across the cycle. These studies generally have found that women taking birth control pills experience less dramatic mood shifts than women not taking the pill (e.g., Kutner & Brown, 1972; Paige, 1971). Significantly, the "combination pill," which regulates hormone titres at the same levels across the cycle, is more effective in reducing premenstrual symptomatology than the "sequential pill," which allows for greater hormonal change (Hamburg, Moos & Yalom, 1968; Kutner & Brown, 1972). Thus, preventing or reducing gonadal hormone changes across the menstrual cycle leads to a decrease in premenstrual symptomatology. This suggests that changes in the levels of the gonadal hormones might play a causal role in the premenstrual syndrome.

However, the pill produces a general regulation of hormone levels, and, even though regulating hormone levels may reduce premenstrual mood shifts, a question still remains concerning the specific relationship between the gonadal hormones and the premenstrual syndrome. That is, why or how do the gonadal hormones affect mood states? Several theories have been proposed, including (1) that the premenstrual syndrome is a response to the presence or absence of specific hormones; (2) that changes in the estrogen/progesterone ratio determine premenstrual symptomatology; and (3) that the premenstrual syndrome is a result of the withdrawal of certain hormones just prior to menstruation (Smith, 1975). This issue has not been settled, although each position has been argued convincingly. For example, progesterone has general anesthetic or tranquilizing properties, and the reduction in the level of this hormone that occurs just prior to menstruation might account for the increase in anxiety that occurs premenstrually. That is, the withdrawal of the tranquilizing effects of progesterone could account for an increase in excitability or anxiety. Significantly, there also is a correlation between the withdrawal of progesterone and the occurrence of depression during both the postpartum period and the involutional period (Hamburg, 1965).

One study by Bäckström and Carstensen (1974) has examined carefully the time course of hormonal changes just prior to and during the premenstrual period, and compared that time course in women who do and do not experience extreme changes in mood premenstrually. The results of that analysis are presented in Figures 8-1 and 8-2. As can be seen from these figures, women who experience premenstrual anxiety (PMT-a) exhibit both higher estrogen levels during the sixth to second premenstrual days and lower progesterone levels during the sixth to fourth premenstrual days than women who do not experience a premenstrual increase in anxiety. Although these findings do not provide a basis for a decision among the alternative explanations outlined above, they do demonstrate clearly that women who experience premenstrual symptomatology exhibit different types of gonadal hormone changes premenstrually than women who do not.

HORMONES AND THE AFFECTIVE DISORDERS

There are some cases where extreme mood states last for long periods of time. When these extremes of mood are both long-lasting and debilitating, they are classified clinically as *affective disorders,* and many studies have examined the relationship between these disorders and endocrine function. Included among the affective disorders are *depression, mania,* and situations where there is cyclicity between depressive and manic states.

The discussion that follows is limited to the relationship between the affective disorders and endocrine function. The vast literature relating central catecholamine and indoleamine levels to the affective disorders will not be reviewed here. The reader interested in pursuing the relationship between central neurotransmitter activity and the affective disorders is referred to the excellent reviews that appear in Freedman (1975), Kline (1974), and Mendels (1973, 1975). It should be noted before proceeding, however, that there have been extensive discussions regarding the role of central catecholamines in the affective disorders, resulting in a variety of "catecholamine hypotheses" about these disorders. The proponents of these hypotheses argue, basically, that depression is

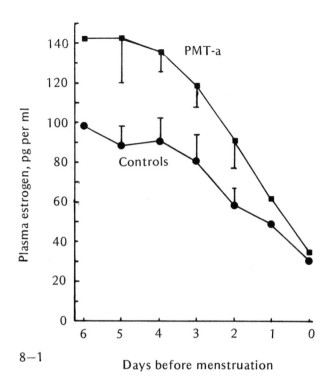

8–1

FIG. 8-1

Mean ± standard error plasma estrogen levels prior to menstruation in women experiencing high anxiety premenstrually and controls (from Bäckström & Carstensen, *Journal of Steroid Biochemistry*, 1974, 5, 258, by permission of Pergamon Press).

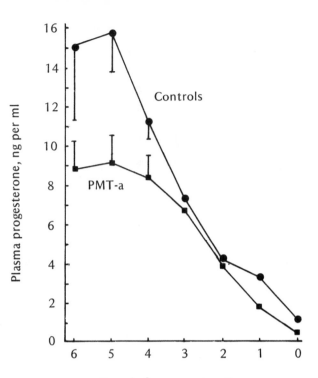

FIG. 8-2

Mean ± standard error plasma progesterone levels prior to menstruation in women experiencing high anxiety premenstrually and controls (from Bäckström & Carstensen, *Journal of Steroid Biochemistry*, 1974, 5, 259, by permission of Pergamon Press).

characterized by decreases in central catecholaminergic activity, whereas mania is characterized by increases in this kind of neurotransmitter activity (see Maas, 1975; Schildkraut & Kety, 1967).

Endocrinopathies and Affective States

Interest in the relationship between the affective disorders and endocrine function seems to have emerged from the clinical observation that there often are marked behavioral changes accompanying endocrine abnormalities or endocrinopathies (see extensive review by Whybrow & Hurwitz, 1976). For example, patients with hyperthyroidism often are quite irritable and excitable, whereas patients with hypothyroidism (myxedema) exhibit symptoms of depression (Sheard, 1975). In addition, patients with Cushing's syndrome, which is characterized by increases in adrenocortical activity, exhibit depression and irritability (Sachar, 1974a; Sheard, 1975). This latter finding would seem to suggest that there is a positive relationship between glucocorticoid secretion and depressive symptoms. However, patients with Addison's disease, which leads to a decrease in glucocorticoid secretion, also exhibit depressive symptoms. Therefore, patients with both increases and decreases in glucocorticoid secretion exhibit symptoms of depression.

Sachar (1974a) has suggested an explanation of this bimodal relationship between glucocorticoid secretion and depression based on ACTH action. Cushing's syndrome can result from at least three kinds of organic disorders, and, although in all three cases glucocorticoid levels are high, each disorder results in a different relationship between ACTH and cortisol levels. First, some Cushing patients have glucocorticoid-secreting tumors that are accompanied by decreases in ACTH levels (via negative feedback effects). Second, some patients have ACTH-secreting tumors that result in increases in both ACTH and cortisol levels. Third, some patients have hypothalamic Cushing's syndrome, where glucocorticoid levels are high, but ACTH levels are normal (because the pituitary can still respond to the inhibitory influences of high glucocorticoid secretion). Now, in Addison's disease, the patient has low glucocorticoid levels but high ACTH levels, presumably because of the lack of the inhibitory influence of the glucocorticoids. Therefore, although Cushing and Addison patients are opposite in terms of glucocorticoid levels, some Cushing patients and all Addison patients have high ACTH levels. On the basis of this kind of similarity in ACTH characteristics, Sachar suggested that the depression associated with pituitary-adrenal endocrinopathies might reflect a psychotropic, depressive action of ACTH itself. Recall from Chapters 3 and 7 that ACTH can exert extra-adrenal effects on a wide range of behaviors, and, therefore, it is not unreasonable to suggest an extra-adrenal action of ACTH in the case of depression. If this hypothesis is correct, however, one would expect to see depression only in those Cushing patients with ACTH-secreting tumors, with no symptoms (or even elation) in patients with glucocorticoid-secreting tumors or hypothalamic Cushing's disease, who do not have abnormally high ACTH levels. Sadly, the clinical data do not seem to have been divided in this way, and, therefore, this ACTH hypothesis must remain speculative.

Caution must be exercised in interpreting the clinical literature on the relationship between endocrine disorders and affective states, because these endocrinopathies lead to a wide range of physical symptoms in addition to their disturbance of endocrine activity. That is, the behavioral changes associated with endocrine disturbances may be side effects of the metabolic abnormalities or general debilitation that these disorders produce. Put simply, patients with endocrine diseases may be depressed because they feel sick. Therefore, a decision about the causal link between endocrine disorders and affective disorders should await more extensive investigations of the specificity of that relationship.

Hormonal Correlates of Affective Disorders

The preceding discussion was concerned with affective disturbances associated with severe endocrine abnormalities. However, most individuals suffering from affective disorders do not have such severe endocrinopathies as Cushing's disease or Addison's disease, and the question remains as to the relationship between affective disorders and endocrine function in these individuals.

Many studies have been directed toward describing the hormonal characteristics typical of severe affective states, and most of those studies have focused on the pituitary-adrenocortical hormones. This literature is vast and will only be summarized here. The interested reader is referred to the very comprehensive reviews by Carrol and Mendels (1976) and Persky (1975).

The earliest studies demonstrated that depressed patients exhibit higher levels of glucocorticoid secretion than do normals (e.g., Bunney, Mason & Hamburg, 1965; Sachar et al., 1963). However, not all depressed patients exhibit high glucocorticoid output; whether or not depressed patients secrete high levels of these adrenocortical hormones seems to depend on the effectiveness of their defenses. If individuals are aware of their depression, they do secrete high levels of the glucocorticoids, but if they seem to deny that depression, their glucocorticoid levels are lower (Bunney, Mason & Hamburg, 1965). In fact, there appears to be a continuum of psychological states and adrenocortical activity: Psychotic individuals secrete more cortisol than anxious individuals, who secrete more cortisol than apathetic individuals (Sachar et al., 1970). In addition, the higher the clinical rating of depression, the greater the cortisol secretion (McClure, 1966).

Depressed individuals also exhibit different dynamics of pituitary-adrenal activity. Although in humans, cortisol is released episodically, there is marked circadian variation in the magnitude of those pulses, and depressed patients exhibit less marked circadian rhythms in cortisol secretion than do normal individuals. Figure 8-3 presents mean hourly plasma cortisol concentrations over a 24-hour period for depressed and normal subjects. Notice that when cortisol levels decline in normals, the levels of this hormone remain elevated in depressives. This diminished circadian variation may account for the increase in cortisol secretion observed in depressive subjects (Sachar, 1975a, 1975b).

Comment: Pituitary-Adrenal Activity and Depression

These discussions have summarized the literature showing, first, that abnormalities of pituitary-adrenal activity are accompanied by disorders of affect, and, second, that disorders of affect, particularly depression, are accompanied by changes in pituitary-adrenal activity. Why are the affective disorders and pituitary-adrenal function related in this way? More specifically, are depression and pituitary-adrenal activity related causally or just coincidentally? There are at least three possible explanations of the relationship between depression and pituitary-adrenal activity: First, the increased pituitary-adrenal activity characteristic of depressives may simply represent a response to the stresses inherent in being depressed. Second, the depressive reaction may be a result of the increase in pituitary-adrenal activity. Third, depression and high pituitary-adrenal activity may both reflect some more complex (neural?) abnormality which, coincidentally, affects them both (Rubin & Mandell, 1966).

There has been no clear decision among these alternative explanations, although it does seem likely that the pituitary-adrenal correlates of depression are more than simply a stress response. The levels of other hormones that usually are altered following stress are not always changed in depression. For example, although stress ordinarily leads to a reduction in androgen levels, depression does not affect these gonadal hormones (Sachar et al., 1973). In addition, growth hormone ordinarily is released in response to stress, and depressives have normal growth hormone levels (Sachar,

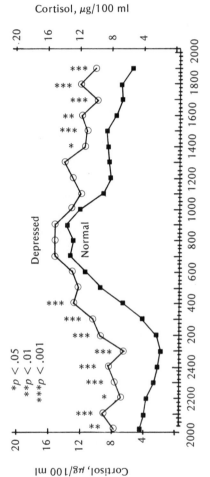

FIG. 8-3

Mean hourly plasma cortisol concentration over a 24-hour period for seven unipolar depressed patients compared with the mean for 54 normal subjects. Each dot represents the mean cortisol concentration during the preceding hour. Asterisks indicate the significance of differences between depressed and normal values for each hour (from chapter by Sachar in *Progress in Brain Research*, 1975, 42, 83, by permission of Elsevier/North Holland).

1974b). Therefore, it seems unlikely that the increased glucocorticoid secretion of depressives is simply a case of a generalized stress response.

Do increases in pituitary-adrenal activity cause depression? The data summarized in our discussion of endocrinopathies and affective states, suggest that modifications in the levels of the hormones of the pituitary-adrenal axis could lead to depression. At least, depression often follows changes in the levels of those hormones. However, the endocrine disorders discussed above have dramatic and pervasive metabolic consequences, and the resultant depression could be due to general debilitation. Therefore, studying endocrinopathies may not be an appropriate method for dissecting the causality in the correlation between depression and pituitary-adrenal activity.

It is tempting to speculate that whether or not changes in pituitary-adrenal activity can *cause* depression, the increases in pituitary-adrenal activity that accompany depression might help to *maintain* the affective state. The pituitary-adrenal hormones have a wide range of behavioral effects in nonhuman animals, including altering levels of aggressiveness, submissiveness, and fearfulness (see Chapters 3 and 7). In each of these cases, we have argued that there probably is a long-chain hormone–behavior interaction operating, wherein the hormonal responses to experience feed back and either modify or maintain ongoing responses. Might it not also be the case that even if the pituitary-adrenal hormones do not cause depression, the increases in the levels of these hormones following the onset of the depressive episode can feed back and help to maintain the affective state? Of course, this kind of suggestion is based solely on indirect evidence, and, therefore, its validity can only be determined through appropriate experimental tests.

SUMMARY AND COMMENT

This chapter was concerned with the relationship of endocrine function to emotion and mood in humans. The first section was concerned with relatively short-term emotional experiences, those most frequently thought of as emotions. That review suggested that hormones affect emotion in only a very general way; specific hormonal manipulations do not affect only specific emotions. However, only the catecholamines have been studied extensively, and, therefore, a general decision about the role of hormones in determining emotional reactions should await further tests.

Having emotional experiences seems to produce fairly dramatic changes in the levels of at least the adrenal medullary and pituitary-adrenocortical hormones. The primary question raised in discussing the hormonal responses to emotional experience concerns the specificity or idiosyncrasy of hormonal responses to specific emotional experiences. Although early studies did support the view that specific emotional experiences are accompanied by specific hormonal responses, later studies have tended to argue that the hormonal responses to emotional experience are really quite general; most emotional experiences seem to lead to similar hormonal responses.

The next section was concerned with the relationship between endocrine function and longer-lasting emotional states, or moods. The discussion focused on one particular case of mood states, the premenstrual syndrome. Correlational studies have shown that many women experience changes in mood across the menstrual cycle, with increases in depression, anxiety, and irritability occurring just prior to menstruation. Studies using the birth control pill to regulate hormone levels have suggested that the premenstrual syndrome may be a result of the dramatic hormonal changes that occur premenstrually. Further studies have suggested that the form of an individual's premenstrual hormonal changes may affect the degree or intensity of the premenstrual mood changes she experiences.

The final section of this chapter was concerned with long-lasting and debilitating extremes of mood, the affective disorders. Certain endocrine diseases appear to result in affective disturbances, and experiencing extremes of affect appears to modify the levels of at least the pituitary-adrenocortical hormones. Whether or not there is a causal relationship between hormones and the affective disorders remains undetermined.

One topic discussed in earlier chapters but not considered here concerns how hormones might be related to behavior. Specifically, how do hormones exert their effects on emotion and mood? It is tempting to speculate that, as in the case of the other classes of behavior discussed in earlier chapters, hormones affect emotion and mood through modifying the state of critical circuits in the brain. However, this may not always be true. In the case of the catecholamines, when these hormones are injected systemically, they do not pass the blood-brain barrier. Therefore, they cannot be affecting emotion through some central action; rather they must be acting through some peripheral mechanism(s).

In the cases of moods and the affective disorders, it is more reasonable to speculate that hormones affect these states by modifying central neural activity. First, both the gonadal hormones (in the case of premenstrual mood changes) and the pituitary-adrenocortical hormones (in the case of the affective disorders) do pass the blood-brain barrier and can get to the brain. Second, these hormones have been shown to affect other classes of behavior (see earlier chapters) through specific actions on the brain. Therefore, although the critical studies have not been conducted (those studies would be difficult using human subjects), it does seem reasonable to hypothesize a central site of action for hormones in mood states.

REFERENCES

Ader, R. Early experience and hormones: emotional behavior and adrenocortical function. In B. E. Eleftheriou and R. L. Sprott (Eds.), *Hormonal Correlates of Behavior*, Vol. 1. New York: Plenum Press, 1975, pp. 7-33.

Archer, J. Tests for emotionality in rats and mice: a review. *Animal Behavior*, 1973, 21, 205-235.

Arnold, M. B. Physiological differentiation of emotional states. *Psychological Review*, 1945, 52, 35-48.

Arnold, M. B. An excitatory theory of emotion. In M. L. Reymert (Ed.), *Feelings and Emotion*. New York: McGraw-Hill, 1950, pp. 11-33.

Arnold, M. B. *Emotion and Personality, Vol. II. Neurological and Physiological Aspects*. New York: Columbia University Press, 1960.

Ax, A. F. The physiological differentiation between fear and anger in humans. *Psychosomatic Medicine*, 1953, 13, 433-442.

Bäckström, T., and Carstensen, H. Estrogen and progesterone in plasma in relation to premenstrual tension. *Journal of Steroid Biochemistry*, 1974, 5, 257-260.

Bindra, D. B. A unified interpretation of emotion and motivation. *Annals of the New York Academy of Sciences*, 1969, 159, 1071-1083.

Black, P. (Ed.). *Physiological Correlates of Emotion*. New York: Academic Press, 1970.

Bunney, W. E., Mason, J. W. & Hamburg, D. A. Correlations between behavioral variables and urinary 17-OHCS in depressed patients. *Psychosomatic Medicine*, 1965, 27, 299-308.

Breggin, P. R. The psychophysiology of anxiety. *Journal of Nervous and Mental Disease*, 1964, 139, 558-568.

Brown, W. A. & Heninger, G. Cortisol, growth hormone, free fatty acids and experimentally evoked affective arousal. *American Journal of Psychiatry*, 1975, 132, 1172-1176.

Candland, D. K. The persistent problems of emotion. In D. K. Candland, J. P. Fell, J. E. Keen, A. I. Leshner, R. Plutchik and R. M. Tarpy, *Emotion*. Monterey: Brooks/Cole, 1977.

Candland, D. K. & Nagy, Z. M. The open field: some comparative data. *Annals of the New York Academy of Sciences*, 1969, 159, 831-851.

Cannon, W. B. *Bodily Changes in Pain, Hunger, Fear and Rage*. New York: Appleton, 1915.

Cannon, W. B. The James-Lange theory of emotion: a critical examination and an alternative theory. *American Journal of Psychology*, 1927, 39, 106-124.

Cannon, W. B. *Bodily Changes in Pain, Hunger, Fear and Rage*. (2nd ed.). New York: D. Appleton, 1929.

Cantril, H. The roles of the situation and adrenalin in the induction of emotion. *American Journal of Psychology*, 1934, 46, 568-579.

Cantril, H. & Hunt, W. A. Emotional effects produced by the injection of adrenalin. *American Journal of Psychology*, 1932, 44, 300-307.

Carroll, B. J. & Mendels, J.   Neuroendocrine regulation in affective disorders. In E. J. Sachar (Ed.), *Hormones, Behavior and Psychopathology*. New York: Raven Press, 1976, pp. 193-224.

Duffy, E.   Emotion: an example of the need for reorientation in psychology. *Psychological Review*, 1934, 41, 184-198.

Elmadjian, F., Hope, J. M. & Lamson, E. T.   Excretion of epinephrine and norepinephrine in various emotional states. *Journal of Clinical Endocrinology*, 1957, 15, 608-620.

Elmadjian, F., Hope, J. M. & Lamson, E. T.   Excretion of epinephrine and norepinephrine under stress. *Recent Progress in Hormone Research*, 1958, 14, 513-553.

Fine, B. J. & Sweeney, D. R.   Personality traits, situational factors and catecholamine excretion. *Journal of Experimental Research in Personality*, 1968, 3, 15-27.

Frankenhaeuser, M.   Experimental approaches to the study of catecholamines and emotion. In L. Levi (Ed.), *Emotions—Their Parameters and Measurement*. New York: Raven Press, 1975, pp. 209-234.

Freedman, M. X. (Ed.).   *Biology of the Major Psychoses*. New York: Raven Press, 1975.

Funkenstein, D. H.   The physiology of fear and anger. *Scientific American*, 1955, 192, 74-80.

Funkenstein, D. H.   Norepinephrine-like and epinephrine-like substances in relation to human behavior. *Journal of Nervous and Mental Disease*, 1956, 124, 58-68.

Gerdes, E. P.   Autonomic arousal as a cognitive cue for subjective report of anxiety and behavior under stress. *Journal of Personality and Social Psychology*, in press.

Hamburg, D. A.   Effects of progesterone on behavior. In Association for Research in Nervous and Mental Disease, *Endocrines and the Central Nervous System*. Baltimore: Williams and Wilkins, 1965, pp. 251-263.

Hamburg, D. A., Moos, R. H. & Yalom, I. D.   Studies of distress in the menstrual cycle and the postpartum period. In R. P. Michael (Ed.), *Endocrinology and Human Behavior*. London: Oxford University Press, 1968, pp. 94-116.

Ivey, M. E. & Bardwick, J. M.   Patterns of affective fluctuation in the menstrual cycle. *Psychosomatic Medicine*, 1968, 30, 336-345.

James, W.   What is an emotion? *Mind*, 1884, 9, 188-205.

James, W.   *Textbook of Psychology*. New York: Henry Holt, 1892.

Kline, N. S. (Ed.).   *Factors in Depression*. New York: Raven Press, 1974.

Kutner, S. J. & Brown, W. L.   Types of oral contraceptives, depression and premenstrual symptoms. *Journal of Nervous and Mental Disease*, 1972, 155, 153-162.

Landis, C. & Hunt, W. A. Adrenalin and emotion. *Psychological Review*, 1932, 39, 467-485.

Leshner, A. I. Hormones and emotion. In D. K. Candland, J. P. Fell, J. E. Keen, A. I. Leshner, R. Plutchik and R. M. Tarpy, *Emotion*. Monterey: Brooks/Cole, 1977.

Levi, L. The urinary output of adrenalin and noradrenalin during pleasant and unpleasant emotional states. *Psychosomatic Medicine*, 1965, 27, 80-85.

Lindemann, E. & Finesinger, J. E. The subjective response of psychoneurotic patients to adrenalin and mecholyl (acetyl-B-methyl-choline). *Psychosomatic Medicine*, 1940, 2, 231-248.

Lindsley, D. B. Emotion. In S. S. Stevens (Ed.), *Handbook of Experimental Psychology*. New York: John Wiley, 1951, pp. 473-516.

Maas, J. W. Catecholamines and depression: a further specification of the catecholamine hypothesis of the affective disorders. In A. J. Friedhoff (Ed.), *Catecholamines and Behavior*, 2. New York: Plenum Press, 1975, pp. 119-133.

McClure, D. J. The diurnal variation of plasma cortisol levels in depression. *Journal of Psychosomatic Research*, 1966, 10, 189-195.

Malmo, R. B. Activation: a neuropsychological dimension. *Psychological Review*, 1959, 66, 367-386.

Marañon, G. Contribution á l'étude de l'action émotive de l'adrénaline. *Revue Francaise d'Endocrinologie*, 1924, 2, 301-325.

Marinari, K. T., Leshner, A. I. & Doyle, M. P. Menstrual cycle status and adrenocortical reactivity to psychological stress. *Psychoneuroendocrinology*, 1976, 1, 213-218.

Mason, J. W. Psychological influences on the pituitary-adrenal cortical system. *Recent Progress in Hormone Research*, 1959, 15, 345-378.

Mendels, J. (Ed.). *Biological Psychiatry*. New York: John Wiley, 1973.

Mendels, J. (Ed.). *The Psychobiology of Depression*. New York: Spectrum, 1975.

Moos, R. H. The development of a menstrual distress questionnaire. *Psychosomatic Medicine*, 1968, 30, 853-867.

Moos, R. H., Kopell, B. S., Melges, F. T., Yalom, I. D., Lunde, D. T., Clayton, R. B. & Hamburg, D. A. Fluctuations in symptoms and moods during the menstrual cycle. *Journal of Psychosomatic Research*, 1969, 13, 37-44.

Paige, K. E. Effects of oral contraceptives on affective fluctuations associated with the menstrual cycle. *Psychosomatic Medicine*, 1971, 33, 515-537.

Parlee, M. B. The premenstrual syndrome. *Psychological Bulletin*, 1973, 80, 454-465.

Persky, H.   Adrenocortical function and anxiety. *Psychoneuroendocrinology*, 1975, 1, 37-44.

Persky, H., Hamburg, D. A., Basowitz, H., Grinker, R. R., Sabshin, M., Korchin, S. J., Herz, M., Board, F. A. & Heath, H. A.   Relation of emotional responses and changes in plasma hydrocortisone level after stressful interview. *Archives of Neurology and Psychiatry*, 1958, 79, 434-447.

Rakoff, A. E.   Endocrine mechanisms in psychogenic amenorrhoea. In R. P. Michael (Ed.), *Endocrinology and Human Behavior*. London: Oxford University Press, 1968, pp. 139-160.

Roessler, R., Burch, N. R. & Mefferd, R. B.   Personality correlates of catecholamine excretion under stress. *Journal of Psychosomatic Research*, 1967, 11, 181-185.

Rogoff, J. M.   A critique of the theory of emergency function of the adrenal glands: implications for psychology. *Journal of General Psychology*, 1945, 32, 249-268.

Rose, R. M., Bourne, P. G., Poe, R. O., Mongey, E. H., Collins, D. R. & Mason, J. W.   Androgen response to stress II. Excretion of testosterone, epitestosterone, androsterone and etiocholanolone during basic combat training and under threat of attack. *Psychosomatic Medicine*, 1969, 31, 418-436.

Rubin, R. T. & Mandell, A. J.   Adrenal cortical activity in pathological emotional states: a review. *American Journal of Psychiatry*, 1966, 123, 387-400.

Sachar, E. J.   Psychiatric disturbances in endocrine disease: some issues for research. In F. Plum (Ed.), *Brain Dysfunction in Metabolic Disorders*. New York: Raven Press, 1974, pp. 239-251. (a)

Sachar, E. J.   Endocrine function in affective disorders. In A. S. Kline (Ed.), *Factors in Depression*. New York: Raven Press, 1974, pp. 115-126. (b)

Sachar, E. J.   Twenty-four-hour cortisol secretory patterns in depressed and manic patients. *Progress in Brain Research*, 1975, 42, 81-91. (a)

Sachar, E. J.   Evidence for neuroendocrine abnormalities in the major mental illnesses. In D. X. Freedman (Ed.), *Biology of the Major Psychoses*. New York: Raven Press, 1975, pp. 347-358. (b)

Sachar, E. J., Halpern, F., Rosenfeld, R. S., Gallagher, T. F. & Hellman, L.   Plasma and urinary testosterone in depressed men. *Archives of General Psychiatry*, 1973, 28, 15-18.

Sachar, E. J., Hellman, L., Fukushima, D. K. & Gallagher, T. F.   Cortisol production in depressive illness. *Archives of General Psychiatry*, 1970, 23, 289-298.

Sachar, E. J., Mason, J. W., Kolmer, H. S. & Artiss, K. L.   Psychoendocrine aspects of acute schizophrenic reactions. *Psychosomatic Medicine*, 1963, 25, 510-537.

Schachter, S. Cognitive effects on bodily functioning: studies of obesity and eating. In D. C. Glass (Ed.), *Neurophysiology and Emotion*. New York: Rockefeller University Press, 1967, pp. 117-144.

Schachter, S. The assumption of identity and peripheralist-centralist controversies in motivation and emotion. In M. B. Arnold (Ed.), *Feelings and Emotions*. New York: Academic Press, 1970, pp. 111-121.

Schachter, S. & Singer, J. E. Cognitive, social and physiological determinants of emotional states. *Psychological Review*, 1962, 69, 379-399.

Schachter, S. & Wheeler, L. Epinephrine, chlorpromazine and amusement. *Journal of Abnormal and Social Psychology*, 1962, 45, 121-128.

Schildkraut, J. J. & Kety, S. S. Biogenic amines and emotion. *Science*, 1967, 156, 21-30.

Selye, H. *The Stress of Life*. New York: McGraw-Hill, 1956.

Sheard, M. H. Endocrines and neuropsychiatric disorders. In B. E. Eleftheriou and R. L. Sprott (Eds.), *Hormonal Correlates of Behavior*, Vol. 1, New York: Plenum Press, 1975, pp. 341-368.

Smith, S. L. Mood and the menstrual cycle. In E. J. Sachar (Ed.), *Topics in Psychoendocrinology*. New York: Grune and Stratton, 1975, pp. 19-58.

Stanley-Jones, D. The biological origin of love and hate. In M. B. Arnold (Ed.), *Feelings and Emotions*. New York: Academic Press, 1970, pp. 25-37.

Stein, M. Some psychophysiological considerations of the relationship between the autonomic nervous system and behavior. In D. C. Glass (Ed.), *Neurophysiology and Emotion*. New York: Rockefeller University Press, 1967, pp. 145-154.

Wenger, M. A. Emotion vs. visceral action: an extension of Lange's theory. In M. L. Reymert (Ed.), *Feelings and Emotions*. New York: McGraw-Hill, 1950, pp. 3-10.

Whybrow, P. C. & Hurwitz, T. Psychological disturbances associated with endocrine disease and hormone therapy. In E. J. Sachar (Ed.), *Hormones, Behavior and Psychopathology*. New York: Raven Press, 1976, pp. 125-143.

Wolff, C. T., Friedman, S. B., Hofer, M. A. & Mason, J. W. Relationship between psychological defenses and mean urinary 17-hydroxy-corticosteroid excretion rates. *Psychosomatic Medicine*, 1964, 26, 576-591.

Chapter 9

CONCLUDING REMARKS

We now have discussed the rather vast literature on hormone–behavior interactions by separate classes of behavior. Although some of the theoretical issues raised in Chapter 1 were discussed in those reviews, no real attempt was made to assess the generality of the form of hormone–behavior interactions across different classes of behavior. The purpose of this chapter is to return to that question. Specifically, we ask here whether we can make generalizations about the multifaceted relationship between hormones and behavior that are appropriate for all of the disparate behaviors discussed in preceding chapters. It should by now be clear that the kinds of models discussed in Chapter 1 do hold in very general ways, as general statements of the role of hormones in behavior. Hormones do affect behavior, many hormonal effects on behavior are neurally mediated, engaging in certain behaviors and having particular experiences do lead to changes in endocrine states, etc. Let us here attempt to refine those very broad generalizations and articulate those relationships more precisely.

HORMONAL EFFECTS ON BEHAVIOR

If we were to start at the beginning again, a first question might be: What do hormones do to behavior? Clearly, hormones do not stimulate behavior directly. In none of the cases discussed here has it been the case that hormones by themselves cause the behavior to occur. Rather, hormones seem to affect whether and how intensely the behavior will occur following exposure to appropriate exciting stimuli. A particularly dramatic example of this distinction can be drawn from the study of hormones and emotion (Chapter 8). Recall that James' early position was that the physiological arousal state accompanying an emotional experience *is* the emotion, and the logical extension of that position is that if the appropriate physiological arousal state is created, the particular emotion should be experienced. However, attempts to accomplish that were summarily unsuccessful. For example, although it is true that injecting epinephrine can affect the intensity of an emotional experience once it is instigated, injecting epinephrine does not lead to genuine emotional experiences in the absence of emotion-provoking stimuli in the environment.

Another example can be seen from the study of hormones and aggression (Chapter 3). Clearly, hormones do not stimulate animals to fight. Fighting only occurs in response to the presence of aggression-provoking stimuli. But, having a particular hormonal state does seem to predispose the individual to be more or less aggressive when exposed to those stimuli. Therefore, we can say that hormones do not *stimulate* or *cause* behavior, although they clearly do *affect* behavioral reactions.

Given that hormones do affect behavior, we might ask further about the nature of that relationship. As discussed in Chapter 1, there are at least two broad types of hormonal effects on behavior. One category includes the effects of the baseline hormonal state on behavior, and the second kind includes those temporally delayed effects of hormones present during certain early developmental stages on adult behavior patterns.

Effects of the Baseline Hormonal State

Let us begin with the effects of the baseline hormonal state. It was suggested in Chapter 1 that the baseline hormonal state affects both the form and intensity of reactions to appropriate environmental stimuli. Although all of its ramifications have not been examined for all of the classes of behavior discussed in this book, that generalization does seem to hold.

Beginning with the question of hormonal effects on the intensity of behavioral reactions, it seems clear that in almost all cases, the baseline hormonal state does affect the intensity of behavioral responses, at least in a gross way. Hormones can affect how much an individual will eat, how much it will fight, how much it will scent mark, how intensely it will react to sexual stimuli, whether or not it will behave maternally, how strong its avoidance reactions will be, and how intensely it will react emotionally.

What of the form of those responses? Do hormones also affect the form of the responses to be exhibited in the presence of certain stimuli? This question has only been studied for some of the behavioral classes discussed here, but in those cases, the answer appears to be "yes." For example, the hormonal state can affect which nutrients will be selected by an individual and in what proportions (Chapter 2). Under some hormonal states, the animal will select more carbohydrates, whereas under others it will select more protein. Although this may be pushing the issue a bit, we can say that the form of responses is affected.

A clearer example can be drawn from the study of hormones and agonistic behavior in mice (Chapter 3). In this case, the hormonal state seems to affect the probabilities that a mouse will react aggressively or submissively to the presence of a novel conspecific. Specifically, an animal with the hormonal characteristics of low androgen levels and high pituitary-adrenocortical hormone levels will not attack a conspecific and will become submissive quite readily when attacked. On the other hand, if the animal has intermediate levels of the androgens and the pituitary-adrenocortical hormones, it will react quite aggressively to a conspecific and will not be submissive readily, even if attacked. Furthermore, during estrous periods, female hamsters will respond to approaches by a male with receptive behaviors, whereas during other times, those approaches are met with aggression. Whether the female will react receptively or aggressively appears to depend on her estrous-cycle status, and, therefore, probably her hormonal state (see Floody & Pfaff, 1974).

There are some cases where the data collected so far suggest that the baseline hormonal state does not affect the form of behavioral responses. The case of emotion just discussed is one example. Here, injections of epinephrine lead to increases in emotional reactions no matter what their form. If the subject is subjected to anger-provoking stimuli, epinephrine injections seem to increase anger reactions, and if the subject is exposed to euphoria-provoking stimuli, the same hormonal treatment seems to increase this type of emotional reaction (see Schachter & Singer, 1962). Of course, as discussed in Chapter 8, epinephrine produces a very general increase in arousal, and if other hormones were studied, we might see different kinds of effects.

Although the effects of hormones on different behaviors are in some ways quite similar, it is important to mention that there are some differences between hormones and between behaviors. One important difference is in the duration of time that the particular baseline hormonal state must be extant before hormonal effects are evident (compare Young, 1961). For example, as discussed in Chapter 5, the androgens' effects on male sexual behavior usually require quite long periods of hormonal exposure before behavioral changes are seen. On the other hand, as discussed in Chapter 7, single injections producing only short-lasting elevations in ACTH levels can have dramatic effects on avoidance responses. Thus, there can be marked differences in the duration of exposure needed to cause hormonal effects to become evident.

There also appear to be differences in the form of hormonal effects. Specifically, in some cases, hormones appear to exert some degree of fine-grain control over how much or how intensely the behavior will be exhibited. We have seen dose-response relationships between experimentally controlled baseline hormone levels and levels of responding in many cases, including glucocorticoid levels and running activity, pituitary-adrenocortical hormone levels and aggressiveness, estrogen levels and some measures of female sexual behavior, ACTH levels and avoidance responding, and others. These hormonal effects can be considered "directive"; the amount of hormone present contributes to the determination of how intensely the behavior will be displayed. It should be remembered, however, that although some hormonal effects seem to be directive, we have not seen many examples where differences in hormone levels can account for such fine-grain differences in behavior as those between individuals. Thus, even though some hormonal effects may be generally directive, they are not totally determining. In addition, many hormones only direct behavior to a limit. Recall that in Chapter 5 we discussed the fact that increases in androgen or estrogen levels above the dosage level needed to induce "normal" sexual responding usually do not lead to further increases in sexual responding.

In other cases, hormonal effects appear to be only "all-or-none" or "permissive." The presence or absence of the hormone is important, but the amount of the hormone present does not affect the amount of responding. For example, this seems to be the case in the relationship between androgen levels and aggressiveness in mice (Chapter 3): if androgens are present in a threshold amount, aggression will be displayed. If, however, the androgen level is below that threshold, the mouse will not react aggressively. Furthermore, gradations of androgen levels do not seem to be associated with gradations in aggressiveness. Another example of this kind of permissive hormonal effect was discussed in Chapter 5, when we discussed the facilitatory effects of progesterone on sexual responding in female guinea pigs and rats. Here again, the hormonal effect is only permissive: the amount of progesterone does not seem to affect the intensity of sexual responses, so long as a threshold amount of that hormone is present. Thus, in some cases hormone levels do directly affect the amount of the behavior displayed; that is, there is a dose-response relationship between hormone levels and levels of behavioral responding. However, in other cases, hormones only affect behavior in an all-or-none way: if the hormone is present in a sufficient amount, the behavior is affected. If the threshold amount of hormone is not present, the behavior is not affected.

In summary, the proposition raised in Chapter 1 that the baseline hormonal state can affect the form and intensity of behavioral responses does seem appropriate as a generalization. However, that statement must be refined for particular classes of hormone–behavior interactions.

Organizing Effects of the Hormonal State Early in Development

We have seen repeated examples of temporally delayed effects of the hormonal state during early developmental stages on both the form and intensity of adult behavioral responses. We have seen these organizational effects expressed in the cases of the regulatory behaviors (Chapter 2), agonistic behaviors (Chapter 3), sexual behavior (Chapter 5), and avoidance reactions (Chapter 7). Clearly, then, the effects of the early hormonal state are both pervasive and dramatic. Interestingly, most of the effects of hormones present early in development that have been studied are those related to gender differences in adult behavior patterns. Perhaps this bias toward gender differences in behavior is a result of the fact that most investigators have been interested in the dramatic effects of early gonadal hormone manipulations. However, there have been some studies examining early hormonal effects on adult behaviors that are not gender dimorphic in the same way, such as the effects of early thyroid manipulations on adult learning abilities (e.g., Davenport & Dorcey, 1972). Therefore, it is important to remember that hormones present during early developmental stages can exert temporally delayed but profound effects on many adult behavior patterns.

What is the nature of these organizational effects of hormones on behavior? Do early hormonal states affect only the intensity or frequency of adult reactions, or do they, like the adult hormonal states just discussed, also determine the form of adult responses? As discussed extensively in Chapter 5, hormones present early in development clearly can affect both parameters. For example, the early hormonal environment seems to determine whether dogs will adopt the male-like or the female-like urination posture (Beach, 1975), thereby affecting the form of at least one adult response. In addition, early hormonal manipulations can affect the intensity of adult reactions. Examples can be seen in Chapters 5 and 7, where we discussed the effects of the early hormonal state on adult sexual and avoidance reactions, respectively. In both cases, we saw that the intensity of adult responses was affected. Therefore, the early hormonal environment can affect both the form and the intensity of adult behavior patterns.

As discussed in Chapter 5, there has been much discussion about what it is that those early hormonal states do to the organism so as to affect its adult responses. Recall from that discussion, that the original *organization hypothesis* suggested that the gonadal hormones present early in development organize the brain, functionally and/or structurally, in a more male-like or a more female-like way (Phoenix et al., 1959). Alternative arguments have been that hormones present early in development only affect the sensitivity of the individual to hormones circulating in adulthood. The data reviewed throughout this book show that in some cases, the effects of hormones early in development might be sensitizing or desensitizing the individual to hormones present in adulthood (as in some cases of early hormonal effects on adult sexual behavior), but clearly there are other cases where a sensitivity explanation would not be sufficient. For example, in the case of gonadal hormone effects on adult avoidance responses (Chapter 7), we saw that the adult gonadal hormone state is not important in the determination of sex differences in avoidance responding, but treating female rats neonatally with testosterone does masculinize their avoidance performance in adulthood (see Beatty & Beatty, 1970). Therefore, it would seem unlikely that these early hormonal effects simply are a result of changes in sensitivity to hormones circulating in adulthood, because the presence or absence of those adult hormones is irrelevant. Thus, although in some cases it may be that the early hormonal state does sensitize or desensitize the individual to hormones circulating in adulthood, those early hormones also must be operating in other ways in other cases.

Some Additional Comments About Hormonal Effects on Behavior

Before leaving a discussion of hormonal effects on behavior, we should mention some additional aspects of this relationship that have not been discussed explicitly in earlier sections. Interestingly, these points were made in Beach's 1948 book, *Hormones and Behavior*, although very little attention has been directed toward studying their implications directly.

First, although we have discussed behaviors separately, it should be clear by now that no hormone has a single behavioral effect. For example, even though the gonadal hormones are often called the "sex hormones," they are important in a wider range of behaviors, including the regulatory behaviors, agonistic behaviors, parental behaviors, and emotional reactions. The pituitary-adrenocortical hormones affect an equally wide range of behaviors. Thus, although we may study behaviors separately, it is important to remember that the behavior under study is only one of many that a particular hormone can affect.

Second, it is important to mention that no behavior depends totally on the actions of one hormone. We have said that hormones do not "own" any behavior, but, more importantly, it should be emphasized that there usually are many hormones involved in the control of any single behavior. The interested reader should be able to find examples supporting both of these generalizations throughout the preceding chapters.

MEDIATION OF HORMONAL EFFECTS ON BEHAVIOR

In Chapter 1 we discussed many ways in which hormones can affect behavior. Since, with the possible exception of the effects of oxytocin on the uterus, hormones cannot make muscles move, they can only affect behavior through mediating mechanisms. Throughout this book we have discussed a range of possibilities, and in each chapter we have considered the role of specific mechanisms in mediating specific hormonal affects on behavior. As a summary statement, it seems clear that there are many operative mediating mechanisms including hormonal effects on the general metabolic state of the organism, on peripheral structures (such as sensory receptors), and on the state of circuits in the brain that are critical to the control of behavioral activity. These mechanisms seem to be important to the effects of both the baseline hormonal state and the hormonal state present early in development on adult behavior patterns. Significantly, for each class of behaviors discussed, it was noted that hormones always seem to affect that behavior in many ways. For example, it was suggested that hormones affect the regulatory behaviors through modifying both peripheral body tissue stores and the neural "set-point" for body weight and/or composition. In discussing sexual behavior, it was pointed out that the estrogens could affect female sexual behavior both by affecting the state of the receptor area around the vagina and by affecting critical brain circuits. Therefore, another generalization suggested by Beach in 1948 is still appropriate after more of the relevant data have been collected; that is, that hormones do not affect behavior through any one mechanism but through a variety of mechanisms. Interestingly, all of the mechanisms that have been studied and identified were proposed as possibilities in Beach's early book.

Yet another question about the mediation of or mechanisms of hormonal effects on behavior deserves mention. Throughout this book we have considered primarily physiological mediating mechanisms. Clearly, much has been learned in this area. However, behaviorists might ask different kinds of questions about the mediation of hormonal effects on behavior than the physiologist would ask: questions concerned with the behavioral processes that hormones affect. Relatively little attention has been devoted to those issues, but they are important nonetheless. (Their importance became apparent through a discussion with R. W. Goy.) For example, do hormones affect the perception of stimuli, the integration of responses, or some intervening mechanism often labeled "motivation"? These issues have been raised repeatedly (e.g., Diamond, 1968; Leshner, 1975; Meyerson & Lindstrom, 1971), but they seem to be left quickly. Surely, there have been some limited attempts to study the effects of hormones on "sexual motivation" (see review by Meyerson & Lindstrom, 1971), and, in some sense, we are studying motivational processes in studying avoidance learning or bar-pressing for food (see discussions of hormonal effects on these behaviors in Chapters 2 and 7). But, by focusing so heavily on the brain or other structures as mediators of hormonal effects on behavior, we somehow seem to ignore the other groups of mediational questions that psychologists might ask. In some cases we seem to infer processes like perception from the behavior of our animals, such as perceiving an agonistic stimulus as "aggression-provoking" or "fear-provoking" (see Leshner, 1975), but we certainly are not studying perception directly. We may avoid these kinds of questions because, as behavioral endocrinologists (emphasis on endocrinologist?), we find intervening variables, such as perception and motivation, uncomfortable or ephemeral.

But, that discomfort does not diminish the importance of those questions. As the study of the mediation of hormonal effects on behavior progresses, it is hoped that there will be some investigators who move not only in more molecular directions, such as to the mediational issues discussed in Chapter 5, but also to the more molar "psychological" questions that are important to a more complete understanding of the effects of hormones on behavior.

THE EFFECTS OF EXPERIENCE
ON ENDOCRINE FUNCTION

Not only do hormones affect behavior, but engaging in certain behaviors and having certain kinds of experiences lead to changes in endocrine function. This bimodal kind of relationship has been discussed in each of the preceding chapters. In Chapter 1, we discussed models proposing that these hormonal responses to experience or behaving might also have consequences for continuing or subsequent behavioral reactions, and in each chapter we have discussed the possibility that there are long-chain hormone–behavior interactions in the specific behavioral case. In some cases, those interactions have been studied explicitly, although in others they are not yet clear. For example, in Chapter 2, we discussed the potential long-chain hormone–behavior interaction in the relationship between glucocorticoid levels and levels of running activity. In that case, it was suggested that the glucocorticoid responses to engaging in activity might feed back and determine the subsequent activity level.

Another kind of feedback effect can be seen from the study of the role of the gastrointestinal hormones in feeding (also discussed in Chapter 2). In this case, it has been suggested that the hormonal responses to stomach loading (whether natural (by eating), or experimentally induced) feed back and terminate feeding.

Long-chain hormone–behavior interactions also have been

studied explicitly for the cases of agonistic reactions (Chapter 3) and parental behaviors (Chapter 6). These kinds of interactions were discussed extensively in the appropriate chapters and will not be reiterated here. What is important is that in both cases, long-chain hormone–behavior interactions have been identified.

Suggestions of additional cases of feedback effects have been made for the cases of pheromonal communication (Chapter 4) and avoidance and emotional reactions (Chapters 7 and 8). Unfortunately, those feedback effects have not been studied directly.

In Chapter 5 we discussed the possibility that sexual behavior might provide an exception to the generality of long-chain hormone–behavior interactions. Recall that attempts to discover those interactions have been relatively unsuccessful. However, those studies have focused only on rather short-term potential feedback effects that would be seen relatively soon after the hormonal response has been emitted. It could be that the hormonal responses to sexual contact do feed back and affect sexual responses, but only in subsequent similar situations; those feedback effects may be too slow to affect the pattern of ongoing sexual responses.

In summary, we can make the generalization that in all cases discussed in this book, there are examples of experiential effects on endocrine function. In some cases those hormonal responses to experience appear to feed back and modify ongoing or subsequent behavioral responses, whereas in other cases they may not. Because there have been so few attempts to study long-chain hormone–behavior interactions directly, an evaluation of whether these kinds of interactions are a general characteristic of the relationship between hormones and behavior will have to await further study.

Another suggestion, presented in Chapter 1, concerned the possible effects of the hormonal responses to experience on the effectiveness of an individual as a stimulus to the behavior of other individuals—feedback effects on the individual's *stimulus quality*. This hypothesis has not been studied directly, and, therefore, we cannot make any generalizations. However, the arguments used to form that hypothesis remain sound: The quality of an animal as a stimulus does appear to depend at least partly on its hormonal state (see extensive discussions in Chapter 4). Furthermore, the form of the hormonal responses to experience are such that if they had been made experimentally, they would have altered the individual's stimulus qualities. Some limited support for this notion has been provided by the study of parental behavior in ring doves (see Chapter 6 and Lehrman, 1961, 1965). In this case, there is a dynamic interaction between the behavioral and hormonal states of both partners in a reproductive interaction. Because the behavior of each individual depends on the behavior of the other individual, and because in each individual there is a long-chain hormone–behavior interaction between its hormonal responses to stimulation and its behavioral responses to that stimulation, one could argue that as the individual's hormonal state changes, so does its stimulus quality. That is, because the behavior pattern of each individual depends on the behavior of the other individual, as one individual's behavior changes, as a result of its hormonal responses, these behavioral changes represent alterations in its stimulus qualities. However, this kind of analysis has not been carried out in any general way and, therefore, we cannot determine whether this kind of feedback effect on stimulus quality is typical.

MODELS REVISITED

In Chapter 1 we discussed some of the models previously proposed as general descriptions of the role of endocrine functions in behavior, and a new model was suggested to include some aspects of that relationship that were not included in those earlier models. It now seems appropriate to return to that general model and ask about its adequacy. It should be made clear at the outset that the model proposed in Chapter 1 is very general and, therefore, is in some sense "safe." It was developed to account for or describe all of the relationships to be discussed in this book. Therefore, rather than ask whether it includes all of the relationships discussed for each behavior, it might be more useful to ask whether we would modify the model when speaking of a particular class of behaviors.

There are some cases, such as the regulatory behaviors (Chapter 2) and some avoidance and emotional reactions (Chapters 7 and 8), where the exciting stimulus is inanimate, and, presumably, an inanimate stimulus would not be affected by the state of the individual being studied. Therefore, the element "stimulus quality" might be extraneous in discussing the relationship of hormones to these classes of behavior.

There also are some cases, such as avoidance reactions (Chapter 7), where the baseline hormonal state may not be important. As previously discussed, this issue is unsettled, but the absence of reliable correlations between baseline hormonal states and levels of avoidance responding argues against a role for this factor in avoidance reactions. Thus, we might eventually choose to delete "baseline hormonal state" from the model when discussing avoidance reactions.

In addition, the data presented in Chapter 5 argue against there being long-chain hormone–behavior interactions, at least in the case of ongoing sexual responses. Recall, for example, that the progesterone responses to copulation do not seem to feed back and alter the female's sexual responding. But, again, this feedback function of the hormonal responses to sexual activity has not been studied in great detail. Furthermore, it could be that although the hormonal responses to sexual contact may not feed back and modify ongoing sexual responses, they may affect future sexual responses. Therefore, a decision to delete that feedback element from the model would seem to be premature.

In addition to there being cases where elements of the model might be deleted, there may be cases where we would want to add to the model. One such case seems obvious. If we wanted to provide a truly accurate and complete description of the role of hor-

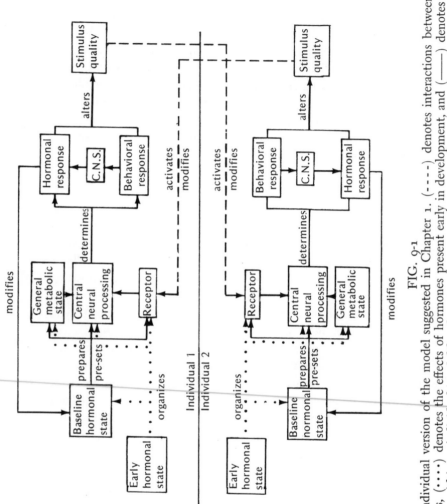

FIG. 9-1

A two-individual version of the model suggested in Chapter 1. (- - - -) denotes interactions between individuals, (••••) denotes the effects of hormones present early in development, and (———) denotes relationships within an individual in adulthood.

mones in social or sexual interactions, would we not want to specify hormone–behavior relationships for all individuals involved in a particular situation? These kinds of multiple-individual descriptions have been suggested for specific kinds of behavioral interactions (e.g., Adler, 1974, Floody & Pfaff, 1977, for sexual interactions; Floody & Pfaff, 1974, Leshner, 1975, for agonistic interactions). A model showing the interactions between two individuals is presented in Figure 9-1, which simply incorporates mirror images of the model presented in Figure 1-2. Only two individuals are included in order to provide an easy means for visualizing the dynamic interactions between individuals and their respective hormonal states, but we could describe a model including hormone–behavior interactions in any number of individuals.

Given that we might want to modify our general model when considering specific classes of behavior or specific interactions, the reader might question why we would want to have such a general model at all. Clearly one cannot have a model that can both incorporate all aspects of hormone–behavior interactions and be a totally accurate description of what happens in one specific case. It can be argued that this kind of general model can serve two functions: First, it does provide a means for stating the role(s) of hormones in behavior in a simple way. Second, and perhaps more importantly, it can serve the heuristic purpose of articulating the range of possible relationships that might exist in a particular case, thereby generating hypotheses and directing research concerned with the relationships between specific hormones and specific behaviors.

EPILOGUE

We now have reviewed much of what is known and what is believed about the relationship between hormones and behavior. A fitting final question seems to be: Where will we go from here? Although much has been learned, we also have discussed many areas where additional research in behavioral endocrinology is needed to articulate suspected relationships. Examples of these proposed but not heavily studied problems can be found in each chapter of this book. Therefore, in some ways we can expect more of the same kinds of studies that we already have seen.

The reader may have noticed that the typical questions asked by behavioral endocrinologists concern the relationships between single hormones and single behaviors. However, individuals do not live in such controlled conditions that they only engage in single behaviors, and no endocrine gland functions independently of other endocrine glands. A remaining important question, then, concerns the interactions among the various hormone–behavior relationships as studied in their dynamic forms in subjects engaging in multiple behaviors and affected by multiple endocrine secretions.

It also seems that many investigators are moving their research activities into more molecular analyses of hormone–behavior relationships. This is particularly evident in the search for the mechanisms that mediate hormonal effects on behavior. It is hoped that some investigators also will turn to the more molar, psychological questions about the mediation of hormonal effects that were discussed earlier in this chapter—questions about the behavioral processes that hormones affect.

Surely, as this relatively young field develops, much of what has been believed will be discarded. Many seemingly clear relationships will be called into question, and many new relationships will be discovered. It is hoped that this book will serve as a basis from which those interested in hormone–behavior interactions can move forward.

REFERENCES

Adler, N. T. The behavioral control of reproductive physiology. In W. Montagna & W. A. Sadler (Eds.), *Reproductive Behavior*. New York: Plenum Press, 1974, pp. 259-286.

Beach, F. A. *Hormones and Behavior*. New York: Paul B. Hoeber, Inc., 1948.

Beach, F. A. Hormonal modification of sexually dimorphic behavior. *Psychoneuroendocrinology*, 1975, 1, 3-23.

Beatty, W. W. & Beatty, P. A. Hormonal determinants of sex differences in avoidance behavior and reactivity to electric shock in the rat. *Journal of Comparative and Physiological Psychology*, 1970, 73, 446-455.

Davenport, J. W. & Dorcey, T. P. Hypothyroidism: learning deficit induced in rats by early exposure to thiouracil. *Hormones and Behavior*, 1972, 3, 97-112.

Diamond, M. Perspectives in reproduction and sexual behavior: an afterword. In M. Diamond (Ed.), *Perspectives in Reproduction and Sexual Behavior*. Bloomington: Indiana University Press, 1968, pp. 461-479.

Floody, O. R. & Pfaff, D. W. Steroid hormones and aggressive behavior: approaches to the study of hormone sensitive brain mechanisms for behavior. *Research Publications of the Association for Research in Nervous and Mental Disease*, 1974, 52, 149-185.

Floody, O. R. & Pfaff, D. W. Communication among hamsters by high-frequency acoustic signals III. responses evoked by playbacks of natural and synthetic "ultrasounds". *Journal of Comparative and Physiological Psychology*, 1977, in press.

Lehrman, D. S. Hormonal regulation of parental behavior in birds and infrahuman mammals. In W. C. Young (Ed.), *Sex and Internal Secretions*. Baltimore: Williams & Wilkins, 1961, pp. 1268-1382.

Lehrman, D. S. Interaction between internal and external environments in the regulation of the reproductive cycle of the ring dove. In F. A. Beach (Ed.), *Sex and Behavior*. New York: John Wiley, 1965, pp. 355-380.

Leshner, A. I. A model of hormones and agonistic behavior. *Physiology and Behavior*, 1975, 15, 225-235.

Meyerson, B. J. & Lindstrom, L. Sexual motivation in the estrogen treated ovariectomized rat. In V. H. T. James & L. Martini (Eds.), *Hormonal Steroids*. Amsterdam: Excerpta Medica, 1971, pp. 731-737.

Phoenix, C. H., Goy, R. W., Gerall, A. A. & Young, W. C. Organizing action of prenatally administered testosterone propionate on the tissues mediating mating behavior in the female guinea pig. *Endocrinology*, 1959, 65, 369-382.

Schachter, S. & Singer, J. E. Cognitive, social and physiological determinants of emotional states. *Psychological Review*, 1962, 69, 379-399.

Young, W. C. The hormones and mating behavior. In W. C. Young (Ed.), *Sex and Internal Secretions*. Baltimore: Williams & Wilkins, 1961, pp. 1173-1239.

Appendix

BASIC CONCEPTS IN
ENDOCRINOLOGY

The purpose of this appendix is to provide the reader who has little experience in endocrinology with a set of fundamental terms and principles that should be useful in reading this book. Since little detail is provided, the reader interested in further information should consult the list of recommended texts provided at the end of the appendix.

The *endocrine system* consists of a group of specialized ductless glands, whose primary function is to secrete *hormones*. Hormones are secreted directly into the bloodstream, and they constitute an important signaling system within the body; they serve primarily to modify the rates and/or directions of cellular functions.

Some hormones or hormone-like substances also are secreted by parts of the body that typically are not considered to be endocrine glands, because they have other important functions. These structures include certain parts of the brain, the stomach and small intestine, the placenta, and others. The locations of hormone-secreting structures can be seen in Figure A-1. The discussion that follows will be restricted primarily to those organs traditionally considered as endocrine glands: the pituitary, the thyroid, the parathyroids, the pancreas, the adrenals, and the gonads.

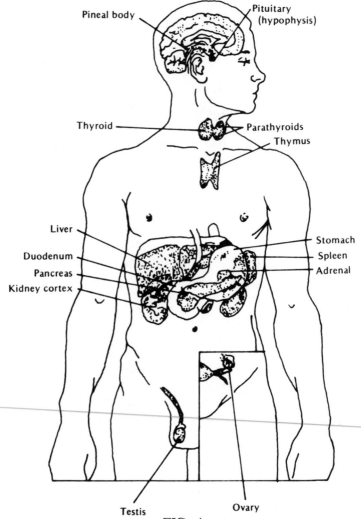

FIG. A-1

Approximate locations of the endocrine glands in human beings. Although the liver, kidneys, and spleen add important materials to the blood they are not definitely known to be organs of internal secretion (from Turner & Bagnara, *General Endocrinology* 6th ed. Phila.: W. B. Saunders, 1976, p. 29, by permission).

SOME GENERAL PRINCIPLES

Before considering specific endocrine glands and specific hormones, it might be useful to mention some principles that apply to endocrine function in general.

Control of Endocrine Secretion: Neuroendocrine Regulation

The endocrine system does not function independently from the rest of the organism, and, in fact, many endocrine activities are closely integrated with and dependent on the activities of the nervous system. In some cases, such as that of the adrenal medullary hormones, endocrine secretions are released following direct neural stimulation of endocrine tissues. In other cases, however, such secretions are controlled through relatively intricate feedback systems involving the brain. Some brain sites that are important to endocrine function, and are pertinent to discussions in this book, are diagrammed in Figure A-2.

The three known kinds of neuroendocrine feedback systems are illustrated in Figure A-3. One kind of arrangement is characteristic of the posterior pituitary hormones, oxytocin and vasopressin (first-order arrangement in Fig. A-3). In this case, the hormones to be released from the posterior pituitary actually are produced in the brain, and they then pass via neurosecretory neurons to the posterior pituitary, from which they are released. Thus, although oxytocin and vasopressin are called "posterior pituitary hormones," they actually are produced in the brain and are only released from the posterior pituitary.

In addition to their effects on target tissues, such as the kidney (vasopressin) and the uterus (oxytocin), the posterior pituitary hormones also affect the brain sites that produce them. When the levels of these hormones become sufficiently high, as sensed via these effects on the brain, their production and/or release is diminished. Therefore, this system exemplifies a neuroendocrine

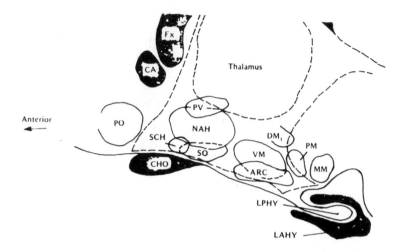

FIG. A-2

Schematic, saggital drawing of the area around the hypothalamus. Fx, fornix; CA anterior commissure; PV, paraventricular nucleus; NAH, anterior hypothalamic area; PO, preoptic area; SCH, suprachiasmatic nucleus; SO, supraoptic nucleus; CHO, optic chiasm; DM, dorsomedial nucleus; VM, ventromedial nucleus; ARC, arcuate nucleus; PM, premammilary nucleus; MM, medial mammilar nucleus; LPHY, posterior lobe of pituitary; LAHY, anterior lobe of pituitary (from chapter by Flerkó in Martini, Motta & Fraschini's *The Hypothalamus*. New York: Academic Press, 1970, p. 355, by permission).

negative feedback system, whereby the level of a hormone feeds back and controls its own rate of secretion.

A second kind of neuroendocrine interaction is characteristic of growth hormone and prolactin, which are secreted from the anterior pituitary (second-order arrangement in Fig. A-3). The secretion of these hormones is dependent on the levels of appropriate *releasing and inhibiting factors* (neurohormones), which are pro-

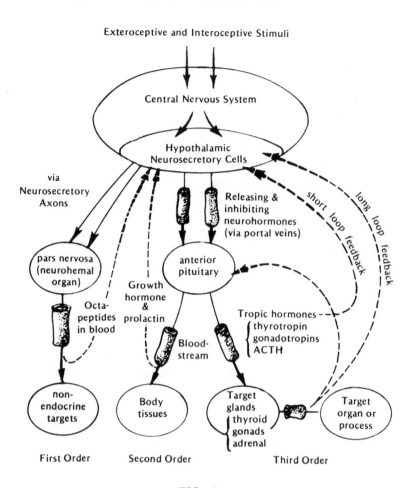

FIG. A-3

Three orders of neuroendocrine arrangements. The broken lines indicate negative feedback; the actions may be directly on the anterior pituitary, more indirectly on the neurosecretory cells in the periventricular brain, or on both (from Turner & Bagnara, *General Endocrinology*, 6th ed. Phila.: W. B. Saunders, 1976, p. 67, by permission).

duced in and released from the hypothalamus. For example, growth hormone is secreted from the anterior pituitary following stimulation of that gland by *growth hormone release factor* (GHRF), which is produced in and secreted from the hypothalamus.

As growth hormone and prolactin levels in the circulation rise, that rise is sensed by hormone-sensitive areas in the brain. Then, as the circulating levels of these hormones get to be quite high, as sensed by the brain, the secretion of the hypothalamic releasing and inhibiting factors is altered. Thus, there is a negative feedback arrangement where growth hormone and prolactin can feed back and modify their own release through affecting the production and release of the hypothalamic neurohormones that control them.

The third kind of neuroendocrine integration is typified by the thyroid, gonadal, and adrenocortical hormones; and it is even more complex than the arrangements just discussed (see third-order arrangement in Fig. A-3). These hormones are under the control of *tropic hormones* released by the anterior pituitary. In turn, these tropic hormones are under the control of releasing and inhibiting factors secreted from the hypothalamus, much in the same way that prolactin and growth hormone are. Thus, the sequence of signals is as follows: Neurohormonal signals are released from the hypothalamus, which cause the release of tropic hormone signals from the anterior pituitary. These pituitary signals then cause the release of hormones from target glands—in this case, the thyroid, the adrenal cortices, and the gonads.

But, in the same way that prolactin and growth hormone can feed back and modify their own secretion rates through affecting the brain and, thereby, the relevant releasing and inhibiting factors, so can the tropic hormones feed back and affect the release of the hypothalamic neurohormones on which they depend (the short loop feedback in Fig. A-3). Furthermore, the hormones secreted by the target glands also can feed back and affect the hypothalamic release of the relevant neurohormones (long loop feedback in Fig. A-3). And, the hormones from the target glands also can feed back and modify the release of the tropic hormones from the anterior pituitary. Thus, there are three kinds of feedback effects in this "third order" arrangement of neuroendocrine interactions: (1) The tropic hormones from the anterior pituitary can feed back and affect the levels of the hypothalamic neurohormones on which the tropic hormones depend; (2) the hormones from the target gland can feed back and influence the levels of the hypothalamic releasing and inhibiting factors; and (3) the hormones from the target glands can feed back to the pituitary directly and affect the release of the tropic hormones on which the hormones of the target gland depend.

These kinds of neuroendocrine arrangements may seem complex or unwieldy, but, actually, they are organized much in the same way as is any homeostatic system. (1) There is a constancy being maintained: in this case, the level of the hormone in question. (2) There is a "sensor" for monitoring deviation from that set-point or constancy level: In some cases the sensor consists of hormone-sensitive neurons in the brain; in other cases, it is in the pituitary. (3) There are mechanisms for correcting deviations from the set-point: In a second-order system, the correcting mechanism is the hypothalamic releasing and inhibiting factors. In a third-order arrangement, the mechanism includes both the hypothalamic neurohormones and the tropic hormones from the anterior pituitary. Of course, dramatic changes in the level of any of these hormones (of whichever type) can be brought about by overriding the feedback systems with prolonged or intense stimulation (such as might occur during stress exposure, when extremely high levels of ACTH and the glucocorticoids are required).

Before leaving a discussion of the control of endocrine secretions, it should be emphasized that not all hormones are dependent on neural stimulation (either directly or indirectly). In particular, the hormones of the pancreas and the parathyroids are released in response to changes in blood levels of the products of intermediary metabolic processes—those of the pancreas are controlled by blood glucose levels, and those of the parathyroids are controlled by blood calcium levels.

Organization of the Endocrine System

Although the endocrine glands typically are studied separately, it is important to keep in mind that the endocrine system really functions in a rather integrated way. The activity of any single gland can have marked effects on the activity of the rest of the endocrine system. This kind of interdependence or interaction among endocrine secretions can be expressed in a variety of ways. The most obvious case is the interaction between pituitary function and the secretory activities of the rest of the endocrine system. As just discussed, the anterior pituitary secretes a variety of tropic hormones that directly stimulate the secretion of other hormones from other endocrine glands. Thus, one kind of intrasystem integration involves the direct stimulation or causation of the release of some hormones by other hormones.

A second kind of endocrine interaction involves the facilitation or inhibition of the activity of one gland by hormones secreted by another gland. In this case, although one hormone may not directly stimulate or inhibit the release of the other hormone, the first hormone does affect the activity of the gland producing the second hormone. An example is the relationship between thyroid function and the secretion of adrenocortical hormones, growth hormone, and insulin. Hypothyroid individuals also have hypofunctioning adrenal cortices, reduced growth hormone secretion levels, and altered insulin metabolism. These characteristics probably are a consequence of the pervasive metabolic effects of changes in thyroid gland activity (see below).

The third kind of endocrine interaction is the result of most hormones having effects that are either similar to or opposite from those of other hormones. That is, very few hormones have effects that are not either partly mimicked by or counteracted by the effects of other hormones. For example, glucagon, growth hormone, cortisol, and the thyroid hormones all lead to increases in carbohydrate breakdown and hyperglycemia. Similarly, insulin, growth hormone, the thyroid hormones, and the androgens all increase protein synthesis. One example of opposite hormonal effects may suffice. When the secretion of the glucocorticoids is increased during periods of stress, there is a consequent increase in blood sugar levels. Following this increase, there is a consequent release of insulin from the pancreas. This increase in insulin secretion promotes the uptake of sugars from the bloodstream into tissues, thereby serving to counteract the effects of the initial increase in glucocorticoid secretion. This example, of course, is also a case where the effects of one hormone are indirectly causing the release of another. That is, the increase in glucocorticoid levels leads to an increase in insulin secretion, but only because the glucocorticoids lead to an increase in the level of sugars in the blood, on which insulin secretion depends.

Mechanisms of Hormone Action

Hormones typically are either protein, modified amino acid, or steroid structures. Although it is not yet totally clear, the evidence collected so far suggests that the protein and modified amino acid hormones exert their effects in a different way from that of the steroid hormones. Both kinds of effects involve the interaction of hormones with specialized receptors in target cells, and preliminary evidence suggests that the specialized hormone receptors are proteins either on the cell surface or inside the cell.

The most common theory is that the protein and modified amino acid hormones first interact with receptors on the cell surface. Following receptor stimulation, an intracellular *second messenger* is elaborated, which then acts within the cell to produce the appropriate physiological change. In most cases, this second messenger appears to be cyclic AMP, which is present in all tissues; significantly, many hormonal effects can be mimicked by local application of this substance.

For the steroid hormones, the current theory is that they first react or couple with a receptor protein inside the cell, in the cytosol. The hormone, now bound, is then carried to the cell nucleus where it modifies protein synthesis at the level of the genome. This modification of protein synthesis then results in changes in enzyme structure or activity, such that the rates and/or directions of physiological reactions are altered.

ENDOCRINE GLANDS AND THEIR SECRETIONS

The Pituitary

The pituitary gland, or hypophysis, is located at the base of the brain and consists of three lobes: the *anterior pituitary* or *adenohypophysis*, the *intermediate lobe* or *pars intermedia*, and the *posterior pituitary* or *neurohypophysis*. Although the functioning of each lobe can affect the functioning of the others, each can be viewed as a separate gland.

ANTERIOR PITUITARY The anterior lobe of the pituitary gland secretes six hormones discussed in this book all of which are proteins or glycoproteins. *Growth hormone* (GH) or *somatotropic hormone* (STH) has as its major metabolic action the stimulation of protein synthesis throughout the body. It also has some marked catabolic effects on lipid and carbohydrate metabolisms. *Thyroid-stimulating hormone* (TSH or *thyrotropic hormone* has as its primary action stimulating the release of thyroid hormones from the thyroid gland. *Adrenocorticotropic hormone* (ACTH) or *corticotropin* stimulates the release of the glucocorticoids (and the adrenal sex hormones) from the adrenal cortex. ACTH also appears to have some extra-adrenal effects on lipid metabolism. *Follicle-stimulating hormone* (FSH) and *luteinizing hormone* (LH) are classified as *gonadotro-*

pins because they stimulate activity within the gonads. The gonadotropins act in both the ovaries and testes to stimulate gamete production and steroidogenesis. The exact functions of and division of labor between the gonadotropins have not yet been explicitly delineated. Finally, *prolactin* exerts its primary effects on lactation, although it also seems to affect some other aspects of reproductive physiology.

As discussed above, the secretion of all of the anterior pituitary hormones is controlled by the hypothalamus through its release of neurohormones called *releasing* and *inhibiting factors*. Thus, ACTH is under the control of *corticotropin releasing factor* (CRF), TSH is under the control of *thyrotropin releasing factor* (TRF), etc.

INTERMEDIATE LOBE The major hormone of the intermediate lobe is *melanophore-stimulating hormone* (MSH), a protein hormone. Although MSH has many secondary effects, its primary effect is the stimulation of pigment cells (chromatophores).

POSTERIOR PITUITARY The posterior lobe of the pituitary is directly connected with the hypothalamus. As discussed above, although the hormones of the posterior pituitary are released from the neurohypophysis, they in fact are produced within the hypothalamus. The hormones stored in and secreted by the posterior pituitary are proteins and are called *oxytocin* and *vasopressin*. Oxytocin is a potent stimulator of uterine contractions and causes milk ejection from the mammaries. Vasopressin, also called antidiuretic hormone (ADH), has as its major function stimulating the retention of water by the kidney.

The Thyroid

The mammalian thyroid is an H-shaped structure located over the trachea. The active thyroid hormones are *thyroxine* (T_4) and *triiodothyronine* (T_3). The thyroid hormones are stored in the form of *thyroglobulin* in the follicles of thyroid tissue. Upon stimulation by TSH, thyroglobulin is hydrolyzed into the series of iodonated amino acids that are the thyroid hormones. Iodine is crucial to the activity of the thyroid, and this gland accumulates iodine in a concentration 20 times greater than the concentration in the plasma.

The actions of the thyroid hormones may be divided into two classes: metabolic effects and growth-promoting effects. Metabolic effects include the production of heat (calorigenesis), which is accomplished through increasing oxygen consumption and energy production, which, in turn, is accomplished primarily by increasing fat and carbohydrate breakdown. The other, growth-promoting actions of the thyroid hormones involve synergism with growth hormone in its protein anabolic action.

The Parathyroids

Little work has been done relating parathyroid activity and behavior, so we shall not devote much attention to this gland. The parathyroids are located on top of the thyroid gland. These glands produce and release *parathyroid hormone* (PTH), whose primary action is in calcium and phosphorus metabolism.

The Adrenals

The adrenal glands are located just above the kidneys in most mammals, and they often are referred to as the *suprarenal glands.* The adrenal is a compound structure consisting of an outer *cortex* and an inner *medulla*. Although these two parts of the adrenal are contained within the same capsule, they really are separate glands.

ADRENAL MEDULLA The tissue of the adrenal medulla is embryologically neural tissue, and its secretions are under the control of the nervous system. The adrenal medulla is made up of *chromaffin tissue*, which is found in other parts of the body. Most accessory chromaffin tissue is located around the sympathetic-chain ganglia, which are parallel to the spinal cord. The adrenal medulla secretes modified amino acid hormones which are called *catecholamines*. These include *epinephrine* (adrenalin) and *norepinephrine* (noradrenalin). Because the actions of these hormones are similar to stimulating the sympathetic nervous system, they are termed *sympathomimetic* substances. In fact, norepinephrine is one of the neurotransmitter substances of the sympathetic nervous system, in addition to being a hormone of the adrenal medulla.

Epinephrine and norepinephrine have profound, though somewhat different, effects on the circulatory system. For example, epinephrine has marked effects on cardiac output, but little effect on blood pressure. On the other hand, norepinephrine has dramatic effects on blood pressure, but little effect on the heart itself. Epinephrine also has dramatic hyperglycemic effects, whereas norepinephrine has little effect on carbohydrate metabolism. The hyperglycemic effect of epinephrine makes the release of this hormone an efficient means of producing energy in emergency situations.

ADRENAL CORTEX The outer layer of the adrenal gland, the adrenal cortex, is divided into three layers, each of which produces a different class of steroid hormones. The outermost layer, the *zona glomerulosa*, produces a class of hormones, the *mineralocorticoids*, which have marked effects on mineral metabolism. The mineralocorticoids promote the retention of sodium and the excretion of potassium. The two major mineralocorticoids are *aldosterone* and *deoxycorticosterone*, a precursor of aldosterone. The mineralocorticoids are released in response to chemical stimulation received from the kidney following decreases in plasma sodium levels.

The middle layer of the adrenal cortex, the *zona fasciculata*, produces the *glucocorticoids*. The primary glucocorticoids are *corticosterone* and *cortisol* (often called *hydrocortisone*). Some species, such as mice and rats, secrete primarily corticosterone, whereas others, such as primates, secrete primarily cortisol.

The glucocorticoids do have some mineralocorticoid activity, although their major actions are on protein, carbohydrate, and fat metabolisms. They promote deposition of glycogen in the liver, facilitate gluconeogenesis (the conversion of protein to carbohydrate), suppress protein synthesis, and increase the release of fatty acids from adipose tissue. The net effect of these metabolic actions is to provide energy that may be used in stressful situations. These glucocorticoids are under the control of ACTH secreted from the anterior pituitary.

The *zona reticularis* secretes the *adrenal sex hormones*, which resemble the gonadal sex steroids. These hormones also are released following stimulation by ACTH, and they appear to act synergistically with the gonadal sex hormones.

The Pancreas

The pancreas is both an endocrine gland and an exocrine gland. Its exocrine function is to produce enzymes used in digestion. Our interest, of course, is with its endocrine functions. The pancreas secretes two protein hormones, *insulin* and *glucagon*, from structures called the *islets of Langerhans*. Insulin is produced in the beta cells and glucagon in the alpha cells of these islets. Both hormones are responsive to the levels of carbohydrates in the bloodstream. Insulin produces hypoglycemia by stimulating the uptake of carbohydrates from the blood into cells. It also has some dramatic anabolic effects on protein and fat metabolisms. Glucagon acts opposite to insulin, producing hyperglycemia through facilitating the breakdown of carbohydrates and fats.

The Gonads

THE OVARY The primary reproductive gland of the female, the ovary, functions chiefly in the production of eggs and in the elaboration of steroid hormones, which condition the reproductive tract and the secondary sex characteristics. The ovary produces two major classes of hormones: the *estrogens*, which include *estradiol*,

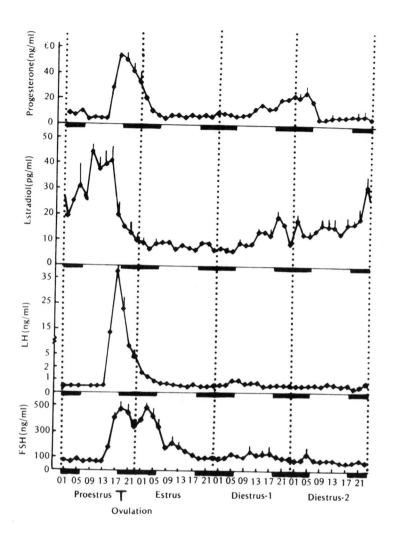

FIG. A-4
The pattern of progesterone, estradiol, LH, and FSH levels throughout
the 4-day estrous cycle of the rat. The numbers along the abscissa
represent the time of day in hours, and the black bars represent the
dark portion of the light/dark cycle (modified from Smith, Freeman &
Neill, *Endocrinology*, 1975, 96, 222, by permission of J. B. Lippincott
Company).

estrone, and *estriol;* and the *progestogens,* primary of which is *progesterone.* Ovarian activity is under the control of the gonadotropins FSH and LH, which are secreted from the anterior pituitary. Because frequent mention is made of cycles of ovarian activity throughout this book, it might be useful to show the levels of the ovarian hormones and the gonadotropins across a reproductive (estrous) cycle. These changes, as seen in the rat, are shown in Figure A-4. Although there is some variation among species, the *general* pattern of pituitary-ovarian secretions is as shown here.

THE TESTES The male reproductive glands, the testes, secrete a class of steroid hormones called *androgens.* Some of the major androgens are *testosterone, dihydrotestosterone,* and *androstenedione.* The primary functions of the androgens are the support of spermatogenesis in the seminiferous tubules of the testes and the regulation of the male secondary sex characteristics. The most important metabolic effect of the androgens is a facilitation of protein synthesis. As in the case of the ovaries, testicular function is under the control of the gonadotropins secreted from the anterior pituitary.

REFERENCES AND SUGGESTED READINGS

Barrington, E. J. W.   *An Introduction to General and Comparative Endocrinology,* 2nd ed. London: Oxford University Press, 1975.

Flerkó, B.   Control of follicle-stimulating hormone and luteinizing hormone secretion. In L. Martini, M. Motta & F. Fraschini (Eds.), *The Hypothalamus.* New York: Academic Press, 1970, pp. 351-363.

Ganong, W. F. & Martini, L. (Eds.), *Frontiers in Neuroendocrinology.* New York: Oxford University Press, a series beginning in 1969.

Lissák, K. (Ed.), *Hormones and Brain Function.* New York: Plenum Press, 1973.

Martini, L. & James, H. V. T. (Eds.), *Current Topics in Experimental Endocrinology.* New York: Academic Press, series beginning in 1971.

Naftolin, F., Ryan, K. J. & Davies, I. J. (Eds.), *Subcellular Mecha-*

nisms in Reproductive Neuroendocrinology. Amsterdam: Elsevier, 1976.

Rickenberg, H. V. (Ed.), *Biochemistry of Hormones.* Baltimore: University Park Press, 1974.

Sawyer, C. H. & Gorski, R. A. (Eds.), *Steroid Hormones and Brain Function.* Berkeley: University of California Press, 1971.

Smith, M. S., Freeman, M. E. & Neill, J. D.   The control of progesterone secretion during the estrous cycle and early pseudopregnancy in the rat: prolactin, gonadotropin and steroid levels associated with rescue of the corpus luteum of pseudopregnancy. *Endocrinology,* 1975, 96, 219-226.

Turner, C. D. & Bagnara, J. T.   *General Endocrinology,* 6th ed. Philadelphia: W. B. Saunders, 1976.

Williams, R. H. (Ed.), *Textbook of Endocrinology,* 5th ed. Philadelphia: W. B. Saunders, 1974.

INDEX

272-274; hormonal responses to, 246-268; injected catecholamines and, 251-254; mechanisms of pituitary-adrenal hormone effects on, 264-267; MSH and, 268-269; pituitary-adrenal responses to engaging in, 257-258; vasopressin and, 269-271
Avoidance responding, 32, 87-89. *See also* Avoidance behavior
Avoidance-of-shock. *See* Avoidance behavior
Avoidance testing, hormonal responses to, 25. *See also* Avoidance behavior

Baseline hormonal state, 5-8, 315-319, 327
Birth control pill, 296-298
Bisexuality, 173-186. *See also* Sexual behavior-heterotypical
Blood-brain barrier, 308
Body composition, 56-57. *See also* Set-point for body weight/composition
Body weight, 47. *See also* Set-point for body weight/composition; hormones and, 40-41
Brattleboro rat, 269-270
Buss-Durkee Hostility Inventory, 102-103

Caecotrophe, 130-131
Carbohydrate intake. *See* Dietary self-selection
Castration, 3, 31. *See also* An-

drogens; activity and, 66; dietary self-selection and, 56; early in life and adult sexual responses, 180-182; sexual behavior and, 8
Catecholamines, 94-95, 345. *See also* Epinephrine, Norepinephrine; affective disorders and, 298-299; avoidance behavior and, 249-254; preference for novelty and, 252
Central neural processing, 15-16, 19
Central nervous system. *See also specific neural structures;* as mediator of early hormonal effects, 9-10; as mediator of hormonal effects on agonistic behavior, 91-92; as mediator of hormonal effects on behavior, 7-8, 14, 322-324; as mediator of hormonal effects on sexual behavior, 169-173; as mediator of pituitary-adrenal hormone effects on avoidance behaviors, 265-267; excitability, 267
Cholecystokinin, 54
Circadian rhythms: in avoidance responding, 257; in corticosterone, 257; in cortisol, 303-305
Coitus. *See* Copulation, Sexual behavior
Cold emotions, 288
Concaveation, 217, 221-223
Conditioned emotional response (CER), 245; adrenal demedullation and, 251; gender differences in, 272; injected catecholamines and, 252
Conditioned stimulus (CS), 245